Children with Cancer

Children with Cancer

A Reference Guide for Parents

REVISED AND UPDATED EDITION

JEANNE MUNN BRACKEN

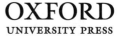

OXFORD
UNIVERSITY PRESS

2010

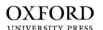

OXFORD
UNIVERSITY PRESS

Oxford University Press, Inc., publishes works that further
Oxford University's objective of excellence
in research, scholarship, and education.

Oxford   New York
Auckland   Cape Town   Dar es Salaam   Hong Kong   Karachi
Kuala Lumpur   Madrid   Melbourne   Mexico City   Nairobi
New Delhi   Shanghai   Taipei   Toronto

With offices in
Argentina   Austria   Brazil   Chile   Czech Republic   France   Greece
Guatemala   Hungary   Italy   Japan Poland   Portugal   Singapore
South Korea   Switzerland   Thailand   Turkey   Ukraine   Vietnam

Published by Oxford University Press, Inc.
198 Madison Avenue, New York, New York 10016
www.oup.com

Oxford is a registered trademark of Oxford University Press

Library of Congress Cataloging-in-Publication Data

Bracken, Jeanne Munn.
  Children with cancer: a reference guide for parents / Jeanne Munn Bracken. –
  Rev. and updated ed.
    p.; cm.
  Includes bibliographical references and index.
  Summary: "Children with Cancer draws together a wealth of up-to-date information
essential for anyone who wishes to help a child or family through this ordeal—including
relatives, friends, teachers, and clergymen, as well as doctors, nurses, and other health care
professionals"—Provided by publisher.
    ISBN 978-0-19-514739-1 (pbk. : alk. paper)   1. Cancer in children—Popular works.   I. Title.
  [DNLM: 1. Neoplasms—Popular Works.   2. Adolescent.   3. Child.   4. Infant.
    QZ 201 B797C 2010]
    RC281.C4B73 2010
  618.92'994–dc22   2009052038

1 3 5 7 9 8 6 4 2
Typeset by Glyph International, Bangalore, India
Printed in the United States of America
on acid-free paper

This is for Lisa and Amy. You're why I do this.

Preface to the New Edition

There is never a "good" time for your child to be diagnosed with childhood cancer, of course, but now there is infinitely more help available—in print, online, and in person—than there was when I went through this ordeal in 1977, as well as generally more hope for long-term survival.

Since the first edition of *Children with Cancer* was published in 1986, there has been both good and bad news in the field of pediatric oncology. The good news is that survival rates have increased gratifyingly until, on average, three of four patients now live at least 5 years after diagnosis. The bad news is that no "silver bullet" has been discovered that will wipe out cancer in a flash. No single agent or procedure has appeared that signals the end of cancer as we know it.

With improvements in the area of supportive care, children are experiencing less pain and (especially with ports and Broviac catheters) far fewer finger sticks and venipunctures than in the past. A new generation of antiemetics has helped ease some of the nausea, while other complementary therapies like acupuncture and guided imagery help children handle their fear and symptoms.

Another major change that has occurred over the past two decades is the explosion of information available to the public on childhood cancer and its treatment. The first edition of this book was written because there was virtually no book or other source for the layperson—parent, teacher, clergyman, friend, relative, and others who are vital in helping child patients through therapy and beyond.

By contrast, today there is almost too much information. Books, the World Wide Web/Internet sites, articles, organizations—the range is astounding. The purpose of this edition of *Children with Cancer*, therefore, is to provide up-to-date basic information and to point the way to more detailed data or assistance for those who need it. Parents with a newly diagnosed child who try to sort through all the offerings on their own are likely to be overwhelmed at a time when simple yet accurate facts are essential. With my reference librarian's eye and experience, I have tried to provide that streamlined gateway to the world of childhood cancer.

I must emphasize here that I am not a doctor. I have gathered material in this book from many published and online sources, but it is not my intention to provide a scholarly review with footnotes and an extensive bibliography of professional reading. For those who wish to have such information, publications are available through public and medical libraries and on the Internet. Be forewarned that these books contain photographs that are upsetting, and the language is scholarly English. Facts are stated dispassionately, almost brutally, because the specialists are writing impersonally about cases—but you are reading about a child much like yours. If you do want to look for more information, you may wish to delay until you have regained your emotional equilibrium, perhaps until the child is well into remission. I am glad now I did not begin my own research until a year after diagnosis.

For the sake of clarity, I have used masculine pronouns throughout the book when I am referring to patients, avoiding the awkward "him or her" and "he or she" phrases.

I would be remiss as a parent and author if I did not update my daughter Lisa's current status. After diagnosis in 1977 and 2 years of intensive chemotherapy, numerous surgical procedures over the years, and escalating urinary tract problems, she endured over 5 years of hemodialysis. On Valentine's Day 2005, a generous, anonymous family in Louisiana donated a kidney that was a perfect match for Lisa. Nor is this her only late effect. Her secondary teeth didn't form properly, requiring oral surgery and orthodontia (which she says now was worse than most of the other procedures she had to bear). She has migraine headaches, although (fingers crossed) recent reconstructive surgery seems to have overcome her recurrent urinary infections. She took growth hormones to reach a respectable 5 feet in height. Mostly because of the kidney transplant, she takes a number of medications each day. She is, overall, a wonderful young woman and an amazing person who works at the library, loves horror movies, and enjoys close friendships. We count each anniversary as a blessing, noting that she is now almost 33 years post-diagnosis.

I echo my wish from the first edition: that there was no need for this book. That cancer was, like the dinosaurs, extinct. Maybe soon. But in the meantime, I hope this book will smooth your path through the maze of childhood cancer.

J.M.B.
Littleton, Massachusetts
October 2009

Acknowledgments

A t the extraordinarily patient Oxford University Press, Jeff House, Lauren Enck, Carrie Pedersen, once again the astute and supportive Shelley Reinhardt, and Sarah Harrington; the Write Stuff critique group at the Lincoln Public Library; the Schmoozers at the Poland Spring Camp Ground; the "Loonies" retreat group, especially Patty Schremmer for her electronic pep talks; the ever-faithful Nancy "Coop" Cooper without whose support this book would never have been finished; the staff of the Lincoln (MA) Public Library and other Minuteman Library Network librarians; Merlene and Bob Smith and Amy Smith Golisano; my late mother Laura Losefsky, who believed again that I could do it; my daughters Lisa and Mollie Bracken, and my husband Ray (who can cook a lot better now than in 1986).

Contents

Appendices

Children with Cancer

What We're Up Against: The Diseases

Introduction

The American Cancer Society and the National Cancer Institute estimate that about 12,400 children in the United States under the age of 20 are diagnosed each year with cancer. This represents about 1% of all cancer cases diagnosed in the United States. However, childhood cancer is the second leading cause of death (after accidents) for children between the ages of 5 and 14, and the third leading cause of death (after accidents and congenital anomalies) for children from birth to age 4.

While this is an increased incidence over the past 20 years, the higher numbers may be partly a function of improved diagnostic and reporting measures. At any rate, while the number of patients has increased, the number of deaths due to childhood cancer has fallen dramatically. From a 20% survival rate in 1950–1954, the rate has climbed to 76.5% in 1989–1996. Boys have a higher overall incidence than girls, and black children are affected at a rate lower than whites.

What is Cancer?

We usually speak of cancer as one disease, but in reality it appears in over 100 forms. There are common factors among the varieties, the most important one being the uncontrolled growth of abnormal body cells. All human bodies are constantly creating new cells and discarding old ones. The difference with cancer is that the growth of the new cancer cells greatly exceeds the rate at which the old ones are being retired. As a result, the cancer cells interfere with the body's functions, either by blocking other organ systems or by displacing the normal cells. Some of these cells grow into masses called tumors that spread into adjacent areas of the body.

Just as a person has a life cycle from birth, through youth, maturity, and old age, our individual body cells, too, pass through several stages from "birth" until, as "adult" cells, they can perform work useful to the body. Cancer begins when a cell gets stuck in an immature stage and reproduces repeatedly. The type of cancer that strikes depends on the kind of cell and the life stage it is in when it becomes malignant and begins to multiply out of control.

Benign tumors have several characteristics that set them apart from malignant ones. They are usually slow-growing, are localized, have few cells dividing at one time, look a lot like normal tissue, are encapsulated, and do not spread to other tissue. In contrast, malignant tumors grow quickly, spread into nearby tissue and organs with many cells dividing at one time, and do not look very much like normal tissue.

Malignant cells wander around the body, either within cavities such as the abdomen or through the blood or lymphatic system. Wherever they land, they may begin to grow new masses. These distant growths are called metastases. Cancer may begin to spread, or metastasize, when the tumor is small, a fact that explains why half of patients already have metastases when their cancer is first detected. Even a benign tumor, depending on its location, may be cause for concern as a threat to the life of the child. If it is placed so that it cannot be removed without endangering vital organs like the brain, it is very serious indeed.

What Kinds of Cancer Do Children Get?

Various forms of cancer attack different body systems, and the forms that strike children are usually not the same ones that adults develop. It is estimated that one quarter of all Americans will eventually contract some form of cancer, a percentage that has increased as other fatal diseases, such as polio and measles, have been controlled or eradicated. Because more of us are living long enough to get cancer, which is essentially a disease of the elderly, more of us are affected by it. Most adult cancers are carcinomas—that is, cancers that arise from the tissues that line the lungs, breast, bladder, intestines, and other organs. Apparently, most of these have environmental triggers.

But children usually haven't lived long enough to contract disease through lengthy exposure to chemicals or other agents. Only 10% of cancers in children and adolescents are carcinomas. Youngsters most commonly develop malignancies of the brain, blood-forming tissues (leukemia), lymph system (lymphoma), sympathetic nervous system (neuroblastoma), and kidneys (Wilms tumor). They are also susceptible to sarcomas—tumors arising from bone, muscle, cartilage, fat, and connective tissue.

These childhood cancers are often embryonic in nature, arising from immature cells common in prenatal life that go awry from some yet unknown cause or causes. In fact, full-sized Wilms and neuroblastoma tumors are sometimes present at birth. The stimuli involved might be genetically transmitted by either parent. The activating factor might also be environmental or even a virus. Embryonic cells are naturally programmed to become more specialized (blood cells, kidney cells, etc.). Because of this, they are also more susceptible to change from chemotherapy and radiation, which direct them back from a malignant course. As a result many childhood cancers are easier to treat effectively than those adults develop, which grow from cells not normally adapted to change.

What Causes Childhood Cancer?

Parents may feel guilty because they fear they have caused their child's cancer by some act or through neglect. Experts agree that this is not true. While several suspected causative agents have been identified, the mechanism by which they work has not been. Thousands of children are exposed to polluted water, or to x-rays, yet only a tiny proportion of them contract cancer.

Genetic Causes

One aspect of childhood cancer that has seen great strides in understanding is the contribution of genetics to the development of cancer. There are a few hereditary diseases that predispose children to certain forms of cancer. One that has received some attention is neurofibromatosis type 1 (NF-1), or von Recklinghausen disease, which is characterized by numerous benign growths arising in the skin or nerves that occasionally become malignant. Sometimes the skin cancer melanoma occurs in a cluster in a given family. Other genetic disorders that can factor into childhood cancers are Beckwith-Wiedemann syndrome or Down syndrome.

Another form of cancer that is hereditary in some cases is retinoblastoma, an eye tumor that often strikes the very young. In a significant proportion of cases, the disease occurs in the children of those who suffered from the disease themselves. These parents often had disease in both eyes. It is usually recommended that anyone who has recovered from this form of cancer and is contemplating having children seek advice from a genetics counselor.

So much progress has been made in the science of genetics as it relates to childhood cancer that the topic warrants its own discussion; see Chapter 2 for more on this subject.

Medicines and Medical Procedures

Research has singled out x-rays as a factor in causing cancer in children. Pregnant women who undergo medical x-rays can give birth to children with a higher subsequent incidence of childhood cancer. Women of childbearing age must be carefully screened before medical x-rays are taken, although fetal ultrasound is considered safe.

Chemotherapy and radiation given to young cancer patients who survive their disease may eventually cause a second malignancy in a few of them. Chemotherapy drugs may in themselves be carcinogenic, and it is known that radiation can cause cancer. However, this small incidence is by all reasonable standards an acceptable risk when we consider that the child would have died of the original disease were no conventional treatment given. Clinical trials constantly seek to determine what doses of therapy are most effective with the fewest negative side effects. Some researchers suspect that these second malignancies are actually caused by new disease in a person somehow more susceptible to cancer.

We are just beginning to learn what the effects will be on the children of those youngsters who are now surviving cancer and giving birth to or fathering babies. The increased survival rate is a relatively recent phenomenon, so few long-term study results are available. Still, some studies have concluded that excepting hereditary cancers like retinoblastoma, there is no evidence that this subsequent generation is at any greater risk of cancer than those born to other parents.

The role of the immune system in warding off cancer is suggested by the increased incidence of malignancies in children who have been on immunosuppressive treatment to reduce the risk of organ rejection after transplant.

Chemical Causes and Environmental Pollution

We have learned a lot about chemicals and childhood cancer in recent decades. Whereas in the mid-1980s parents were concerned about flameproof sleepwear treated with TRIS, today the field has widened a great deal. TRIS, for all the fear, probably caused few if any cases of childhood cancer; it was banned from use in the United States, but realistically it probably did more good in preventing burns than harm in causing cancer.

Some chemicals are passed on to the infant through breastfeeding. Environmental contaminants such as DDT and PCBs are stored in human body fat and passed from mother to child. (Cow's milk accumulates these contaminants at a low level because of the cow's regular, lifelong giving of milk.) Formulas may be no safer if prepared with contaminated drinking water. However, researchers have not determined yet whether these substances cause cancer in children.

What about nuclear accidents like the one at Three Mile Island in Pennsylvania in 1979? Some independent studies have shown that the release of radioactive material into the atmosphere did not demonstrably cause an increase in cancer in children. Others disagree. The accident at Chernobyl in the Ukraine in 1986 was a different matter: vast amounts of radioactivity were released and spread over many countries, contaminating agricultural land and causing an increased incidence of cancer, childhood and other. Greece, for example, had a temporary increase in infant leukemia attributed to the

Chernobyl release. The nearby state of Belarus suffered the greatest contamination from the accident, resulting in increased numbers of childhood thyroid (mostly), bone, lung, and soft tissue cancers. In Belarus before Chernobyl, there were two cases of thyroid cancer in 1986; in 1992 there were 66, and in 1994 there were 82. The capital city of Minsk documented increased numbers of brain, bone, and kidney tumors. European studies of proximity to nuclear power plants have found a slight increase in childhood leukemia, although the results are limited to variations in design.

For the past decade or more, activists have insisted that power lines and related electromagnetic fields (EMF) are causing cancer in children and others. These fears have been expressed internationally, resulting in many studies to prove or disprove the notion. Results in the United Kingdom, Sweden, Australia, and the United States have not shown EMF to pose any significant danger. Even those who most vocally speak out against EMF agree that the number of children affected is tiny—in Western Australia, three extra cases of leukemia and one death over 50 years. (Of course, if one of those few cases is your child, your perspective changes radically.)

Realistically, experts note, over the past 50 years the incidence of childhood leukemia and other cancers has crept up, while the use of electricity in the home and elsewhere has increased exponentially. If EMF were indeed such a health danger, there should be an epidemic of ills, and there is not.

The use of pesticides in the home, garden, and workplace has grown to a huge volume. Experts suggest there is a modest risk of Wilms tumor, Ewing sarcoma, or germ cell tumors from these substances. Children living on farms, who are more exposed to these pesticides, have an increased risk of some cancers. More research is needed to clarify the danger of these chemicals, but in the meantime it would be wise to avoid them wherever possible. This includes those sticky pest-catching strips we hang around the house to snag flies and the like.

Water pollution is often regarded as the cause of cancer clusters, a group of cases of similar cancers that arise in a strict geographical area within a limited time. While these clusters are suspect, few are proven to be the result of contaminated water. One example is the Woburn, Massachusetts, case reported in Jonathan Harr's *A Civil Action*, where a determined mother and an obsessed lawyer appealed in court after court until the owners of the polluted properties were found guilty. A similar case in Toms River, New Jersey, litigated by the same lawyer, resulted in a negotiated settlement that avoided court action.

Occupational exposure to some chemicals carries a risk for children in the household. Benzene and similar substances used in painting, automotive work, and the like should be avoided as much as possible.

In yet another indictment of tobacco, paternal smoking has been shown to lead to an increased incidence of Burkitt lymphoma, acute lymphocytic leukemia (ALL), and brain tumors. The longer the father smoked and the more cigarettes he consumed, the greater the risk. The actual cause is not yet known, although damage to sperm is suggested.

An interesting study in China bears out this risk. Children of smoking fathers were more likely to contract ALL, lymphoma, and brain tumors. Because the cultural norm in China is for men but not women to smoke, these results are not related to maternal smoking. The effects of passive smoke during and after pregnancy have not been determined. Studies in the United Kingdom support these findings.

A study in France agrees with these findings too—paternal smoking is significantly associated with childhood ALL, acute myelocytic leukemia, and Burkitt lymphoma, while maternal smoking and alcohol consumption do not seem to carry this risk.

Viruses

A virus has been identified as a probable factor in the development of some types of leukemia. However, this does not mean that leukemia or lymphomas are contagious in the common sense. There has been a great deal of research over the past few years on RNA tumor viruses, or retroviruses. Subsequent mutations and the anomalies they cause are the subject of much speculation and clinical work.

Recently researchers have discovered the link between human papillomavirus (HPV) and cervical cancer, leading to a preventive vaccine for adolescent girls. HPV may cause 10% to 15% of adult cancers, including cervical carcinomas. The majority of HPV carriers do not get these cancers, so additional factors are required for malignant change.

Epstein-Barr virus (EBV), a herpes virus, is more strongly related to the development of cancer, including Burkitt lymphoma in Africa and Hodgkin lymphoma and other lymphomas in patients with compromised immune systems, like those with HIV or organ transplants.

Congenital Problems

Some congenital problems increase the tendency to develop certain malignancies. A disorder of unusual growths such as an enlarged tongue and umbilical hernia called Beckwith syndrome is sometimes found in conjunction with Wilms tumor and hepatoblastoma (a kidney tumor and a liver tumor, respectively). Children with Down syndrome are more likely to contract cancers such as neuroblastoma and leukemia.

What Are the Odds?

Those involved with childhood cancer, whether patients, parents, or specialists, talk a lot about statistics. Maybe it's easier to have a number to cling to, whether or not it really means anything. Certainly the chances of contracting a malignancy in childhood are mercifully small, but our pediatrician put it in perspective. Most parents ask about SIDS (crib death), she said, yet she had never had a case in her practice, although she had at that time three young patients with cancer.

In terms of survival, the statistics are educated guesses at best. A specialist on my daughter's treatment team noted that when he entered the field 40 years ago, most of the patients died. Now the majority live. Prognosis is based on generalities derived from past experience with the particular tumor involved.

Improvements in therapy have increased the odds significantly in the child's favor. While a few decades ago there was perhaps a 20% overall survival rate, today three in four cancer patients recover and live a normal life span. The percentage is much higher for several childhood forms of cancer, such as Wilms tumor and Hodgkin disease as well as ALL.

Many people delay going to the doctor because they fear the worst, that they or someone they love has cancer. Having a child referred from a general practitioner is particularly terrifying for the family.

Still, it would be comforting for those awaiting diagnosis at a clinic to know that between 80% and 90% of the children referred for evaluation do not have cancer. Nobody told me this when I was sitting there. But I have a vivid memory of more than one lucky mother who had heard the good news that her child didn't have cancer, gathering her things and almost running out of the clinic, never looking back.

Parents and others also want to know how long they will have to wait to find out if their child will be one of the survivors. One doctor says that we will know for sure that they are cured when they die at the age of 72 of some other cause. In the meantime, some experts consider 5-year survivors to be cured; in other words, if a child lives for 5 years after diagnosis in remission or without evidence of disease, it is less likely that there will be a relapse of the original malignancy. Other experts discount this notion and are waiting until the dust of recent advances in treatments has settled to see if the 5-year-period theory still holds.

Still other specialists have confidence in the so-called period of risk. This theory holds that certain tumors grow at a uniform rate, and that the maximum period of growth can only be the length of time the person has been alive plus the period of gestation. For adults this obviously does not help much, but for children the theory is useful. For example, if a child of 12 months is diagnosed with Wilms tumor, the longest the tumor could have been growing is 21 months (the age plus 9 months prenatal life). Therefore, it is assumed that if the original tumor is removed, any new tumor growth would reach the same size as the original mass by the time the youngster is 33 months old (12 months plus 21 months), and if at that age the child still has no new evidence of disease, it is unlikely that there will be further masses.

The child's age at diagnosis is also an important factor in some diseases like neuroblastoma in determining who has a better chance of survival, a very young age being a clear advantage.

What Will Happen and Who Will Help?

Childhood cancer has been called a family disease, because the impact on the child inevitably affects everyone in the family. Therapy usually consumes many hours or days over long months and years, disrupting the household routine not only for the patient and his parents but for everyone else, too. Schoolwork may be neglected, siblings feel slighted, money may be a problem, and always there is fear, whether or not it is discussed.

Cancer is particularly devastating in adolescents, who are old enough to understand what is happening to them, in whom the hair loss that is often a temporary side effect of chemotherapy is particularly embarrassing, and whose struggles for independence are inhibited by their need for special care.

Children can be cruel and may sometimes single out the cancer patient for ridicule or abuse. In other instances teachers may feel uncomfortable or reluctant to have a child with cancer in the classroom. Some uninformed people still fear that cancer is contagious and ostracize the victim and his or her family. Fortunately, this is not always the case, and for those seeking help, it is available through support groups such as Candlelighters, whose members have "been there, done that." Some clinics have formal parents' groups, and in others, those waiting for treatments can shore each other up informally. The advent of the Internet has been another boon, with numerous online chat or discussion groups specific to the various forms of cancer. The World Wide Web is such a valuable resource that it gets a separate chapter in this book.

We were extremely fortunate in meeting many parents who helped us through some rough times and others whom we could help later. Some of them are still close friends. I am in regular contact with a mother I met in what was to be one of the darkest hours of Lisa's ordeal, when we were all exhausted and afraid. This marvelous woman has been my salvation on more occasions than I can count, and I hope I have been able to reciprocate. We discovered that no matter how wonderful and helpful your friends are (and ours were), it is not the same as having someone beside you who is going through the same thing. Parents who cannot attend any groups might ask at their clinic if there is a family living near them who has been through a similar situation and who might be willing to lend reassurance and advice.

How Does Cancer Affect the Body?

Even given all this, children still die of cancer—the American Cancer Society estimated that 1700 youngsters would die of malignancies in the year 2002. In fact, over the past 30 years cancer has risen from the tenth ranking killer of children to the second. This is not because there has been a surge of cancer; rather, it is a result of advances in diagnosis and in preventing and curing such traditional killers as measles and polio.

Cancer kills the victim in several ways, often in combination. Many children die of overwhelming infection when the body loses its ability to fight off disease, whether because of the cancer itself or because of lowered resistance from chemotherapy; the latter risk, however, is not sufficient to stop the therapy. High-risk periods can usually be anticipated and the dosages can be altered to minimize the danger or to protect the child in other ways (keeping him out of crowds, for example).

Tumors can also invade organ systems and inhibit vital functions. If the stomach is blocked, for example, the patient can starve to death. If the kidneys are blocked, the child can die of the poisoning that results when the body cannot cleanse itself of waste. If the tumor metastasizes to the lungs, the body does not get enough oxygen to survive. Invasion of the brain or liver stops other vital life-support systems. Some patients succumb to severe anemia or, if the cancer eats through a major blood vessel, massive bleeding. The tumor may press on nerves or block intestines or other body passages, but doctors can ease any resulting pain with powerful sedatives and painkillers.

What About the Survivors?

What will happen to the survivors? We are just learning whether they will face discrimination in obtaining an education, a good job, or insurance benefits as they mature. Late consequences of cancer are being studied. There may be future physical effects caused by the radiation, chemotherapy, or surgery, including a second cancer. Some may have serious social or psychological disorders as a result of having had such a serious illness in childhood. Delayed physical development may occur.

Long-term survivors will have to be followed throughout their lives to seek the answers to these questions and to care for any recurrence or late effects that surface. It is certainly a blessing that there are enough long-term survivors to warrant a special chapter in this edition.

Who Treats Childhood Cancer?

The question of where to go for help brings up a very important point. These diseases are rare; with thousands of pediatricians and general or family practitioners in the United States and only 12,400 or so children diagnosed annually with a wide variety of cancers, it is immediately obvious that regular pediatricians and family doctors will see very few cases in a lifetime of medical practice. As shown in Section II of this book, the treatments are continually changing and improving rapidly, which also makes it difficult for the generalist trying to keep up with the field.

For these reasons, the National Cancer Institute and the American Academy of Pediatrics strongly recommend, almost insist, that children with cancer go to centers or clinics where they can be diagnosed and treated by specialists in pediatric oncology (the study of tumors) or hematology. Here they will receive the best, most up-to-date care by a team of people intimately familiar with the disease and its therapies. Studies have shown that the survival rate of children cared for at these centers is double and possibly triple that of those treated by local physicians. This improved rate reflects not only the specialists' knowledge of state-of-the-art treatment, but also the availability of special facilities and support services at these cancer centers as well as access to cutting-edge clinical trials. The most important question in interviewing a physician is, "How many times have you seen and treated this illness, and what was the outcome?"

Using a cancer center is not without its problems. Costs not covered by insurance can escalate: transportation, parking, housing, meals, and so on. Also, being some distance from your own local support system, whether friends, neighbors, place of worship, or family, can be very difficult when your needs are so great. Still, the results overbalance the problems at these "centers of excellence."

This is not to say that the local pediatrician or practitioner should be discarded. Far from it! We were in regular contact with our pediatrician throughout Lisa's treatment. She was kept up to date by the clinic and by the surgeon, and when the ordeal was over we resumed regular checkups and immunizations with her, traveling to the clinic on an increasingly infrequent basis.

Fortunately we could handle Lisa's illness this way because we live within an hour's drive of several major cancer centers. For families who must commute much longer distances, centers can often evaluate and stabilize the patient, then arrange for some treatments to be continued by local doctors close to home and supervised by the long-distance specialists, who perform infrequent examinations but provide advice and expertise as required. This happy collaboration, when it is possible, allows the family to live as normally as possible and still receive optimal care.

Amy and Tommy

Recently, treatments have saved some youngsters with advanced disease. I didn't know Amy when, at the age of 11 months, she was dying from widely metastasized stage IV neuroblastoma. Test after test was made, each result worse than the one before it. Her parents were given no reason to hope for her survival. Yet today she is a college graduate; we danced at her wedding and we fuss over her son and her daughter.

On the other hand, I did meet Tommy and his parents when he was about 2 months old. This beautiful infant was diagnosed as having stage I (localized) Wilms tumor, described as "almost as curable as the common cold" with 90% survival. The affected kidney was removed, treatment was begun, and his relieved family settled down to a semblance of normal life. Then, inexplicably, a tumor began to grow in his brain and metastases appeared elsewhere in his body. Tragically, he died at the age of 5.5 months.

Both of these children received the best care available and the newest treatments at pediatric centers of excellence. We may never understand in our lifetimes why one lived and one died.

How to Use This Book

The first section of *Children with Cancer* is devoted to the types of cancers that children develop. The next part explains the different therapies that the family will encounter as well as some experimental treatments. Use the later parts of the book to find sources of support, to cope with the emotional as well as physical and practical aspects of the childhood cancer experience. Finally, check the appendices for names, addresses, Web sites, and other contact information for those who will help the patient and the family. Rather than read cover to cover, use the index to pinpoint the section you need. Over the course of the child's treatment, various aspects and developing issues will come up that are addressed here, so use the index to zero in on topics as you need them. Also, the appendices and glossary have a huge amount of information. Check there for definitions of unfamiliar words or for descriptions of medical tests you encounter.

Further Resources

A note about Further Resources: I have kept the most important resources for each type of cancer or each therapy together at the ends of the chapters. In some cases, where the organization or resource relates specifically to a chapter's topic, I have included complete contact information at the chapter end and omitted a duplicate listing from the appendices at the end of the book. Again I stress: this book is intended to support you and your child, but it is no substitute for the best medical advice you can get. I can clarify your doctor's advice, but in no way can I replace it.

Most hospital and clinic libraries will cooperate with parents, helping them find information, perhaps preparing a computer-generated list of reading. The Candlelighters Foundation also provides an excellent bibliography of materials. Other booklets are available from the American Cancer Society and the National Cancer Institute as well as online.

READING

Berglund, Rita. *An Alphabet About Kids With Cancer*. Denver, CO: The Children's Legacy, 1994 (P. O. Box 300305, Denver, CO 80203; 303-830-7595)

Not an ABC book per se, but cleverly designed using the familiar format to explain to elementary-aged children about their illness from A (an ache) through diagnosis and treatment to Z (Zowee!). Comes with blank alphabet pages at the back for the patient to use. Artistic black-and-white photos. Multicultural kids, generations of loved ones, and poetic text. A classy source. Not an "easy reader" but a "read-to-me" level book—an excellent conversation starter. A couple of very graphic pictures of surgery are in the front, but they can be glossed over because of their small size.

Cefrey, Holly. *Coping With Cancer*. New York: Rosen Publishing Group, Inc, 2000.
For junior high readers and up. Covers various types of cancer and body systems, and explains with black-and-white drawings. Good chapter on risks and causes, including a discussion of genetics.

Chamberlain, Shannon. *My ABC Book of Cancer*. San Francisco: Synergistic Press, 1990.
Written and illustrated by a 10-year-old fighting rhabdomyosarcoma, it includes hospital, clinic and camp experiences, faith, and more. For Grade 1 up, to open discussion or dialog.

Chan, Helen S. L. *Understanding Cancer Therapies; a Practical and Hopeful Guide to the Many Treatments Available*. Jackson, MS: University Press of Mississippi, 2007.
Written for knowledgeable adults, an educated explanation of cancer treatments. This volume covers childhood cancer well.

Coleman, C. Norman. *Understanding Cancer: A Patient's Guide to Diagnosis, Prognosis and Treatment*. Baltimore: Johns Hopkins University Press, 1998.
Really almost an attack plan for families who intellectualize treatments. There is little disease-specific information, but this is an excellent early source for in-depth information on treatment theories and practices overall, with checklists and case studies. Especially good discussion of clinical research trials—the whys and hows. Adult reading level.

Janes-Hodder, Honna, Nancy Keene. *Childhood Cancer: A Parents' Guide to Solid Tumor Cancer*. Sebastopol, CA: O'Reilly & Associates, Inc., 1999.
Readable information liberally sprinkled with been-there, done-that anecdotes.

Keene, Nancy, and Trevor Romain. *Chemo, Craziness and Comfort: My Book about Childhood Cancer*. Candlelighters Childhood Cancer Foundation, 2003.
It would be impossible to recommend this book too highly. Simply put, every cancer patient, especially between elementary and middle school ages, should have a copy of it. Medical writer Nancy Keene, mother of a leukemia survivor, here explains the whole process, from healthy body through the end of treatments, in a journal format for kids to add their own pictures and

notes. Romain's cartoon-like illustrations brighten and clarify the text with humor and understanding. Copies are free to families with children between the ages of 6 and 12 with a cancer diagnosis.

Klett, Am, and Dave Klett. *The Amazing Hannah: Look at Everything I Can Do*. Candlelighters Childhood Cancer Foundation, 2003.
For children between 1 and 5 diagnosed with cancer. Picture book with photos sick children can identify with. Free from Candlelighters. Also available in Spanish.

Lyons, Lyman. *Diagnosis and Treatment of Cancer (The Biology of Cancer Series)*. New York: Chelsea House, 2007.
This is a clearly written discussion of cancer in its various forms and modern treatments, including stem cell transplantation. Not specific to pediatric malignancies. Readable for high school age up.

Sarg, Michael. *The Cancer Dictionary*. New York: Facts on File, 3d edition, 2007.
Not a simple defining dictionary, this title includes drugs, tests, surgical procedures, staging, and much more. The newer edition also has Internet addresses.

Stern, Grant, PhD, and Joseph Mirro, MD, eds. *Childhood Cancer—A Handbook from St. Jude Children's Research Hospital*. Cambridge, MA: Perseus Pub., 2000.
Written by professionals in the health care field, this is packed with solid, readable information, sometimes in question-and-answer format. Has an excellent chapter on "Spiritual Support for Children and Families."

This Battle Which I Must Fight: Cancer in Canada's Children and Teenagers. Ottawa: Minister of Supply and Services Canada, 1996.
This excellent, basic book has solid, accessible information especially but not exclusively for Canadians. Incidence, types of disease, feelings, resources. Also available in French.
Available online at www.phar-aspc.gc.ca/publicat/tbwimf-mcplv

ORGANIZATIONS/WEB RESOURCES

American Cancer Society
www.cancer.org (lots of publications and information)

The Cancer Survival Toolbox
National Coalition for Cancer Survivors (see Appendix B for address). Free 6-CD audio program designed to help families face cancer, from communicating with the medical team to finding financial help. An excellent

way to fill some of those innumerable waiting room and bedside hours. Also available from www.cancersurvivaltoolbox.org.

Childhood Cancer Guides

www.childhoodcancerguides.org. This Web site, from a nonprofit organization, has a lot of links to useful information and all aspects of the pediatric cancer experience. Also sells some highly regarded books.

Children's Oncology Group

www.curesearch.org. Combines the resources of the National Childhood Cancer Foundation and the Children's Oncology Group. An excellent gateway for all families.

U. S. National Cancer Institute

www.cancer.gov (includes an excellent discussion of cancer clusters). From this site you can also access Physicians Data Query, an outstanding selection of disease- and treatment-specific fact sheets written separately for professionals and laypersons. A subsite, http://seer.cancer.gov/, has a wealth of statistical information on incidence and outcome, although the latest numbers may be embargoed.

University of Pennsylvania

www.oncolink.org. A good portal for cancer information, including breaking news in the field from Reuters.

2

Genetics of Childhood Cancer

For years researchers hoped to find a "magic bullet" that would cure all types of cancer. Today, with few exceptions, that magic bullet is a faded dream, but the search has uncovered a wealth of other information. One very important area of discovery is the role genes play in causing and, we hope, treating cancer. Armed with the growing knowledge of genetics, researchers are discovering ways to detect, treat, and sometimes even predict cancer. It's not a magic bullet, but it is a promising new weapon in the arsenal.

There have been a number of discoveries in the study of cancer genes. The gene is the basic building block of each cell's heredity, and is contained in the DNA and strung together into chromosomes. All of us have oncogenes, or cancer genes, but we do not yet understand what activates them. An oncogene may break off from its normal chromosome position and trade places with another gene. An oncogene is not exactly a chromosomal abnormality; it is an area on the chromosome that, if activated somehow, can direct a cell to grow abnormally and undergo malignant change. In fact, oncogenes have been related to viruses that cause cancer in animals (which does not mean that cancers are spread from one person to another like, say, influenza). So far many human oncogenes have been found, and by studying them and seeking others, we may learn to identify people who are more susceptible to carcinogens like tobacco and industrial chemicals.

We now know that cancer is, simply speaking, a genetic abnormality gone wild. The defects might be inherited or perhaps acquired through environmental factors (e.g., diet, the aging process, radiation, chemicals). An in-depth discussion of the human genome project and the genetics of cancer is beyond the scope of this book. Interested readers can check out the resources listed in the appendices for further information.

If genetic defects are causing the cancer, theorists are thinking, fixing those defects should be an effective form of treatment. There are three parts to the equation. First, we have to identify the genetic "mistake" that is causing the problem. Then we have to learn how to make a "patch" that will fix it. And finally (and far from the easiest step) we have to figure out a vector, or a go-between, to carry the "patch" to the damaged cell and stick there while it goes to work.

Experts think that genes might be able to control cancer in different ways:

- By killing malignant cells directly
- By protecting the bone marrow from tumors
- By improving the patient's immunity and with it enhancing the ability to "fight off" malignancies

Researchers have made a lot of progress figuring out which genes have gone awry in the various types of cancer. Presence or absence of the Philadelphia chromosome, for example, is important in staging chronic leukemias. (*Staging* means to determine the spread of the disease in order to select the most effective treatment for the patient.) Brain tumors in very young children often show an abnormal 22 chromosome. The RB1 gene is also damaged or absent in many cancers. Changes in the INI1 gene may be passed from parent to child and form a risk factor for some very rare brain tumors, especially in children under the age of 3. Abnormalities in chromosome 1 are found in well over half of all neuroblastoma patients. Some genetic defects, called *trisomies*, are related to the acute leukemias, helping to determine the best therapy.

Chemotherapy for malignancies has for many years targeted cancer cells at various stages in their development. Genetic therapy may work the same way, with drugs that attach to malignant cells at specific phases in the development or reproduction cycle. As researchers learn more, they are working to develop new drugs to target the genetic abnormality and teach the cells to stop reproducing wildly. The body's tumor suppressor genes, if defective, don't stop the wild cell growth. Scientists are looking for ways to replace the faulty gene with normal ones that function properly. This is like finding the "off" switch for a crazily reproducing cancer cell that is stuck in the "on" position.

Some drugs that target genetic abnormalities are already being used on human patients, although there are no approved gene therapies for childhood cancer. Imatinib (Gleevec) has been approved for use against chronic myeloid leukemia (CML) and is being studied for use with glioblastoma (brain tumor) patients.

An article in *Cure* notes that new developments in cancer therapy will include "molecular chemotherapy, where genes that encode toxic proteins are delivered to tumors…" One problem remains: "the limitation of current methods for delivering the therapeutic genes to tumor cells."

Genetics can help determine which patients with acute lymphocytic leukemia (ALL) have more treatment-resistant disease. Since doctors will have more difficulty in curing these children's diseases, they can then be treated more aggressively On the other hand, those with more indolent (or slow-growing) types can be spared therapies (and side effects) that they don't need to beat their leukemia. Knowing a child's genetic makeup will tell doctors which drugs will be more effective in his case and which combination is optimal for him.

Ideally, all patients will some day have a "molecular diagnostics test" included in the arsenal of studies used to identify and stage their cancer. Knowing which genes are causing (or not stopping) the abnormal cell growth and division will be a big step in planning effective treatment in the future. A lot of research is needed to understand the *30,000 genes* found in every human cell!

Experts estimate that fewer than 5% of all childhood malignancies are clearly inherited. About a third of all cases of retinoblastoma are considered familial, as well as 1% to 2% of Wilms tumors, 3% of leukemia cases (Down syndrome), and 2% of brain tumors (related to type 1 neurofibromatosis). Xeroderma pigmentosum is an inherited syndrome that carries a thousand-fold incidence of skin cancers at an early age; these children must be protected from the sun.

The body has different types of genes that affect cancer. Some of them promote rapid cell division and the growth of malignancies. Some of them are tumor suppressors, stopping that rapid cell division and growth in its tracks.

As more and more children survive their cancers, late-effects clinics are looking at their offspring. Overall their children seem no more likely to develop a malignancy than children in the general population. Certainly many survivors consult with geneticists before starting their own families. It is important to insure that the heritable aspects of cancer in identified individuals are used in legal and ethical ways in terms of risks, insurability, and employability. This is a touchy subject that needs a great deal more research so that the positive side of genetics research doesn't backfire on those who seek help.

Further Resources

READING

Bozzone, Donna M. *Cancer Genetics (Biology of Cancer Series)*. New York: Chelsea House, 2007. A particularly lucid explanation of the genetic causes of cancer, written for high school students and adults.

Curiel, Daniel T., and Casey Cunningham. "Gene therapy: a targeted therapeutic." *Cure*, vol. 3 (1) (Spring 2004), p. 53.

"Working toward tailored therapy for cancer." *The Lancet* vol. 357 (9267) (May 12, 2001), p. 1508.

ORGANIZATIONS/WEB RESOURCES

The National Cancer Institute Web site (http://www.cancer.gov) has a clear, thorough discussion of genes and cancer.

TARGET (Childhood Cancer Therapeutically Applicable Research to Generate Effective Treatments) from the U.S. National Cancer Institute and the Foundation for the National Institutes of Health (www.fnih.org) aims to study genetic applications to fight pediatric malignancies.

3

Leukemia

As noted earlier, cancer begins when a cell gets stuck in an immature stage of its life cycle and reproduces repeatedly. In the case
of leukemia and lymphoma, the form of cancer that develops is especially dependent on the life stage the cell is in when it becomes malignant and begins to multiply out of control, because these diseases
arise from the same basic cell at different "ages."

The Differences between Leukemia and Lymphoma

Leukemia and lymphoma both arise from immature blood cells, usually those destined to become white cells. Some of the types of white
blood cells are lymphocytes, granulocytes, and monocytes.

Because of recent research, we now understand more about cells in
general and cancer cells in particular. Specialists studying tumor cells
have learned that some types of white blood cells affected in leukemia
are similar to those that cause non-Hodgkin lymphoma. The identifying surface markers (antigens) on the cells are alike, as are the
symptoms for some forms of chronic leukemia and lymphoma.

In lymphoma patients, tumor masses grow when cancer cells swell
the lymph nodes and related organs such as the liver and spleen.

Sometimes leukemia patients develop tumor masses too, when cancer cells "catch" in the lymph nodes and collect there.

Doctors sometimes have trouble telling whether a child has leukemia or non-Hodgkin lymphoma, both of which involve lymphocytes. There are several types of acute lymphoblastic leukemia (B cell, T cell, null cell, and undifferentiated), depending on the cell and its degree of maturity. There are also several subgroups of non-Hodgkin lymphoma. Whether a child is diagnosed as having leukemia or non-Hodgkin lymphoma might vary from one treatment center to another, depending on the extent of bone marrow involvement and whether or not malignant cells are found circulating in the bloodstream.

Some children with non-Hodgkin lymphoma relapse with leukemia. Those with a known risk of that happening receive treatments similar to those for leukemia.

Leukemia

Descriptions of leukemia date back as far as Hippocrates. It received its current name in 1847 when the German pathologist Rudolf Virchow identified it by the Greek words meaning "white blood." With about 3250 new cases of childhood leukemia diagnosed annually in the United States, it accounts for about 25% of all malignancies before the age of 20. Of these, about 75% will be acute lymphocytic (or lymphoblastic) leukemia (ALL). There has been an increased incidence over the past 20 years, mostly with ALL, but not in younger or black children.

Leukemia is a cancer of the blood-forming organs, including the bone marrow, the spleen, and the lymph nodes. When leukemia strikes, the body starts cranking out a vast number of immature cells that do not mature or perform their proper functions. They also interfere with the manufacture of the correct proportion of red cells, white cells, and platelets.

All blood cells begin life as identical cells and then mature in the bone marrow into three types of blood cells, which are suspended in the liquid portion of blood called plasma:

- *Red blood cells* (erythrocytes) collect oxygen from the lungs for distribution to the tissues, then help return carbon dioxide waste to the lungs to be exhaled.

- *Platelets* (thrombocytes) are cells that form little plugs to stop bleeding and help clots form.
- *White blood cells* (leukocytes) fight infection.

The white blood cells (WBCs) are called the body's defense department, and for good reason. They seek out bacteria, viruses, and other foreign matter and produce substances to destroy them. When there is an infection in the body, the number of white cells increases naturally to combat the intruder.

There are different kinds of white cells. Granulocytes, particularly the neutrophils, are the body's "PacMan": formed in the bone marrow, they engulf and destroy bacteria and cellular wastes. Lymphocytes act in other ways to destroy viruses, fungi (yeast-like organisms), and some bacteria.

There are different types of lymphocytes. Some T lymphocytes control the immune response by recognizing a foreign invader and ordering another group of lymphocytes, B cells, to create antibodies to attack the invader. Other T lymphocytes act directly on foreign cells (including those in transplanted organs).

In leukemia, the immature white blood cells multiply so prolifically that they fill the bone marrow. Crowding out healthy cells, they eventually spill out into the circulating blood. The child with leukemia becomes listless, tired, and pale because the number of red cells in the bloodstream is reduced. The nose or gums may bleed because the child has fewer platelets than normal. Since there aren't enough mature white cells, the child may be unable to fight off an infection. Blood tests and bone marrow examinations help to identify exactly which type of WBC is involved.

The type of leukemia depends on the type of cell involved. The two major types are ALL and acute nonlymphocytic leukemia (ANNL). The term "ANLL" is often used to classify the other less common types of acute leukemia, such as acute myelocytic leukemia (AML), acute monomyelocytic leukemia (AMML), acute monocytic leukemia (AMOL), acute promyelocytic leukemia (APL), and acute erythroid leukemia (AEL). Sometimes the cell involved is too immature to determine what it would have become normally. This form of disease is called acute undifferentiated leukemia.

After the doctors determine what type of leukemia the child has, they carefully study the abnormal cells to identify the specific

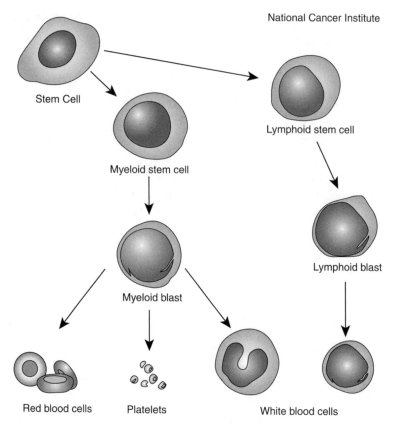

National Cancer Institute

Stem Cell

Myeloid stem cell

Lymphoid stem cell

Myeloid blast

Lymphoid blast

Red blood cells   Platelets

White blood cells

FIGURE 3.1   Blood cells maturing from stem cells

subgroup (like B cell or T cell). This close examination of cells, using antibodies to differentiate cell surface antigens, is crucial in planning individualized therapy.

WHAT CAUSES LEUKEMIA?

Sometimes parents are afraid that a fall or an earlier illness caused the leukemia. This is not so. Probably no single factor causes leukemia. As with other kinds of cancer, a number of factors appear to trigger the disease. Until these factors are better understood, we will not know why, exactly, our children fall ill.

One factor that is known to be involved in the development of some cases of leukemia in children is radiation. There is a lag of 10 to 15 years between exposure and the onset of leukemia. One in six survivors of the atomic bomb in Hiroshima who were within 1000 meters of the explosion contracted leukemia over the following 12 years. Still, the vast majority of those exposed to radiation do not develop leukemia.

Parental exposure to ionizing radiation is another risk factor, which is one reason for all those signs in x-ray departments about pregnant women notifying their doctors before being tested. A lot of media coverage has been given to the theory that high-voltage electric lines cause leukemia or other cancers, but studies have not shown this to be true. Some tap water contaminants (zinc, arsenic, chloroform, and cadmium among them) have been implicated in the development of some cases of leukemia.

Another known factor is exposure to the solvent benzene, a petroleum derivative that is used in the paint and chemical industries. Benzene is emitted by refineries and is a common gasoline additive to which large numbers of people are exposed daily. Paternal tobacco consumption is also a risk factor for AML.

Because some animal leukemias are caused by viruses, a viral cause has long been sought for the human disease. Researchers have, in fact, isolated the human T-cell leukemia virus that causes a rare form of cancer. A viral cause does *not* mean that human leukemia is contagious, however. If it were, the family of leukemia patients would "catch it," and they do not, nor do people "get" leukemia through blood transfusions from a donor who subsequently develops the disease. Indeed, pregnant women with leukemia give birth to babies without the disease, and there is no apparent link to breastfeeding, except for a suggestion that nursing your child might protect against leukemia somehow.

Previous treatment with chemotherapy or radiation also opens the door to second malignancies, which often surface as leukemia. The drug most commonly associated with treatment-related leukemia is etoposide.

Certain genetic disorders increase the risk of leukemia. In individuals with Down syndrome there is clearly an increased incidence of leukemia. Still, only about 6% of children with Down syndrome develop leukemia, divided equally between ALL and ANLL.

If one identical twin develops leukemia, there is a one-in-five chance that the other twin will develop it too, usually within a few months. It is even more likely if the first child contracts leukemia before the age of 5. The likelihood that the second twin will have leukemia decreases as the age of onset in the first twin increases.

If one child in a family develops leukemia, his brothers and sisters are more likely to get it, too, than are unrelated children their age with healthy siblings. The risk is still small—one sibling in 720 developed leukemia in one study. The cause is thought to be genetic, not contagion.

As discussed earlier, researchers believe that no single factor leads to leukemia. Rather, a combination of factors—genetic, environmental, and viral—probably sets the stage for a particular child to develop leukemia or, indeed, other cancers. Risk factors for specific forms of leukemia will be discussed later in this chapter.

Acute Lymphocytic Leukemia

In 75% of childhood leukemia cases, the lymphocyte production goes haywire, leading to the form of leukemia called ALL. The lymphoblasts (immature lymphocytes, or "blasts") stay immature, reproducing when they should not and crowding the bone marrow so that normal cells, while not killed, do not have enough room to multiply and mature.

Since the early signs and symptoms of ALL may be vague and seemingly nonthreatening, they are often shrugged off by parents and sometimes even by doctors as a minor illness. The pediatrician might be fooled initially into thinking the youngster is suffering from arthritis, infectious mononucleosis, or a blood infection because early ALL symptoms can mimic these diseases.

SYMPTOMS

Children with ALL suffer from a number of symptoms. Most have:

- Fatigue
- A low-grade fever
- Easy bruising
- Pallor

Some others suffer:

- Bleeding
- Severe infections

- Irritability
- Loss of appetite
- Weight loss
- Slow recovery from colds or other infections

Less commonly, the leukemia mimics other diseases with a number of puzzling symptoms:

- Restricted, painful movement in bones and joints
- Swollen abdomen due to enlarged spleen or liver
- Swollen lymph nodes in neck, groin, underarms
- Headaches
- Unexplained vomiting
- Sore mouth and gums
- Puffy eyes and face (particularly in infants)

INCIDENCE

Who gets ALL? The vast majority of all ALL cases are seen in children, with more boys than girls affected. The incidence peaks between the ages of 2 and 6, around puberty, and, in women, after menopause. In the United States blacks develop ALL much less frequently than do whites. Children of Latino and Filipino descent have the highest American rate of ALL, Asian-Americans the lowest. Internationally, ALL is more common in the developed world.

DIAGNOSIS

A series of tests confirms a diagnosis of leukemia. A complete blood count (or CBC) checks the ratio of the various types of blood cells. A smear of blood is studied under a microscope to see whether any of the cells look abnormal. Finally, a bone marrow sample is examined. If it reveals a large number of immature leukemia blast cells, the diagnosis is certain.

Tests are then made to determine the extent of the disease and to look for complications. Depending on the symptoms, cultures of blood, urine, nose, and throat identify any underlying infections, and kidney and liver function tests assess the health of those vital organs. An examination of cerebrospinal fluid (CSF) obtained by a spinal tap assesses the involvement of the central nervous system (CNS). The results will be compared with those of later tests to document the child's response to treatment.

One very important step is immunophenotyping, testing to identify the type of cell involved, whether T cell or B cell, because that determines the child's risk and therefore the treatments. The chromosomes of the blasts are analyzed for telltale genetic changes.

TREATMENT

Treatment is started as soon as possible, the aim being to induce a remission. This means that leukemia cells are no longer detectable, although some will remain in the body. Remission may be attained quickly or over a period of weeks. When the patient is in remission, the blood counts are normal and there are no leukemia symptoms. Successful treatment of ALL has become a model for treating other types of cancer with drugs; it is *the* big success story in chemotherapy advances.

Current phases of leukemia treatment are induction (of remission), consolidation, interim maintenance, and delayed and maintenance. The induction phase uses drugs like vincristine, asparaginase, daunomycin, and prednisone. In the consolidation phase, cytosine arabinoside (ara-C), cyclophosphamide, methotrexate, mercaptopurine, and doxorubicin may be added in varying blends. If the child relapses, another remission is sought with different drug combinations, quite possibly followed by a bone marrow or stem cell transplant. The maintenance phase continues for 18 to 30 months.

During the consolidation phase, steps are taken to prevent the leukemia cells from invading and hiding in the CNS, out of the reach of most chemotherapy drugs. Successful treatment requires measures to eradicate the cells that might seek sanctuary there. This is important in prolonging remission in children with ALL and curing them.

Traditionally two approaches have been used to combat this problem. Some protocols used drugs injected into the CSF during a spinal tap. Others had used radiation to kill the leukemia cells. Still others combined the two. Some centers inject very high doses of methotrexate into the bloodstream, then rescue the body with injections of citrovorum before too much healthy tissue is damaged. All of these strategies have sparked controversy as to the best way to reduce side effects, and experts still do not agree on the best course of action to prevent relapse in the CNS, although the use of radiation is much less common today. However, they do agree that some step must be taken to prevent the leukemia from entering the CSF. It is becoming evident that some children with ALL require more intensive or different treatment both to control the disease in the CNS and to eradicate leukemic cells elsewhere.

Because cranial radiation was shown to cause learning and other disabilities, especially when given to children under the age of 5, that therapy is not used as much today as in the past. Even most high-risk patients who go into remission quickly are less likely to have CNS radiation. Children who are older than 10, have T-cell markers, and are diagnosed with a white blood cell count over 50,000/microliter are more likely to receive radiation in addition to chemotherapy to prevent spread to the CNS.

Recent studies have shown that patients with a higher-than-average level of interleukin-15 in their bone marrow at diagnosis are at greater risk of CNS involvement. This discovery could lead to therapies that are personally tailored for each patient.

Instead of staging leukemia like other cancers, specialists determine each patient's risk group. Experts recognize groups of leukemic children for whom the prognosis is not as good, based on age, the white blood count at the time of diagnosis, and other factors, which help determine which therapy is most appropriate for each child.

The two major risk groups are T-cell and B-cell ALL. B-cell ALL is much more common, especially in children, and at diagnosis they have leukemic cells in their blood, lymph nodes, spleen, liver, and possibly the CNS. T-cell leukemia is potentially in all those sites at diagnosis, plus the thymus gland.

Standard-risk ALL includes:

- Patient aged 1 to 9
- Total white blood count less than 50,000/microliter at diagnosis
- B-cell precursor leukemia

Higher-risk ALL includes:

- Patient under the age of 1 or over the age of 9
- White blood count over 50,000/microliter at diagnosis
- T-cell leukemia
- Presence of genetic marker Philadelphia chromosome (5% of pediatric ALL cases)

COMPLICATIONS

A number of complications can make fighting leukemia more difficult. The most common problems are infection or bleeding, which fortunately can be treated with antibiotics and red cell or platelet transfusions. Common illnesses such as measles or chickenpox can be lethal for patients with ALL, requiring a hospital stay. However, most children are able to handle common infections such as colds without much problem.

Patients failing to go into remission with regular induction therapies can still be successfully treated, as can patients who relapse after achieving a complete remission.

Children who survive leukemia usually experience long-term effects. Some survivors will develop a second cancer in the dozen or so years following remission. Some may have a slowing of growth that may not correct itself when therapy is completed. Certain treatments may cause sterility, such as radiation therapy when a boy's testicles show evidence of leukemia. Learning disabilities are common with leukemia survivors who have had radiation for CNS preventive therapy. As more children survive for longer periods, researchers can find out how great the risks of these long-term effects are. Whatever the risks, there is no doubt that they are preferable to an uncontested death.

PROGNOSIS

Using treatment plans with several drugs and in some cases radiation, more than 95% of all ALL patients achieve remission. A majority remain disease-free during the therapy period of 18 to 30 months. Treatment can then be stopped. The overall survival rate is 80%, girls having a slightly better rate than boys. Broken down, the 5-year survival rate for children ages 1 to 9 at diagnosis is 80% to 85%. Diagnosis before age 1 yields a 37% 5-year survival rate, and 75% of children diagnosed between ages 15 and 19 are long-term survivors. Blacks may have a lower survival rate than whites, whether because of genetic considerations, poorer access to optimal health care, or other reasons. Research indicates that measuring absolute lymphocyte counts at the time of diagnosis can help predict survival and risk of relapse. Those with low absolute lymphocyte counts (normal cells) in the early days of chemotherapy did not fare as well as those with higher counts at that stage. This holds true for both ALL and AML patients.

If relapse occurs within the first 6 months of therapy, a bone marrow or stem cell transplant can achieve a 20% to 50% rate of long-term survival. If relapse occurs within 2 to 3 years of therapy, more chemotherapy is given, then a bone marrow transplant in the event of a second relapse; in these circumstances 40% to 50 % of children still become long-term survivors. To be sure that children who survive are truly cured, they must be examined regularly throughout their lives. Hospitals should be referring these patients to long-term survivor clinics. Studies will help determine whether the 5-year mark used to indicate cures in other forms of cancer applies to leukemia. Some experts feel that late recurrences might be new disease in a somehow susceptible individual.

Acute Nonlymphocytic Leukemia

Most often found in adults, ANLL accounts for about a quarter of leukemia cases in children. ANLL develops when a blast different from the one involved in ALL proliferates. The incidence of ANLL peaks in the first 2 years of life, with the lowest juvenile incidence about age 9, followed by slowly increasing frequency in adolescence. One risk factor is prior treatment with chemotherapy or radiation. Whites and blacks have similar rates, although Hispanics have an elevated risk. Children with Down syndrome have a higher risk of ANLL, as do siblings of children with leukemia (especially twins). There is a potential link with alcohol and tobacco use in pregnancy.

SYMPTOMS

Symptoms are similar to those seen in ALL, with bleeding, anemia, and infections. Doctors perform the same diagnostic tests for ANLL. ANLL patients are more likely to have involvement of the gums (which may be swollen and spongy to the point of covering the teeth) and infections of the skin, anus, and vulva. They may have joint or bone pain or painless lumps in the neck or elsewhere (which may be blue or purple).

TREATMENT

Primary therapy requires much more intensive chemotherapy than in ALL. Supportive therapy consists of antibiotics and transfusions of platelets, white blood cells or red blood cells as needed. ANLL patients also have phases of therapy, beginning with induction (including CNS preventive measures), then consolidation and intensification, followed by maintenance.

One form, acute promyelocytic leukemia, responds well in research settings to standard chemotherapy combined with tretinoin (Vesanoid), with a 70% to 75% survival rate reported. This form of vitamin A or retinoic acid is also used to treat acne.

The drug combinations used in chemotherapy differ from those used in childhood ALL. The aim is to literally wipe out all the marrow cells, in anticipation that normal cells will then repopulate the marrow. Receiving intensive drug therapy in various combinations, about 70% to 80% of children achieve remission; about 40% survive 5 years. Again, girls have a slightly better cure rate than boys, although the outcome for blacks and whites is similar. Recurring ANLL calls for more chemotherapy, followed by a stem cell transplant (which might also be carried out in first remission).

Other Leukemias

Chronic leukemia accounts for less than 3% of childhood leukemia cases; it is much more common in adults. It has a slower onset than acute leukemia and involves a more mature type of cell. In some children it changes into acute leukemia (in a so-called blast crisis). There are two types that occur with about the same frequency in youngsters. For both boys and girls, there is a peak of CML in the first year of life and then in the late teen years; boys, however, have four times the incidence of CML as compared to girls. The adult type, which tends to strike older children, is characterized by white blood cell counts over 100,000 leukocytes per microliter of blood at diagnosis and by an abnormal chromosome pattern, the Philadelphia chromosome.

As a rule the juvenile form develops in the first years of life with the following symptoms:

- Recurrent infections
- Facial rash
- Low platelet count
- Normal or low white cell count
- An enlarged spleen

- Anemia
- Weight loss
- Hemorrhage
- Sweating

A bone marrow or stem cell transplant is the treatment of choice for CML, and results have been gratifying. As with ANLL, CML patients may receive all-trans retinoic acid or arsenic trioxide in clinical trials.

Further Resources

READING

Keene, Nancy. *Childhood Leukemia: a Guide for Families, Friends and Caregivers.* Sebastapol, CA: O'Reilly and Associates, 3d ed., 2002.

Westcott, Patsy. *Living with Leukemia.* Austin, TX: Raintree Steck Vaughan, 2000.
This well-illustrated picture book for middle readers presents three children who have faced leukemia at ages 12, 9, and 5. They are living normal post-therapy lives. The book explains what leukemia is and how it affects the body. It is honest, noting, for example, that some children don't get better. Treatments and side effects are described, with the reassurance that the latter go away after therapy is finished. Bone marrow transplantation, siblings' feelings, the reaction and fears of friends, school re-entry, and support groups are all here, plus an age-appropriate glossary and a list of contacts.

ORGANIZATIONS/WEB SITES

Leukemia and Lymphoma Society (1311 Mamaroneck Avenue, White Plains, NY 10605; 800/955-4572; 914/949-5213; www.lls.org)
This association, with chapters throughout the United States and Canada, provides financial assistance, peer support, and referrals nationwide, as well as information resources ranging from pamphlets to excellent teleconferences. Funds research into causes and cures.

National Cancer Institute SEER Pediatrics Monograph (www.cancer.gov)
This online resource has incidence and survival statistics for leukemia.

4

Lymphoma

There are two broad types of lymphoma, Hodgkin disease and non-Hodgkin lymphoma (NHL), both characterized by abnormal masses in the lymph system. While both leukemia and lymphoma are malignancies of the blood-forming tissues, they differ in that leukemia first appears in the bone marrow and lymphoma in the body's lymph system. NHL is a catch-all term used to describe several forms of lymphoma that are not Hodgkin disease. An estimated 800 children under the age of 20 are diagnosed with NHL in the United States annually. Hodgkin disease will be discussed in the next chapter.

The Lymphatic System

The lymphatic system is a network of nodes and tiny tubes or vessels that drain fluid from spaces in the body's tissues. The lymphatic system destroys foreign matter and produces antibodies to fight infection. To put it very simply, think of the immune system as baseball teams. Say your system is the Boston Red Sox. When your Boston Red Sox lymphocytes notice foreign invaders like New York Yankees antigens (protein, bacteria, viruses, pollen, and so on), the

Sox lymphocytes fight back with antibodies to repel the Yankees antigens.

The lymphatic system also produces new lymphocytes, a type of white blood cell, to replenish worn-out cells. Tonsils, adenoids, the spleen, and the thymus are all specialized lymph glands. Lymph nodes are found in the armpits, groin, neck, mid-chest, and abdomen. Other lymphatic tissue, not formed into nodes, lines bone and organs such as the stomach and small intestine.

Classification of Non-Hodgkin Lymphoma

Several classification systems are used to identify NHL. One that is often (but not universally) used groups the diseases by the origin of the malignant cell:

- Lymphoblastic lymphoma
- Small noncleaved cell lymphoma (Burkitt and Burkitt-like lymphoma)
- Diffuse large B-cell lymphoma
- Anaplastic large-cell lymphoma

This is understandably very confusing for patients and their families, but it is somewhat reassuring to know that doctors don't even agree on these names. Some classification systems group the NHL according to the degree of malignancy as low-, intermediate-, and high-grade cancers. These categories are based on the cells' appearance under a microscope, their behavior, and their growth patterns.

Other schemes emphasize the growth pattern and appearance—that is, whether they grow in distinct clumps (nodular) or replace normal lymph tissue more uniformly (diffuse). Unlike adults (who have many more subtypes of NHL), more children develop the diffuse pattern, which is a high-grade, or more aggressive, form of lymphoma. There are many similarities in both symptoms and therapies for the various kinds of NHL, so it makes sense to consider them as a group first, then look at the differences.

All of the subtypes have a genetic component, although different chromosomes are involved in each.

Risk Factors

Exposure to pesticides and herbicides may play a role in the subsequent development of NHL. Presence of the Epstein-Barr virus may also be a factor. Some rare genetic syndromes, inherited within families, are also significant in some NHL diagnoses. These include:

- Bloom syndrome
- Fanconi syndrome
- Ataxia-telangiectasia

Site and Incidence

Depending on the subgroup, NHL in children can arise in the tonsils, thymus, bone, small intestine, or spleen, or in lymph nodes anywhere in the body. The disease can spread to the central nervous system (CNS) and the bone marrow. (Note this similarity to leukemia.)

NHL is more common in younger children than Hodgkin disease. More boys than girls are affected, and the age of onset ranges roughly from 5 to the teens, with a peak in the second decade of life. More whites than blacks contract NHL, more males than females. The disease is rare before the age of 3, although young AIDS patients are more likely to develop NHL before their fourth year.

Symptoms and Signs

Features of NHL vary according to the site of origin but might include:

- Painless swelling of lymph nodes in the armpit, neck, stomach, or groin
- Shortness of breath
- Difficulty swallowing
- Skin lumps
- Swollen tonsils
- Abdominal swelling (in advanced disease this may include bowel obstruction leading to pain, distention, and vomiting)

- Fever
- Loss of appetite
- Weight loss
- Night sweats
- Weakness
- Bone pain
- Fluid retention in tissues of the upper body or in the abdominal cavity
- Swollen liver and spleen
- Effects of bone marrow infiltration, like anemia, infection, or bleeding

Diagnosis

Final diagnosis of NHL is made through biopsy of suspicious nodes or other involved organs. Other tests may help define the extent of the disease:

- Complete blood count
- Computed tomography (CT) scan
- X-rays of chest, skeleton, nose, and throat
- Endoscopy
- Ultrasound
- Magnetic resonance imaging (MRI)
- Body scans (possibly of bone, brain, liver, spleen)
- Positron emission tomography (PET) scan
- Examination of a sample of bone marrow
- Kidney and liver function tests on urine
- Examination of fluid drawn from the chest cavity (thoracentesis)
- Spinal tap

Staging

After diagnosis, doctors must determine how widely the cancer has spread throughout the body. This is called staging, and it is a very important factor in planning optimal treatments. Stage I disease is localized and Stage IV is widespread to adjacent lymph nodes or the bone marrow or into the CNS. About two thirds of children have widespread disease at the time of diagnosis.

Treatment

Treatment of NHL depends on the stage and location of the primary tumor. In the past radiation was a major component of NHL therapy, but the risks and long-term complications were very serious. Researchers are discovering that chemotherapy in varying protocols and combinations can be as effective as radiation, the latter being used primarily for resistant or recurrent disease.

Surgery

If the disease is localized to a single lymph node or a small area, the tumor is removed. This is the only primary role that surgery plays in NHL, other than biopsy.

Radiation

NHL responds well to radiation. Therefore, despite the long-term risks, patients who have CNS involvement or head and neck tumors at the time of diagnosis may receive radiation; so do children with large chest tumors that interfere with lung or heart function. Radiation may be used with children having chemotherapy-resistant or recurrent disease, which must be treated more aggressively.

Chemotherapy

Almost all children with NHL receive a combination of chemotherapy drugs to destroy any spread of the disease, whether or not it can be detected. Over a dozen drugs play a role in treating NHL, primary among them being vincristine, cyclophosphamide, prednisone, and methotrexate. As with leukemia, it is important to protect the CNS against invasion by lymphoma cells, so preventive injections of methotrexate are customarily used, in some circumstances in combination with cranial radiation.

An emergency situation can complicate diagnosis and treatment of NHL. A patient who has a large mass in the chest could be at increased risk of heart or breathing difficulties if he is anesthetized or heavily sedated. Biopsies and other tests must be carefully planned, using light sedation, an upright position, and local anesthesia. If diagnosis is impossible under these conditions, treatment with steroids or local radiation may shrink the mass sufficiently to carry out more invasive procedures. In that case, though, a biopsy should be done as quickly as possible, since those therapies may alter the tissue enough to make a firm diagnosis difficult or impossible.

The immunotherapy drug rituximab, a monoclonal antibody, may be added to the chemotherapy arsenal in clinical trials, providing benefits without the toxic side effects of some other agents.

Children who relapse or who fail to go into remission are candidates for high-dose chemotherapy and total body radiation, followed by stem cell transplantation.

Patterns of Spread

NHL tends to spread to lymph nodes, but any organ of the body can be affected. Some children may relapse with leukemia; in these cases blast cells appear in the bone marrow or in circulating blood.

Prognosis

The child's chance for a full recovery depends on several factors: the type of NHL, the stage, metastasis, and his general overall health. Survival rates have improved dramatically with combination chemotherapy protocols. Overall 80% of children survive at least 5 years after diagnosis, boys and girls at the same rate, blacks and whites also at the same rate. Those with CNS involvement, a lot of chest or abdominal disease, or bone marrow involvement at diagnosis require more intensive therapy for an improved outlook.

Lymphoblastic Lymphoma

About 30% of NHL cases are lymphoblastic lymphoma. A majority (70%) of those patients are boys. Disease may present in the chest, bone marrow, skin, bone, or testes. No age is dominant with this sub-type, although it strikes more preadolescents and adolescents. Since lymphoblastic lymphoma is similar to acute lymphocytic leukemia, the therapy is also very similar. Stages I and II patients are given combination chemotherapy, with CNS therapy if the brain, head, or neck has tumors at diagnosis. Children with stages III and IV receive a combination of drugs, perhaps with radiation to large areas of lymphoma cells in a small area of the body. Patients with recurrent lymphoblastic lymphoma are candidates for allogeneic bone marrow transplant.

Small Noncleaved Cell Lymphoma (Burkitt and Burkitt-like Lymphomas)

About 40% to 50% of NHL patients are diagnosed with small non-cleaved cell lymphoma. Earlier classification schemes singled out the highly malignant Burkitt lymphomas because of their curious patterns in the developed world versus Africa. Both forms predominate in children from ages 5 to 14, with a huge preponderance of boys. Studies in Africa first demonstrated a link with Epstein-Barr virus (EBV). Patients in the developed world have intestinal or abdominal masses, as well as involvement of the nasal sinuses, testes, bone, skin, bone marrow, and CNS. The therapy differs from that for lympho-blastic lymphoma, with shorter periods of treatment and higher doses of chemotherapy drugs. State-of-the-art therapy has led to a greater than 90% survival rates even for advanced Burkitt lymphoma.

Diffuse Large B-Cell Lymphoma

This type of NHL, constituting 20% to 25% of all cases in pediatrics, appears predominantly in teenagers from 15 to 19 (and beyond into young adulthood), with the incidence rising with the age. The lymph nodes, abdomen, bone, and possibly CNS show involvement at diagnosis. Therapy, as with the two previously mentioned subtypes, is stage-related, with combination chemotherapy for all patients, and possibly CNS protective treatments, and the addition in some protocols of the drugs L-asparaginase, rituximab, and monoclonal antibodies.

Anaplastic Large Cell Lymphoma

Anaplastic large cell lymphoma constitutes only a tiny portion of pediatric NHL cases. The sites of origin are variable but the disease is usually systemic at diagnosis, with skin, lymph node, bone, or lung involvement, but not CNS or bone marrow. Therapy is similar to the combination chemotherapy provided for other subtypes of NHL, although the drug vinblastine is often given, along with stem cell transplant and possibly radiation.

Further Resources

ORGANIZATIONS/WEB SITES

Cure for Lymphoma Foundation (215 Lexington Ave., New York, NY 10016-6023; 212-213-6023; 800-235-6848; www.lymphoma.org)

Educational programs and publications, networking, and support for patients and medical professionals.

Leukemia and Lymphoma Society (1311 Mamaroneck Avenue, White Plains, NY 10605-5221; 914-949-5213; 800-955-4572; www.LLS.org)

Publications, research funding, some patient financial aid, school re-entry materials, audiotapes. Some publications in Spanish and French. Excellent booklets available by mail and online. Educational programs online and by teleconference.

5

Childhood Hodgkin lymphoma

Childhood Hodgkin lymphoma (sometimes called Hodgkin disease) and non-Hodgkin lymphoma are the two major divisions of lymph system cancer. The former progresses more slowly, while the latter spreads quickly through the body at an earlier stage. Non-Hodgkin lymphoma, which was discussed in detail the previous chapter, has many similarities with leukemia.

Childhood Hodgkin lymphoma appears in several forms, depending on the specific cell that has become malignant and its behavior. The various forms, however, are a matter for specialists and beyond the scope of this book.

Hodgkin disease, first described in 1832 by the English doctor Thomas Hodgkin, is the most common form of lymphoma. Any lymph node (or gland) that remains swollen for 3 weeks or longer without any other evidence of illness should be examined by a physician, as this is a common feature of the lymphomas. Hodgkin lymphoma tends to affect the peripheral lymph nodes like those in the neck, rather than those in the trunk. Half of patients are under the age of 25 at the time of diagnosis.

Research suggests a viral cause. Up to a third of patients may have asymptomatic Epstein-Barr virus (EBV), especially in children under the age of 10. EBV is also the suspected cause of infectious mononucleosis, a disease that sometimes precedes Hodgkin disease. Environmental and genetic factors may also play a role in the development of this cancer, which accounts for about 6% of childhood malignancies, with about 900 cases diagnosed in the United States annually. HIV-positive patients are at higher risk of Hodgkin lymphoma, although newer therapies are reducing this risk.

Incidence

Generally speaking, Hodgkin lymphoma is rare in young children. Fewer than 15% of all cases appear in children under the age of 14. Especially before the age of 15, boys are affected much more frequently than girls. The predominance of male cases is less obvious among older children and decreases by the mid-teens. This malignancy reportedly peaks in boys before puberty and in girls in late adolescence. Fewer blacks develop Hodgkin lymphoma, although the difference is stronger after the age of 10. Patients who are older at diagnosis usually have a higher risk if they have a better standard of living, while younger patients with a lower socioeconomic status carry a lower risk. For some reason, the incidence of Hodgkin lymphoma seems to be decreasing.

On rare occasions a number of people living in the same region, attending the same school, or married to cancer patients contract the same or a related cancer. This is called a cluster. Clusters of leukemia and the lymphomas have been recorded, but no infectious or environmental basis for the disease has been conclusively proven. Having a sibling with Hodgkin lymphoma is another risk factor, suggesting a genetic aspect. The environmental or genetic factors linking EBV to Hodgkin lymphoma are not clear, although they seem to occur more often in developing countries.

Signs and Symptoms

The major sign of childhood Hodgkin lymphoma is an enlarged, painless lymph node, usually in the neck. Depending on which parts of the lymph system are involved, other signs and symptoms may be:

- An enlarged liver
- An enlarged spleen

- Abdominal pain
- Fatigue
- Sore throat
- Difficulty breathing
- Jaundice (rare in children)
- Pain in the back or legs

Pain is usually a result of enlarged organs or nodes pressing on nerves or interfering with body functions like digestion. Children with a more advanced case of the disease might also suffer:

- Night sweats (B-type symptom)
- Fever (B-type symptom)
- Unexplained weight loss (B-type symptom)
- General weakness
- Anemia
- Itching (less common in children)
- Tumor masses

Diagnosis

Depending on the symptoms, the diagnosis of childhood Hodgkin lymphoma is made by a biopsy of the abnormal nodes or other affected tissues, looking for a special type of cell called Reed-Sternberg that characterizes Hodgkin disease. Other tests might be performed also:

- Blood tests: a complete blood count (CBC), which might show an increased number of leukocytes and platelets
- X-rays of the chest, skeleton, and digestive tract
- Computed tomography (CT) scans of the chest, abdomen, or pelvis
- Magnetic resonance imaging (MRI)
- Positron emission tomography (PET) scan
- Bone scan
- Blood urea nitrogen (BUN)
- Bone marrow aspiration and biopsy
- Liver function tests

Staging

Describing the extent of the disease within the body, or staging, is especially important in Hodgkin lymphoma for planning therapy that will wipe out the disease yet spare normal tissue as much as possible. Stage I is localized disease, while more widespread cases are assigned higher numbers. Stage IV is widely disseminated in the body. Subclasses identify the presence (B type) or absence (A type) of symptoms like a large weight loss, night sweats, and fever. An additional class subdivision indicates E (disease detected outside the lymph system, or extended) and S (disease involving the spleen).

Treatment

Treatment of childhood Hodgkin lymphoma depends on the stage but most often includes chemotherapy (to wipe out cancer cells throughout the body) and radiation (possibly alone for localized disease).

Radiation

Radiation alone may be used to treat very early-stage, limited stage I Hodgkin lymphoma. In earlier years, high doses of radiation to wide areas of the trunk did eradicate the malignancy but led to unacceptable side and late effects. Current radiation and chemotherapy treatments take into account factors such as the B symptoms mentioned above as well as the size of any solid tumors. Clinics individualize therapy for Hodgkin patients perhaps even to a greater degree than with other diagnoses. Modified doses of radiation to closely target areas limit the late effects like breast cancer and heart or lung disease. The designation LD-IFRT is used, meaning "low-dose involved-field radiation therapy."

Chemotherapy

Chemotherapy has proven effective against widespread Hodgkin lymphoma as well. A combination of drugs is commonly used, including cyclophosphamide, procarbazine, vincristine, prednisone or dexamethasone, doxorubicin, bleomycin, dacarbazine, methotrexate, and cytosine arabinoside (ara-C). Other drugs are also used in some instances, such as when initial therapy fails to induce remission or the patient relapses. These include cytarabine (moderate or high dose), carboplatin/cisplatin, ifosfamide, vinorelbine, gemcitabine, and vinblastine. Side effects can be severe: nausea, vomiting, and low blood counts often result from damage to the bone marrow. Because of this toxicity and the need for a team of experienced surgeons, radiologists, and oncologists, treatment should take place in a center specializing in pediatric patients.

Combination Radiation and Chemotherapy

Radiation and/or chemotherapy in a variety of regimens and combinations have effectively cured large numbers of patients with Hodgkin lymphoma. The choice of treatment in a particular case will be determined by the patient's age and extent of disease, taking into account the risk of second cancers and potential side and late effects such as problems with growth and fertility.

Surgery

Surgery may also play a role in treatment, although chemotherapy and possibly radiation are the primary forms of therapy. Besides the biopsy, some affected lymph nodes may be removed, and the pressure or obstruction of a tumor mass might be relieved through surgery. Individual masses that appear in the lungs can also be removed with good results.

In the case of progressive disease (a patient who does not go into remission with initial therapy) or a recurrence after remission, specialists may use high-dose chemotherapy to wipe out the disease, followed by a peripheral blood stem cell transplant (PBSCT). An autologous PBSCT (using the patient's own cells) is preferable to allogeneic PBSCT (using a donor's cells), although the latter may be successful in some circumstances.

Prognosis

The prognosis in childhood Hodgkin lymphoma has improved with the development of better staging, more precise radiation treatments, and multidrug chemotherapy. About 95% of patients survive for 5 or more years after diagnosis. The survival rate is the same for boys and girls, although whites have a slightly higher survival rate than blacks in the United States. Even children with advanced disease who need additional therapy have a survival rate better than 50%. Patients in lower-risk groups include those with lower stages at diagnosis, especially without the B symptoms or bulky tumors. The therapy a child receives may be more important overall than the stage, the type of cell involved, and the patient's gender and age at diagnosis. Major referral centers provide the best chance for patients to beat this cancer. As with other forms of cancer, the more quickly the patient responds to the therapy, the more favorable the outlook.

Special Considerations

The greatest risk of relapse comes in the first 2 years after treatments are stopped, so careful follow-up of patients during these and succeeding years is necessary.

Herpes zoster (shingles, an infection closely related to chickenpox) affects many Hodgkin lymphoma patients who receive aggressive therapy. It may occur before the disease is diagnosed or during therapy, but it is not related to relapse or a poorer prognosis. The infection may be localized or may become widespread. Patients whose Hodgkin disease is under control can usually fight off herpes zoster, but for those in a weakened condition it sometimes proves fatal. Inactivated varicella vaccine can lower the incidence of shingles, particularly in PBSCT patients.

Late Effects

A small percentage of childhood Hodgkin lymphoma survivors later develop a second cancer, although current doses of chemotherapy and radiation are lower than in the past and late effects should be fewer. The treatments may damage the immune system. Perhaps these patients' immune systems were already damaged, leading to both the disease and the second malignancy. Infertility as well as detrimental effects on the thyroid, bone growth, and development may result from the therapy.

Further Resources

READING

Caley, Beverly A. Hodgkin disease: the other side. *Cure*, vol. 4 (1) (Spring 2005), p. 40–47. Available at www.curetoday.com.

ORGANIZATIONS/WEB SITES

Leukemia and Lymphoma Society (1311 Mamaroneck Avenue, Suite 310, White Plains, NY 10605; 800-955-4572; www.LLS.org)

Provides educational materials, excellent pamphlets and booklets, including some in French and Spanish. Web and teleconferences report on new therapies.

6

Neuroblastoma

Neuroblastoma is one of the most common forms of childhood solid tumors. Representing about 10% of childhood cancer cases in the United States, neuroblastoma is the likeliest cancer to strike infants under the age of 1 at diagnosis. Arising in the sympathetic nervous system, it is a highly malignant growth. Until improvements in chemotherapy, it ran an almost universally fatal course in children with advanced disease, with notable exceptions like stage 4S. Since neuroblastoma spreads so quickly, it often comes to the attention of a parent or a pediatrician only after the disease is already widespread. Bruising or hemorrhages around both eyes (like unexplained black eyes) caused by metastases can be the first signs of neuroblastoma.

The Nervous System in Brief

The nervous system is the network of organs and tissues that controls and coordinates all of the body's activities. The autonomic nervous system, which controls involuntary body activities such as sweating, blushing, heartbeat, and blood pressure, consists of a sympathetic division, which stimulates action, and an opposing parasympathetic division, which inhibits action. For example, the sympathetic division dilates the pupils of the eyes by stimulating muscles of the iris, and the parasympathetic branch constricts the same muscles. Most organs of the body are supplied with both sympathetic and parasympathetic involuntary nerves, and it is in the sympathetic nerves that the neuroblastoma arises.

Incidence

Although neuroblastoma is a common childhood cancer, its incidence in the general population is still tiny, with a few hundred new cases in the United States each year. Affected children are very young, with a third of the diagnoses occurring in the first year of life and half in children under the age of 2. Eighty-five percent of cases are diagnosed in the first 5 years of life and only 3% after the age of 10. Boys are affected about 20% more often than girls.

Neuroblastoma can arise in nerve cells anywhere in the body, but the primary tumor site in 70% of cases is the abdomen (50%) or pelvis. Other sites are the chest (30%), neck (10%), and within the skull. The greatest number of cases (35%) begins in the adrenal gland. It is sometimes hard to pinpoint the exact primary site of a large neuroblastoma.

Certain genetic risk factors have been identified by St. Jude Children's Research Hospital that suggest a familial aspect to some cases of neuroblastoma. Maternal exposure to phenytoin for seizure prevention may be a factor, as well as neurofibromatosis, Beckwith-Wiedemann syndrome, and nesidioblastosis (overgrowth of certain pancreatic cells).

A large-scale study is currently looking at the effects of parental exposure to occupational chemicals on the incidence of neuroblastoma in offspring. Maternal exposures don't seem to be associated with the disease, but paternal exposure to hydrocarbons such as diesel fuel, lacquer thinner, and turpentine was associated with an increased risk of neuroblastoma, as were exposures to wood dust and solders.

With the suspicion that neuroblastoma might often be a prenatal development, wouldn't early screening catch cases at an early, very treatable stage, especially since the procedure is so simple? This would seem to be the case, but results so far have been disappointing. Urinary testing of infants in Japan has shown some success at identifying new cases of neuroblastoma. However, a clinical study in Quebec that screened infants at the age of 3 weeks and again at 6 months had a frustrating outcome. Many neuroblastomas with the most favorable characteristics were found that would apparently have spontaneously regressed and never reached a clinical diagnosis. This is a unique feature of neuroblastoma. A study in Germany suggests overdiagnosis of neuroblastoma from screening, with documented spontaneous regression in a significant minority of participants with localized disease. On the other hand, no reduction of high-risk, unfavorable cases occurred, suggesting that screening will not lower the incidence of illness and death from neuroblastoma. These studies have been completed and show that screening is ineffective.

Symptoms

As is the case with all cancers, neuroblastoma symptoms depend on the location of the tumor. A fairly large number of cases are first diagnosed through symptoms of metastases, such as:

- Abdominal swelling or pain
- Listlessness
- High blood pressure
- Loss of appetite
- Rapid heartbeat
- Unexplained weight loss
- Persistent diarrhea
- Black-and-blue marks around the eyes
- Fever
- Excessive sweating
- Weakness of an arm or leg
- Anemia
- Protrusion of an eyeball
- A limp (when bones are involved) or paralysis (when tumor compresses the spinal cord)
- Coughing or shortness of breath (chest tumors)
- Problems with urination or defecation (pelvic tumors)
- Bone pain and swelling

Often the symptoms of neuroblastoma are vague or mimic those of other diseases. When first seen at the clinic, the presentation may be very similar to that of acute lymphatic leukemia of childhood, even in the appearance of bone marrow aspirates (fluid withdrawn from the marrow). The location of a primary site aids in diagnosis.

Diagnosis

Diagnostic procedures vary according to the specific signs and symptoms and include:

- Complete blood count
- Ultrasound (especially if an abdominal mass is present)
- Skeletal x-rays (to check for bone metastases)
- Chest x-rays
- Bone scan
- Computed tomography (CT) scan (to delineate tumor size and relation to other structures)
- Magnetic resonance imaging (MRI)
- Bone marrow aspiration (looking for a specific microscopic cell pattern that distinguishes neuroblastoma from other tumor types)
- Biopsy of tumor tissue (if bone marrow doesn't indicate the presence of neuroblastoma cells in the marrow)
- Assessment of tumor markers in urine or blood (homovanillic acid [HVA] and vanillylmandelic acid [VMA] levels are increased in 90% of neuroblastoma cases)

Staging

The stage of neuroblastoma at the time of diagnosis is important in the planning of treatment as well as in prognosis. Doctors need to know how far the tumor has spread from its primary site. Determining this spread, if any, is called staging. Classification ranges from stage I through stage IV, with the higher numbers representing disease that has spread more widely in the body. Unfortunately, many neuroblastoma patients have stage IV at diagnosis. A special group of very young patients with widely disseminated neuroblastoma but without bone metastases have what is called stage IV-S disease; these tumors can undergo spontaneous regression without any treatment at all. (Do not count on this phenomenon, however, to save your child's life. Seek the best available medical care.)

Treatment

It is important that the child with neuroblastoma be treated aggressively by an experienced team of specialists. A cure by surgery alone is uncommon unless the tumor is localized (stage I) and does not involve vital structures or organs.

There are several quite similar staging systems for neuroblastoma, but rather than dealing in semantics, it is more important here to look at the risk factors that determine a treatment plan for each patient (which is basically stage-related). The following information is drawn from the St. Jude Children's Research Hospital classification.

Treatment of neuroblastoma depends on several factors—the age of the patient at diagnosis, location of the tumor, stage, and microscopic analysis of the tumor cells. These variables constitute the risk for each patient. For an in-depth discussion of the complicated staging system and risk levels for neuroblastoma, see the National Cancer Institute Web site at www.cancer.gov.

Low-risk patients are infants with localized disease or a metastasized but favorable cell type and children over 1 year of age with localized disease. Treatment for these patients is surgical removal of the tumor, followed by observation to see if the disease recurs.

Intermediate-risk patients are infants with metastatic disease of an unfavorable cell type and older children with a local tumor that can't be surgically removed or with nearby spread but only on one side of the body. Therapy for these children includes surgery to remove as much tumor as possible, perhaps radiation to the tumor, and chemotherapy with cyclophosphamide and doxorubicin for 4 to 6 months. Additional drugs may be used to treat resistant tumors.

High-risk patients may be of any age with regional disease and amplification of a specific oncogene (N-myc) in the tumor tissue, or children over the age of 1 with metastases. Therapy for these youngsters depends to a certain extent on the age of the patient: over or under the age of 1 is the most important factor. Surgery, radiation, chemotherapy (cyclophosphamide, ifosfamide, cisplatin, carboplatin, doxorubicin, and/or etoposide) may follow. Radiation is most commonly used in patients over the age of 1.

The highest-risk patients may receive very-high-dose chemotherapy with radiation followed by an autologous stem cell transplant to repair bone marrow. Treatment involving 6 months of cis-retinoic acid therapy (Accutane, a derivative of vitamin A) and an autologous stem cell transplant has increased the duration of disease-free survival. Reports indicate that high-risk patients who receive this state-of-the-art therapy have a 10% to 15% higher survival rate than those who do not. Researchers are investigating the use of monoclonal antibody treatment (a form of immunotherapy) for disseminated neuroblastoma, and clinical trials show this to be effective. This approach does not work in the presence of large tumor bulk. Promising research in Japan suggests that postponing surgery until high-dose chemotherapy has been completed may be an appropriate treatment for patients with high-risk metastatic neuroblastoma.

Other forms of supportive treatment commonly used are blood cell and platelet transfusions and antibiotics.

Metastases

An unfortunate feature of neuroblastoma is its unusual pattern of metastasis. Even a very small primary tumor might spread to distant areas of the body via the bloodstream. Most patients have detectable metastases at the time of diagnosis. The tumor also grows into adjacent areas of the body by invading healthy tissues, and it commonly is found in lymph nodes near the primary site.

Bone metastases in most types of cancer are a relatively late-stage phenomenon, but in neuroblastoma, deposits in the bones and marrow are present in a significant percentage of cases at diagnosis. To some extent metastasis patterns seem to be age-dependent: a pattern of liver, skin, and marrow metastasis is found primarily in children up to 12 months of age, whereas skeletal metastases are common in older children. Neuroblastoma may spread to the brain in late-stage disease.

Prognosis

The prognosis in neuroblastoma is strongly age-related, although it also depends on the site and stage of the primary tumor at diagnosis. The lowest-risk patients are diagnosed at ages younger than 18 months. About 90% of the lowest-risk patients reach the 5-year survival mark. With intermediate-risk patients, 80% to 90% are long-term survivors. The highest-risk patients unfortunately face the most difficult odds, although today the 5-year survival rate overall is 50% to 70%. Survival rates decrease as the age of the patient at diagnosis and the stage of the disease increase.

Prognosis also depends somewhat on the site of the primary tumor. The child's chances are better if the primary tumor is located in the neck, chest, or pelvis rather than the abdomen. It is also more favorable if the primary tumor can be totally removed. Patients with bone metastases do not do as well, especially if they are over 1 year old at diagnosis, but they may still live a long while.

In a very few cases, neuroblastoma patients have relapsed many years after everyone thought they were cured—in a couple of cases 6 to 9 years later. Long-term follow-up is therefore in order.

Further Resources

READING

Childhood Cancer: A Handbook from St. Jude Children's Research Hospital, edited by R. Grant Steen and Joseph Mirro, Jr. Cambridge, MA: Perseus Press, 2000.
  An excellent all-around source of solid information.
DeRoos A. J., et al, "Parental occupational exposures to chemicals and incidence of neuroblastoma in offspring." *American Journal of Epidemiology,* vol. 154 (2) (July 15, 2001), p. 106.
Hero B., et al, "Localized infant neuroblastomas often show spontaneous regression." *Journal of Clinical Oncology,* vol. 26 (9) (March 20, 2008), p. 1504–1510.

"Neuroblastoma: A Handbook for Families," Association of Pediatric Hematology Oncology Nurses; available by e-mailing info@aphon.org

ORGANIZATIONS/WEB SITES

Association of Cancer Online Resources (www.acor.org)

Has a neuroblastoma discussion list as well as a neuroblastoma section in the Ped-Onc Resource Center. Many links to government and other sites, as well as a section on finding new treatments.

Children's Neuroblastoma Cancer Foundation (P.O. Box 6635, Bloomingdale, IL 60108; 866-671-2623 [toll-free]; e-mail: info@cncf-childcancer.org; Web site: www.nbhope.org)

This organization has documents you can download to learn about this disease, including the latest news on treatments.

NANT Universities and Children's Hospitals Consortium (www.nant.org)

Founded by the National Cancer Institute, this professional organization is collaborating to develop new therapies for high-risk neuroblastoma. The Web site has contact information for the 14 U.S. hospitals associated with the program, which is administrated from Children's Hospital in Los Angeles.

National Cancer Institute (www.cancer.gov)

The Patient Data Query (PDQ) section has excellent discussions of each form of cancer as well as therapies, written for both laypersons and for medical professionals.

Neuroblastoma Children's Cancer Society (P. O. Box 957672, Hoffman Estates, IL 60195; 800-532-5162; www.neuroblastomacancer.org)

Publishes quarterly newsletter, has message board, "Resource Survival Handbook" online.

7

Wilms Tumor

Also called cancer of the kidney or congenital nephroblastoma, Wilms tumor is a rare malignant solid tumor usually found in children between the ages of 1 and 5 years. Named after Max Wilms, a turn-of-the-20th-century German surgeon who studied childhood kidney tumors, it is considered a congenital disorder regardless of the age at which it is discovered, since it arises from embryonic tissue (fetal cells that develop early in pregnancy). Wilms tumor may arise in one or both kidneys. Not all primary childhood kidney tumors are Wilms tumors; some varied types of sarcoma also appear and generally have a less favorable outcome. (See the chapter on rare tumors [Chapter 14] for additional information on non-Wilms kidney cancers.)

The Kidneys

The kidneys are two small organs found in the small of the back, one on each side of the spine. They filter the blood, cleansing it of waste products and forming urine. They regulate the amount of water and the proportion of chemicals in the body, a function necessary to maintain life. The kidneys also help regulate the formation of red blood cells by the bone marrow and play a role in maintaining normal blood pressure.

Blood is carried into the kidneys by the renal artery. Urine manufactured in the kidneys is carried through tubes called ureters to the urinary bladder, where it is collected and finally excreted through the urethra.

Incidence

Fewer than 500 new cases are diagnosed each year in the United States. This form of childhood cancer peaks at ages 3 to 4, with deaths peaking at age 5, although it has been seen in youngsters up to the age of 15. Ninety percent of cases are diagnosed before the age of 8. There is little international variation in the incidence of Wilms tumor, although Japanese and other Asian cultures have half the "usual" risk (perhaps because they lack the Wilms tumor genetic changes). More African-American children are affected and more girls than boys. It appears at a somewhat younger age when it is bilateral (in both kidneys) or familial (when it "runs in families").

Genetic Risk

About 10% of Wilms tumors appear in patients with recognized congenital malformations. Aniridia is the partial or complete absence of the iris, the colored part of the eye. This birth defect is caused by a genetic abnormality and may appear in one or both eyes of affected babies. A particularly clear link is seen between a genetic defect on chromosome 11, which produces aniridia, and the subsequent development of Wilms tumor. Perhaps 1 in 50,000 people in the general U.S. population lack one or both irises, but 30% of those whose chromosome 11 has been damaged develop Wilms. (Overall, though, only one child in 70 with Wilms tumor also has aniridia.) The birth of a child with aniridia is a red flag for doctors, who should begin to monitor the child for Wilms tumor using ultrasound of the kidneys. This is alarming news for parents, but they can be reassured that the earliest possible detection and treatment of the tumor provides an excellent likelihood of a long and healthy life for their child.

Children with aniridia and Wilms tumor may have other signs as well, including mental retardation, small heads, and hemihypertrophy, a swelling on one side of the body (limb, face, etc.), with abnormalities of the genitourinary tract or the skeleton, or with benign tumors. Another risk factor is Beckwith-Wiedemann syndrome, which carries a 5% to 10% risk of Wilms tumor.

Hereditary cases can be identified when the tumor develops at several sites within the same kidney simultaneously, or in both kidneys, or in a patient's twin or brother or sister. Other genes that appear to affect the development of Wilms tumor are chromosome 16 and chromosome 1p. Overall only about 1% to 2% of Wilms tumor cases are inherited. The risk of Wilms tumor in the offspring of recovered Wilms patients is less than 2%. Patients at risk due to a recognized syndrome or physical findings should be screened with ultrasound for about 8 years. Families with this risk may want to seek advice from a geneticist.

Signs and Symptoms

The major sign of Wilms tumor is a swelling or lump at one side of the abdomen, often discovered during a bath or routine checkup. *This lump should not be squeezed, poked, or knocked, because it can rupture and scatter tumor cells.* Other symptoms are:

- Fever
- Listlessness, weakness, fatigue
- Pallor and anemia
- Blood in the urine (25% of the time; perhaps invisible to the naked eye but detectable in the laboratory)
- Loss of appetite and weight
- Abdominal pain and vomiting
- Difficulty breathing
- High blood pressure
- Pain (chronic ache rather than sharp stabs)

Diagnosis

If the cancer is not removed at diagnosis, a careful biopsy is usually done. Caution must be used because cancer cells could be seeded into the abdomen during the removal of tissue from this highly malignant mass. Depending again on symptoms, some of the following procedures are carried out to define the nature of the mass and its organ of origin, to determine its extent in relation to other structures, and to look for metastases:

- Blood counts
- Blood urea nitrogen (BUN)
- Serum electrolytes
- X-rays of the chest (to check for metastases)
- Nephrotomography
- Computed tomography (CT) scan
- Magnetic resonance imaging (MRI)
- Bone scans (looking for metastases)
- Ultrasound (to distinguish fluid-filled cysts from solid tumors and to detect cardiac [inferior vena cava] involvement)
- Physical examination
- Urinalysis (measuring certain chemicals to distinguish Wilms tumor from neuroblastoma)

In diagnosing Wilms tumor, doctors also closely examine the cell structure (histology) of the malignant tissue itself to determine which of several subgroups of the disease the child has.

Staging

Solid tumors like Wilms are classified according to how far the disease has spread, ranging from stage I (local and completely removable by surgery) to stage IV (metastasized) and stage V (bilateral at diagnosis). The tumor is also classified according to favorable or unfavorable histology, which distinguishes different cancer cell appearances that play an important factor in planning treatments. The National Cancer Institute's PDQ Web site offers an extensive discussion on the various stages.

Treatment

Treatment of Wilms tumor depends on the size of the tumor, the stage, and the histology. The basic strategy is to remove all or as much of the mass as possible with surgery, to use radiation if needed to kill local residual disease, and to use chemotherapy drugs to eradicate distant spread, or metastasis, whether or not any has been detected. Studies show that patients treated by a team of pediatric oncology experts fare better overall.

Surgery

Surgery is often the first step taken in treating Wilms tumor. The surgical removal of the affected kidney, its surrounding tissues, and nearby lymph nodes is called radical nephrectomy. An encapsulated tumor, one completely contained within the kidney, is a prime candidate for removal. Tumors in stages I and II are usually treated in this manner.

Sometimes the disease is so extensive at the time of diagnosis that removing the tumor and all the detectable spread would require removing too many organs, with serious consequences. In these cases chemotherapy or radiation is given first to shrink the tumor, and surgery is carried out at a later date. Surgery may also play a role later in treatment if metastases in the lungs do not respond to radiation or chemotherapy. During surgery the opposite kidney, liver, and lymph nodes are carefully examined and suspicious areas are biopsied.

Radiation

Wilms tumor often responds well to radiation treatments, which begin soon after surgery. However, radiation is no longer used in patients with stage I disease if the biopsy reveals a more favorable histology. Particularly in young children, radiation can affect the growth of bones in the spine.

Radiation treatment before surgery to shrink a tumor is used less commonly in the United States today. The benefit of preoperative radiation is unproven and there is a danger of radiating a benign tumor. If lung metastases appear, radiation may be effective in eradicating them, but as a rule radiation is used after surgery and chemotherapy.

Chemotherapy

Almost all patients receive drug treatment, starting right after surgery. The drug treatment can last from 18 weeks to 6 months.

Occasionally chemotherapy is begun even before surgery to shrink a large tumor. It is commonly used to destroy metastases or when doctors suspect at the time of surgery that cancer cells have escaped. The duration and frequency of chemotherapy depend on the stage of the tumor, its response to the drugs, the child's tolerance of the side effects, and the cell structure of the tumor. Among the drugs that may be used in combination to treat Wilms tumor patients are vincristine, dactinomycin, and doxorubicin.

Bilateral Wilms Tumor

Special considerations prevail when both kidneys are affected by Wilms tumor; this occurs in about 5% to 10% of all cases. Therapy must be individualized. The kidney more affected by the tumor may be removed completely, while only part of the other is removed. Many patients are now given chemotherapy before surgeons attempt to remove the tumor to save, if possible, part of both kidneys. It is important to realize that a child can still lead a normal life with only part of one kidney and as little as 20% to 25% of normal kidney function. If it is necessary to remove both kidneys completely because of the extent of the disease, a transplant or artificial kidney will be required to cleanse the blood and prevent the poisoning of the body by its own waste products.

Patterns of Metastasis

An encapsulated tumor may break during biopsy, which is why that procedure must be carried out by an experienced surgeon, or it may rupture from poking before or during surgery. Tumor cells can seed elsewhere by traveling through the bloodstream to the lungs, the abdomen, the liver, or the bones. Because most metastases appear within the first 2 years after the primary tumor is removed, chest x-rays or CT scans should be taken for early detection. Surgical removal or radiation can be effective for lung metastases. In the case of local reappearance of the tumor without evidence of any distant spread, surgeons can sometimes remove the new tumor, followed by radiation and different chemotherapy to wipe out undetectable metastases.

Prognosis

Patients with Wilms tumor generally do extremely well and have among the best chances for recovery of any childhood cancer patients. The size of the primary tumor has no bearing on long-term survival. Prognosis depends on the stage at diagnosis, the tumor's histologic pattern, and the age of the patient. Stage I disease with favorable histology is most likely to be cured, although that is not a certainty. Children under the age of 2 have a better prognosis. Older patients and those with higher-stage disease have a somewhat poorer chance for long-term survival; still, more than half live over 3 years, even with stage IV disease. Relapses are early, with 84% in the first year of treatment and 96% within the first 2 years. Even if there have been metastases to other organs, especially the lungs, there is still a 75% cure rate. Patients with stage V, or bilateral, disease have a good cure rate. The overall 5-year survival rate is a reassuring 93%.

Further Resources

READING

Childhood Cancer: a Handbook from St. Jude Children's Research
   Hospital, edited by R. Grant Steen and Joseph Mirro, Jr. Cambridge,
   MA: Perseus Press, 2000.
   This book has a detailed, understandable discussion of the various genetic syndromes that may lead to Wilms tumor and is an excellent all-around source of solid information.

ORGANIZATIONS / WEB SITES

Association of Cancer Online Resources (www.acor.org)
   Includes a Wilms discussion list.

CancerNet (Go to www.cancer.gov and choose the file for Wilms tumor)
   A service of the National Cancer Institute. Constantly updated information from a trusted resource.

Cure Search (www.curesearch.org)
   See "Health Links" for late effects information and follow-up, including a paper on "Keeping your single kidney healthy."

Kidney Cancer Association (Suite 203, 1234 Sherman Avenue, Evanston, IL 60202-1375; 847-332-1051; 800-850-9132; www.kidneycancerassociation. org)

Provides print materials, physician referrals, and support groups. Formerly called the National Kidney Cancer Association. A gateway to information and contacts (message boards, video, podcasts, blogs, etc.) in Chinese, English, and other languages.

8

Bone Cancers

Bone cancer, any malignant tumor in skeletal tissue, accounts for about 6% of childhood cancers. This disease is not new: at the end of the 19th century a million-year-old skeleton was found in Java of *Pithecanthropus erectus*, one of man's ancestors, with the remains of a cancerous bone tumor.

Types

In adults most bone tumors are metastases from cancer arising elsewhere in the body, but in children most are primary tumors. There are two main types of primary childhood bone cancers, osteogenic sarcoma (osteosarcoma) and Ewing tumor, plus some less common, related forms.

Osteogenic Sarcoma

The most common childhood bone cancer is osteogenic sarcoma. The tumor is composed of bone cells that have undergone a malignant change. It appears in the ends of the bones, primarily the leg (tibia and femur) and the arm (humerus), although it may also be found in

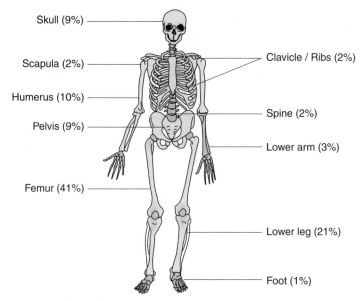

Skull (9%)

Scapula (2%)

Humerus (10%)

Pelvis (9%)

Femur (41%)

Clavicle / Ribs (2%)

Spine (2%)

Lower arm (3%)

Lower leg (21%)

Foot (1%)

FIGURE 8.1 Skeleton showing major sites of osteosarcoma
Voute, P. A., et al, *Cancer in Children: Clinical Management* Oxford
University Press, 1998

any other bone. Half of all tumors arise around the knee. Wherever it
appears, osteogenic sarcoma grows into surrounding muscles and
tendons.

Ewing Tumor

Named after James Ewing (1866–1943), the American pathologist
and tumor authority who first described the disease, Ewing sarcoma,
or Ewing tumor, grows in connective tissue around large bones or in
the marrow spaces inside the mid-shaft of bones. The cells that multiply out of control in this form of cancer are thought to be endothe-
lial, which are non-bone cells that line the shafts of the bones
themselves. Ewing tumor is most common in the proximal end (closer
to the center of the body) of the thigh bone (femur), the leg (tibia and
fibula), pelvis, arm, and ribs.

Less Common Bone Cancers

Chondrosarcoma arises in the cartilage of large bones, the elastic
tissue that covers the ends of bone, especially at the joints. It forms a

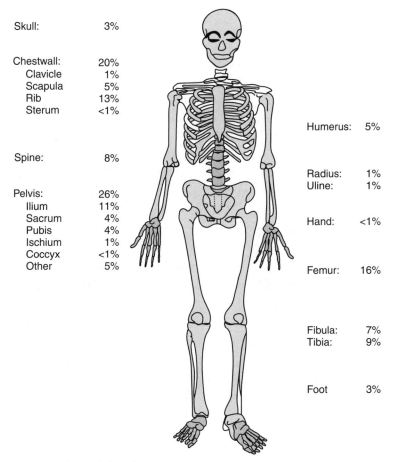

Skull:	3%	
Chestwall:	20%	
Clavicle	1%	
Scapula	5%	
Rib	13%	
Sterum	<1%	
		Humerus: 5%
Spine:	8%	
		Radius: 1%
		Uline: 1%
Pelvis:	26%	
Ilium	11%	
Sacrum	4%	Hand: <1%
Pubis	4%	
Ischium	1%	
Coccyx	<1%	
Other	5%	Femur: 16%
		Fibula: 7%
		Tibia: 9%
		Foot 3%

FIGURE 8.2 Skeletal distribution in Ewing's sarcoma
Voute, P. A., et al, *Cancer in Children: Clinical Management* Oxford
University Press, 1998

mass in the knee (the most common site in children), the pelvis, the
upper ends of the thighs, or the shoulders. This tumor grows slowly
into surrounding tissues. Surgical removal provides the best treatment, and 75% of patients survive if their tumor is completely
excised.

A minority of all fibrosarcoma cases appear before the age of 10.
Diagnosis and treatment of this very rare cancer is individualized.
Adamantinoma (affecting bone and tissue around muscles and nerves)
is a very rare bone tumor.

Multiple myeloma, primarily an adult malignancy, arises in the
bone marrow and acts more like leukemia than a solid bone tumor.

d connective tissue tumors account for only about 6% of all childhood cancers, but in the 10- to 20-year age group, they are the fourth most common cancer. Two thirds of all cases are seen in patients under the age of 20. These tumors seldom appear before the age of 4, and the incidence peaks in early adolescence. There is some suspicion that the growth of bone sarcomas is related to bone growth generally, since the peak incidence coincides with the growth spurt experienced around age 14. A small and inconclusive study suggesting that taller adolescents are more likely to be affected might explain why boys are more affected than girls. Osteogenic sarcoma also arises in sites radiated for earlier cancers, primarily retinoblastoma.

Ewing sarcoma appears to be related to a change on chromosome 22 or chromosome 11, but is not known to be inherited. This factor, however, may lead to a vaccine to target affected cells. Both Li-Fraumeni syndrome and retinoblastoma can be risk factors for osteogenic sarcoma.

A few hundred new cases of bone cancer are diagnosed each year in the United States. Blacks and whites have about the same incidence of osteogenic sarcoma, but the vast majority of Ewing sarcoma cases affect white children.

Signs and Symptoms

The chief symptom of bone cancers is pain, often worse at night. The pain may occur in a location away from the site of the tumor, "referred" there by a nerve. A mass is also commonly present. At first there may be suspicion of arthritis. If the pain persists more than a week or two, medical attention should be sought. Incredibly, one study revealed that pain was tolerated for 9 months or more before a doctor was seen. Some of the tumors grow for a couple of years before they are diagnosed. Malignant tumors present with a weak and painful limb, while nonmalignant tumors generally have a painless, asymptomatic mass.

Other symptoms vary according to the state of the disease, the site, and, to a certain extent, the type. Ewing tumor tends to produce more systemic symptoms like fever, chills, and weakness than do other bone tumors. Unexplained long-term back pain and weight loss are two more potential signs. Occasionally a bone, weakened by tumor, breaks without a fall or as the result of a relatively minor accident. The fall does not cause the tumor but brings it to attention. A tumor affecting joint function may lead to limping. Metastases may appear as lumps in the groin and armpits or, if located in the lungs, may cause coughing and chest pain. These respiratory symptoms, however, are rare at diagnosis and are indicative of far-advanced disease.

Diagnosis

Diagnosis of bone tumors is made by a series of tests and procedures, which are selected according to the symptoms and the location of the mass. First the doctor performs a physical examination and asks about the history of the symptoms. Once bone cancer is suspected, the patient should be referred immediately to a major pediatric cancer center, where the staff is experienced in treating these malignancies. Even the site of a needle biopsy can affect later surgery. A team of specialists consulting from the earliest days is essential for optimal care.

Biopsy tissue may be withdrawn by needle or through an incision, made by cutting into the tumor, and is usually done in the operating room under general anesthesia. Then a series of tests determine whether the tumor has infiltrated nearby tissues or spread elsewhere in the body:

- Blood tests
- Urine tests
- Bone scan (looking for metastases)
- X-rays (bone, skeleton, chest, looking for fractures or metastases)
- Computed tomography (CT) scans (to define site of origin and extent of the disease and to determine if any adjacent soft tissue is involved. Chest CTs identify metastases too small to be seen on x-rays.)
- Magnetic resonance imaging (MRI) (to pinpoint the location and size of the tumor)
- Bone marrow aspiration (any metastases)

Treatment

Again, experts recommend that treatment of bone tumors take place at a large cancer treatment center because of the rarity of the diseases in the general public and the availability of sophisticated techniques now used to combat them.

Saving the patient's life is the primary goal of treating these bone cancers; saving the affected limb when possible is a bonus. For all bone cancer patients, treatments include a combination of surgery and chemotherapy and often radiation (especially with Ewing sarcoma).

Very broadly speaking, the strategies for attacking the two major types of bone cancers are as follows:

- Ewing sarcoma patients first receive chemotherapy to reduce the size of the tumor. Drugs include vincristine, doxorubicin, cyclophosphamide, ifosfamide, and etoposide. This is followed by an individualized plan for radiation and/or surgery. The operation will probably be limb-sparing, saving the arm or leg, with a graft or implant to take the place of the removed bone. Finally, additional chemotherapy is used to "mop up" any remaining cancer cells anywhere in the body. Some high-risk Ewing patients may be candidates for autologous stem cell rescue.
- Osteogenic sarcoma is attacked first by chemotherapy (using cisplatin, doxorubicin, and/or high-dose methotrexate with leucovorin rescue). Preoperative drug therapy increases the number of patients who are candidates for limb-sparing surgery rather than amputation. More than 80% now have the less disfiguring operation. Osteogenic sarcoma is considered radioresistant, so further therapy consists, again, of mop-up chemotherapy.

Surgery

Today, despite major advances, it is not possible to save all arms or legs that have a bone tumor. This applies particularly to osteogenic sarcoma, chondrosarcoma, and fibrosarcoma. The limb is usually amputated about 3 inches above the tumor for safety.

While younger children tend to adjust well to the loss of an arm or leg, teenagers find it harder. For adolescents, who are struggling with their sense of identity, amputation is a severe blow to their body image. Phantom limb pain can be a problem, perhaps for months or years, and the reactions of family, friends, and medical staff can affect how well the teenager deals with this crisis.

A plaster cast is put in place while the patient is still in the operating room to protect the stump and to keep the swelling down. An exercise program is begun soon after to strengthen the remaining muscles. In fact, the patient will probably be out of bed the first day after surgery. The plaster cast is removed in a day or so, replaced with elastic bandages. A regular routine of powdering and airing the stump and changing the stump socks provides a good opportunity for the patient to take part in his own care. Resuming normal activity has both physical and mental benefits for the patient.

Fittings for artificial limbs (prostheses) begin right after surgery. One type of artificial leg is made of willow and plastic, covered with foam rubber and held on with suction. The action of the prosthesis is much like that of a natural joint, and a normally active life is possible. There are different types of devices to attach the limbs—some use suction and others have straps. Physical therapists teach the patient to use the new limb when it is ready.

Modern artificial limbs are very natural in appearance. Careful measurements are taken of every possible dimension of the affected arm or leg before surgery to match the artificial limb to the natural one; skin color is also matched. These limbs are expensive, costing $6500 or more, while equipment to hold the limb in place adds another $5000 a year. The prostheses have to be replaced every year or so. If your health insurance does not cover the whole cost (and most do), contact the American Cancer Society, Candlelighters, or your state rehabilitation service for information on financial aid sources. The social service department of the hospital will also have a list of references to help the family and the patient. Addresses for many helpful organizations are included in Appendices A and B.

It is easy enough to say, "Well, you lost your (fill in the blank—arm, leg...) but we have saved your life." For someone facing this loss, talking (before surgery if possible) with someone else who has had the operation and who is well can be enormously reassuring. If the hospital does not offer for an amputee to visit your child before the operation, ask if there is someone who has successfully faced the same situation with whom you can talk. Your local Candlelighters or similar parents group might also know people who can help, and online discussion groups may work as well.

There are many national figures who have had limb amputations and have overcome the handicap, resuming their normal physical activities such as skiing and jogging. The courage of Ted Kennedy Jr. and Terry Fox (the Canadian youth who undertook a cross-country run to raise money for cancer research) must be inspirational, although offering children heroes to emulate can be overdone.

For amputees who wish to learn or relearn how to ski, note that many ski areas and resorts provide ski lessons for the disabled. A quick check on the World Wide Web turned up this service at Ski8 Apache, New Mexico; Sunday River, Maine (with an annual handicap ski race); Monarch and Winter Park, Colorado; Mt. Sunapee, New Hampshire; Vilars Gryon, Switzerland; Combloux (Mont Blanc), France; Big Bear, California; Aprica, Italy; and Poly-Aktief, a Netherlands-based program with skiing in Austria. Surely there are more. Several organizations for handicap sports in general are noted at the end of this chapter.

Because surgical techniques have improved greatly in recent years, amputation may be avoided. Doctors now remove the tumor and graft replacement bones from the patient himself or from a cadaver to the remaining bone. Metal or plastic tailor-made implants are also used. Long-term function of these limbs generally seems to be good and the emotional value for the patient is enormous, although quality of life for amputees is perhaps even better, a matter under investigation.

New prostheses can be fashioned taking into account potential growth of the patient's bones. Using an expansion mechanism, the salvaged limb does not end up shorter than the corresponding natural one. With up-to-date techniques like "growable" prostheses, children as young as 8 might have limb-salvage surgery. In this case, a metal "bone" replaces the natural one, and the new "bone" can be adjusted over time to "grow" along with the child. These expandable devices may not serve for a lifetime of growth and activity, however. Researchers continue to improve devices and prostheses.

Preoperative radiation and chemotherapy may reduce tumor bulk. If a child's disease is advanced enough that chemotherapy must be continued without interruption, he cannot receive a bone graft.

If, however, the doctors think it is safe to suspend drug therapy temporarily to perform bone graft surgery and allow time for healing, the child may be a candidate for the limb-sparing operation.

In hospital bone banks, bones are taken from cadavers with cartilage still attached. Pretreated and frozen at −70 degrees Celsius, they can be stored for at least 5 years. Cells that might lead to rejection are killed by deep freezing so that the recipient's immune system is more likely to accept the transplant.

Reports in the medical literature suggest that length of survival in osteogenic sarcoma patients is not adversely affected by the limb-sparing procedure, nor is local recurrence a major worry. Patients who have successful limb-salvage operations will require extensive rehabilitation to regain full use of the affected limb. Whether the patient has an amputation or a limb-salvage operation, physical therapy may continue for some time to help him learn to use the new or altered limb.

Amputation is still necessary for some patients. In case of extreme pain the limb may be amputated to relieve the pain, even if such surgery will play no part in curing the patient.

Radiation

Ewing tumor is considered relatively radiosensitive and therefore is attacked efficiently by external beam radiation, while osteogenic sarcoma is not. With Ewing sarcoma, the bone and the nearby tissue are radiated and chemotherapy is used; metastases may also be radiated. In osteogenic sarcoma, radiation might be used to palliate the bone pain.

The long-term effects of radiation on a limb may weaken it, and the high doses needed will retard its growth. Radiation also carries a risk that another cancer will develop in the future. During radiotherapy, an active exercise program should either be started or continued to maintain use of the limb. Tight-fitting clothes that rub on the radiation site should be avoided.

Chemotherapy

Surgery and radiation control local disease, but used alone they cure only a small percentage of patients. The majority of patients have micrometastases at the time of diagnosis, so today drug therapy plays a major role in treating bone cancers. Several drugs are given at specified intervals over a period of months, beginning as soon as possible after surgery. Often chemotherapy is used before surgery as well as afterwards.

If the patient relapses after chemotherapy has been stopped, it is started again with different drugs. If there is a relapse during treatments, the drugs used are also switched. Drugs may also be changed to avoid enhancing the side effects of radiation. For example, if the urinary bladder is in the target zone, Cytoxan (which can damage the urinary tract) may be replaced with another drug. Many drug combinations have yielded good results.

Oncologists recommend routine chemotherapy in patients with osteosarcoma. An effective treatment for osteogenic sarcoma is the use of very high doses of methotrexate, given intravenously to the hospitalized patient. After a period ranging from 2 to 24 hours, the methotrexate is stopped and the body is "rescued" by injection of leucovorin. In this way the tumor is bombarded with a much larger amount of tumor-killing medication than would ordinarily be administered or tolerated, and the body is saved from dangerous side effects.

Complementary Therapies

Acupuncture may help with pain relief, while guided imagery, hypnosis, or relaxation techniques can alleviate some nausea and vomiting, not to mention anxiety.

Patterns of Metastasis

Bone sarcomas tend to metastasize at an early stage, generally to the lungs. There is a good chance that osteogenic sarcoma patients will have undetectable lung metastases at the time of diagnosis; many Ewing tumor patients have early metastases, too. While most lung metastasis takes place in the first year, late spread to the lungs is possible. Besides appearing in the lungs, some metastases may crop up in other bones. Lymph nodes are affected in only a small proportion of cases.

Frequent chest x-rays and/or CT scans are required to locate these metastases as early as possible. Radiation may be effective in destroying the Ewing lung tumors, and a chest operation or repeated operations to remove one or even several lung tumors may be performed, especially in patients with osteogenic sarcoma.

Prognosis

Modern therapy, both drugs and surgical techniques, has improved the survival rate for bone cancer patients enormously. In the past, perhaps 10% of youngsters with Ewing sarcoma lived for a couple of years, and 80% of osteogenic sarcoma patients died in the first 2 years. Now, using combination treatments, there is an overall 5-year survival of over 66% for those with bone sarcomas, although relapses even 10 years later have been seen. The chances are the poorest for those who are diagnosed after the onset of such late symptoms as fever and weight loss.

Localized Ewing sarcoma has a 60% survival rate. Those with primary tumors at the far ends of bones (distal) or in a central location do better than patients with primaries in the bones closer to the trunk (proximal). Younger patients fare better, as do girls. Still, 10% to 40% of those with metastases survive if they receive state-of-the-art chemotherapy and radiation. The overall survival rate for Ewing sarcoma is 50%. National Cancer Institute researchers are studying a monoclonal antibody, R1507, in relapsed Ewing patients who have not responded to earlier therapies. Results are promising.

Osteogenic sarcoma patients with localized disease at diagnosis have a 60% to 75% long-term survival rate. There is no difference in long-term survival between patients with amputations and those who have limb-sparing surgery.

Further Resources

READING

Childhood Cancer: A Handbook from St. Jude Children's Research Hospital, edited by R. Grant Steen and Joseph Mirro, Jr. Cambridge, MA: Perseus Press, 2000.
    A wealth of information for bone cancer treatments and general support, written by seasoned experts.

ORGANIZATIONS/WEB SITES

ABLEDATA (8630 Fenton St., Suite 930, Silver Spring MD 20910; 800-227-0216; www.abledata.com)

This commercial site provides a gateway to assistive device manufacturers for various sports and activities.

American Academy of Orthopedic Surgeons (6300 North River Road, Rosemont, IL 60018; 847-823-7186; www.aaos.org)

This organization provides lots of self-help fact sheets for patients and various other informational services.

Amputee Coalition of America (900 East Hill Ave., Suite 205, Knoxville, TN 37915; 888-267-5669; www.amputee-coalition.org)

Provides a broad range of services for amputees and their families. Also in Spanish.

CureSearch from the Children's Oncology Group (www.curesearch.org)

Provides many resources for bone cancer patients.

Disabled Sports USA (451 Hungerford Drive, Suite 100, Rockville, MD 20850; 301-217-0960; www.dsusa.org)

Programs and equipment resources. Lots of links to regional and national organizations.

International Child Amputee Network (I-CAN) (P.O. Box 514, Abilene, TX 79604; www.child-amputee.net)

International conferences, mentor program, resources for patients and families, school issues, lots more.

ÖSSUR (www.ossur.com)

The website of this Iceland-based manufacturer of prostheses and other medical devices has a wealth of international contacts and links to many aspects of amputee life.

Physician Data Query (PDQ) (www.cancer.gov)_

The National Cancer Institute's Comprehensive Cancer Database, updated regularly.

Sarcoma Alliance (775 East Blithedale, #334, Mill Valley, CA 94941; 415-381-7236; www.sarcomaalliance.org)

Has a list of institutions with sarcoma expertise, leaders in treatment of these tumors.

Sarcoma Foundation of America (9884 Main St., P.O. Box 458, Damascus, MD 20872; 301-253-8687; www.curesarcoma.org)

Advocates for optimal therapy for sarcoma patients. Funds research. One of their fundraisers is a special series of Willow Crest wines.

9

Brain and Central Nervous System Tumors

Tumors of the brain and spinal cord, or central nervous system (CNS), are the most common type of primary solid tumor in children. Leukemia is the only malignancy more prevalent in young patients. CNS metastases are more common than primary tumors. There has been less dramatic progress in treating these tumors than with most other childhood malignancies because the therapies that might cure it can be so devastating to the child. Not only is the rapidly growing brain of a newborn or young child especially susceptible to damage from the tumor and the treatments, but fluid may collect in the brain (a condition known as hydrocephalus) when normal fluid circulation pathways are blocked, causing additional problems.

Improvements in neurologic techniques and radiation therapy have increased the length of survival, so that diagnosis of a brain tumor is not the end of hope today.

Incidence

There are about 2000 to 3000 new diagnoses of brain and CNS tumors in children under the age of 16 in the United States each year. Twenty percent of all primary brain tumors arise in children in this age group, somewhat more in boys than in girls, with a higher incidence in white children. There is a peak between the ages of 5 and 10.

Children with certain genetic disorders are more likely to develop a CNS tumor. These disorders include neurofibromatosis type 1 and von Hippel-Lindau syndrome. These children still account for only a tiny minority of CNS tumor patients.

Another important risk factor for a brain tumor is prior CNS radiation therapy for cancer, especially leukemia. The higher the radiation dose the patient received, the greater the possibility of a secondary CNS tumor developing. Pediatric cancer specialists are well aware of this possible consequence and plan therapy with this in mind. Recent European research suggests that paternal smoking prior to conception and a high intake of caffeine (coffee and tea) during pregnancy may contribute to the development of CNS tumors.

Researchers have spent many years looking for causative factors like electrical power lines in the environment, but nothing conclusive has resulted so far. Results have flip-flopped with a number of frightening stories in the mass media, but no definitive reports have risen above the rest.

Signs and Symptoms

The symptoms of a CNS tumor can be caused by the growth of the tumor into brain tissue or, more frequently, by increased intracranial pressure resulting from tumor growth elsewhere in the brain or from fluid buildup. In other words, it may not be the direct invasion of normal tissue that causes the symptoms but the squeezing of that tissue by excess growth somewhere else within the skull's limited space. These symptoms are hard to pin down, particularly in a young child who can't communicate his discomfort. A parent's "gut feeling" that something is wrong is vital in these cases and should be heeded.

- *Headache* is a major symptom of a brain tumor. The pain is often worse in the morning. If a headache is so severe that the child lies down holding his head, the doctor should be phoned at once. If a headache interferes with the child's activities for over an hour, the physician should also be notified.
- *Vomiting*, worse in the morning and unexplained, particularly if unaccompanied by nausea, is an important sign.

- *Blurred vision or seeing double* are common symptoms. Swelling of the optic nerve, which can be detected during a routine examination, is often present.
- *Personality changes* may include irritability in a normally even-tempered child, crankiness, the slowing down of an energetic child, a thriving toddler's loss of appetite, behavior problems, changes in sleeping patterns, lethargy, untidiness, and a poor memory. In an older child, temper tantrums and poor schoolwork are possible symptoms.
- *Regression in motor skills*, especially under the age of 2. Some children may stumble or seem clumsy.
- *Endocrine changes* such as diabetes insipidus (a disease marked by excessive thirst and passing huge amounts of urine) or precocious puberty (onset of sexual maturation at too early an age).
- *Increased head size* in infants whose skulls have not yet closed
- *Seizures*, although a tumor is an uncommon cause of seizures in children
- *Coma or change in level of consciousness* is very rare at the time of diagnosis, although possible.

Diagnosis

The diagnosis of CNS tumors is confirmed by various techniques.

- X-rays (skull)
- Computed tomography (CT) scans—often the first test and the most valuable diagnostic tool for localizing the tumor—can detect tumors of 1 to 2 cm or more (less than 1 inch in diameter). It is most useful in making the initial diagnosis; after treatment has started, it may show that tumor is still present.
- Magnetic resonance imaging (MRI) provides an excellent picture of brain structures without radiation and locates even smaller tumors.
- Positron emission tomography (PET), a new tool, is used for more precise tumor location, and finding recurrences or metastases.
- Electroencephalogram (EEG; brain wave reading) if the child is having seizures

- Cerebral arteriography (to study the blood supply to the tumor)
- Examination of cerebrospinal fluid (CSF) drawn by spinal tap (lumbar puncture) for staging the disease
- Biopsy (by operation or through a needle if the tumor is deep and inaccessible). In some cases the tumor is located in a critical area of the brain where biopsy by any method is impossible.
- Body scans to locate the primary site of the tumor if the brain mass is a metastasis

Brain Tumors

The most common site for children's brain tumors is the cerebellum, the portion of the brain responsible for regulating and coordinating voluntary muscular movements and equilibrium. The types of tumors most often found in the region of the cerebellum are astrocytoma, medulloblastoma, brain stem glioma, and ependymoma.

Because the flow of CSF is usually obstructed in early stages of the tumor development, signs and symptoms of increased pressure

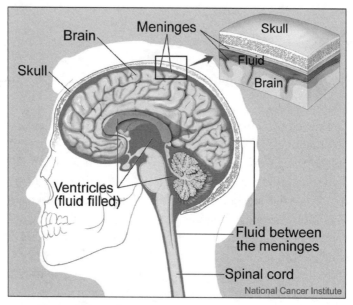

FIGURE 9.1 Brain and nearby structures

within the skull are common. These include headache, irritability, and vomiting.

Gliomas, astrocytomas, and ependymomas are also found elsewhere in the brain, along with rarer tumors like pineoblastoma.

Cerebellar Astrocytoma (Also called Glioma)

When located in the cerebellum, these tumors appear almost exclusively in childhood and early adolescence. Signs and symptoms may have been present for a long time before diagnosis: hydrocephalus, morning headache, vomiting, lethargy, head tilt, double vision, and lack of limb muscle coordination. Diagnosed by CT scan, they are treated by surgery, which may be curative in more than half of all patients if the tumor is completely removed. If it is not, the surgery can be repeated. Radiation may follow, especially if nearby tissues have been invaded. This slow-growing tumor is likely to recur or spread if it is not totally resected (removed by surgery). Varying in degree of malignancy, cerebellar astrocytoma has the most favorable prognosis of brain tumors.

Medulloblastoma

Medulloblastoma, which accounts for 20% of all pediatric CNS tumors, arises in the cerebellum or the fourth ventricle. More boys than girls are affected up to the age of 10; half of diagnoses come before the age of 5, including some infants. Signs and symptoms include headache, vomiting, muscle problems, personality changes, squint or double vision, neck stiffness, papilledema, lack of coordination in the trunk, rhythmic eyeball motion, and hydrocephalus. Diagnosis is by biopsy. Treatment includes surgery to remove as much tumor as possible, although medulloblastoma is not curable by surgery alone. Radiation to the entire brain and spine increases survival time, and chemotherapy may be effective as well. Rarely, patients develop metastases, mostly in the spine, and the bone marrow tumor may seed into the CSF and spread into the rest of the body. Other metastases may appear in the skeleton. Recurrences may happen even after 5 years. Carboplatin used with radiation can increase the radiosensitivity and therefore effectiveness.

Researchers are studying the use of intrathecal chemotherapy as a preventive measure (as in leukemia) to treat undetectable metastasis. Spinal taps can be dangerous except under carefully controlled conditions with this highly malignant, rapidly growing tumor. Some patients with metastatic disease may benefit from peripheral blood stem cell transplants. Prognosis is poorer if the tumor has spread before diagnosis; overall, half of the children survive 5 years. Children under the age of 3 at diagnosis are especially difficult to treat because the standard cranial radiation can lead to severe neurologic and cognitive problems.

Medulloblastoma is one cancer that has been studied in the use of anti-angiogenesis drugs, designed to interrupt the flow of blood to the tumor, starving it. This research is still in early stages.

Primitive Neuroectodermal Tumors (PNET)

PNETs are similar in location, appearance, biology, and treatment to medulloblastoma. PNETs are fast-growing tumors that form in brain cells in the cerebrum, which is the largest part of the brain and is located at the top of the head. This part of the brain controls thinking, learning, problem-solving, emotions, speech, reading, writing, and

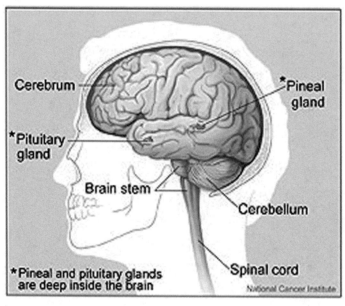

FIGURE 9.2 Major parts of the brain

voluntary movement. Because these tumors are treated with chemotherapy and high doses of radiation, brain injury and learning disabilities are likely as a result of the treatment. The prognosis is especially poor if the disease is widespread at the time of diagnosis.

Pineoblastoma (pineal blastoma) tumors occur in the midline of the brain in both young children and adolescents, more boys than girls being affected. Signs and symptoms include delayed or precocious puberty, diabetes insipidus, and endocrine abnormalities from the tumor's invasion into the hypothalamus. Diagnosis is by MRI and biopsy. Treatment may include placement of a shunt to relieve hydrocephalus. Most pinealomas are radiosensitive, so radiation therapy is helpful. Surgery is rarely possible because of the inaccessible location of these tumors. Pinealomas may seed into the spine. Some studies show about 70% survival, although the prognosis is poorer if the tumor is disseminated at diagnosis or when it strikes very young children, in whom radiation may not be used because side and late effects are too disabling.

Ependymoma

Ependymoma arises in cells that line the spaces in the brain or spinal cord. Slightly more males than females are affected, and with a peak in the second year of life; more than half of diagnoses are before the age of 5. Signs and symptoms include hydrocephalus, vomiting, headache, personality change, papilledema, and lack of muscle coordination. Treatment includes surgery if possible to remove all or most of this tumor. Postoperative radiation to the brain or spine follows if there is evidence of residual primary tumor, and patients with disseminated disease at diagnosis may also require radiation therapy to the spine or spinal cord. This tumor may be highly malignant yet lie dormant for years. Surgery alone seldom cures it, and it may recur even after 5 years. Survival rates vary according to the degree of surgical removal of the tumor, with about half of all patients remaining disease-free 10 years after diagnosis.

Glioma of the Optic Nerve

This tumor appears in the optic nerve, sometimes in adolescents but with a peak occurrence between the ages of 2 and 6. Signs and symptoms include rapid side-to-side eyeball motion, crossed eyes, early puberty, fading vision, headache, and morning vomiting. Diagnosis by biopsy may be too risky. This slow-growing tumor may be present without symptoms for 20 years. The role of surgery is controversial except to relieve hydrocephalus or when the tumor is in only one optic nerve and completely resectable. Some experts advocate radiation, which does seem to decrease the incidence of recurrence. Chemotherapy is used in most patients, especially those younger than 10. Long-term survival is expected even when only part of the tumor can be removed. Many patients have the genetic disorder neurofibromatosis type 1.

Brain Stem Gliomas

Appearing in the brain stem, these gliomas have a poorer prognosis than those located elsewhere in the brain. The incidence among girls and boys is equal, with a peak between the ages of 3 and 10 and rare occurrence before the age of 3. Signs and symptoms include facial palsy, difficulty in speaking or swallowing, lack of coordination, limb weakness, squint or double vision, personality changes, headache, and seizures. Diagnosis is by MRI. Surgery may not be an option on diffuse pontine glioma (located in the pons, which is part of the brain stem) because of the high probability of neurologic damage, and biopsy is rarely done. However, some low-grade brain stem gliomas can be removed surgically. Radiation increases survival time. Chemotherapy is used in some protocols. These pontine gliomas may extend into the hypothalamus and tissue connecting to the cerebellum. Tumors of the pons and medulla have a poor prognosis, a 20% 5-year survival rate, although brain stem gliomas that do not involve the pons have a much better prognosis; some can be cured by surgery alone.

Treatment

Hydrocephalus, the accumulation of fluid in the brain, causes many CNS tumor symptoms and poses a major threat to life. Thus, an early goal of treatment is to decrease the pressure of excess fluid in the brain. Next, an attempt is made to remove all or part of the tumor if feasible, followed by radiation and possibly chemotherapy to eradicate residual disease. When cure is not possible, the same techniques can relieve the symptoms and permit the patient to live comfortably for a time.

Surgery

The first line of action in treatment is often surgery. Opening the skull to expose the brain is called a craniotomy; with microneurosurgical techniques, these operations can now be performed more often than previously was the case. During the operation the surgeon will try to remove the tumor either completely or to the greatest extent possible. A biopsy to identify the tumor type may be carried out if the tumor cannot be removed in whole or in part.

During a craniotomy, the surgeon may put a shunt in place to drain fluid from the center of the brain into the abdomen or to the bloodstream, where it is harmlessly removed. Newer techniques provide CT/MRI images during surgery to target the site precisely.

After surgery the patient may need special nurses or may be put in intensive care. He may be restless or confused.

Some tumors cannot be removed surgically because the location is too dangerous. Cures by surgery alone are rare and depend on the nature of the tumor, its location, and its relationship to vital structures. Sometimes the location of the tumor precludes even a biopsy.

Radiation

Radiation is an important tool in the treatment of children with brain tumors. Although radiation of the spinal cord and brain in the developing child can stunt growth and disturb the endocrine system, in many cases these risks must be taken because of the greater dangers posed by an untreated brain tumor.

Because the nervous system cannot always tolerate the level of radiation needed to kill the entire tumor, it is vital to have a skilled pediatric specialist determine the dosage size and the precise area to be treated. Modern therapy may include use intensity-modulated radiation therapy (IMRT), a type of scan called SRS that uses an injected radioactive drug, or proton beam therapy.

Children must lie still for radiation treatments, and they generally adapt well. Doctors, wishing to avoid repeated use of sedation or anesthesia, create a special restraint to immobilize the child. Some children still require anesthesia every day of their treatments. A moving target is not acceptable for these delicate treatments, which require pinpoint accuracy.

A new therapy called "stereotactic radiosurgery" uses a number of beams of ionizing radiation, coming from many directions around the patient's head and meeting at a precise point (where the tumor is located), although this is not standard.

Chemotherapy

The role of chemotherapy in treating CNS tumors was long disputed, but it has become part of standard therapy. Getting chemotherapy drugs to the target is difficult because many drugs, when given orally or intravenously, are unable to cross the blood–brain barrier. In leukemia therapy, the drugs are injected directly into the CNS to bypass the barrier. This route is used to administer some drugs in treating brain tumors as well, but studies have shown that other drugs pass the blood–brain barrier easily. One drug, BCNU, can be used as a wafer placed in the tumor site during surgery. Other drugs used in brain tumor therapy include cisplatin, carboplatin, etoposide, methotrexate, cyclophosphamide, and vinblastine.

Chemotherapy works best on fast-growing cells. Although not all CNS tumors grow quickly enough to be affected by the drugs, certain brain tumors are sometimes quite sensitive to them. Other drugs may be used to treat the symptoms of CNS tumors as well as the side effects of treatments such as radiation. Dexamethasone or other steroids are sometimes given to relieve the fluid pressure in the skull. Anticonvulsants may be required on those rare occasions when seizures occur.

Children with some recurrent brain tumors may respond to high-dose chemotherapy followed by an autologous stem cell transplant.

Rehabilitation

Either the tumor itself or therapy may interfere with normal functioning of the body. Rehabilitation may be required to regain use of affected limbs or senses like smell or hearing, or to overcome other physical impairments. Planned by the hospital's physical therapy department, an exercise program carried out at home is an important investment in the child's future.

Prognosis

The prognosis of CNS tumors depends on the type and location of the tumor. Previously, the outlook for these diseases was grim and little was attempted in the way of treatment. Now, with CT scans and MRI, diagnosis is improved and less risky. Better surgical techniques are also leading to an improved quality and length of life for these children. With prompt diagnosis and treatment by a team of skilled specialists, the odds are favorable for a full recovery. According to Roger Packer, MD, three quarters of children live 5 years from diagnosis and more than half are probably cured. White children have a higher survival rate.

Spinal Cord Tumors

Spinal cord tumors are relatively rare in children, accounting for less than 5% of all CNS tumors. When they do occur, they are often metastases from primary tumors located elsewhere that are first diagnosed after the spine has been invaded.

Symptoms are constant or intermittent pain in the neck, shoulder, chest, abdomen, pelvis, and extremities. The pain is worse when the child is at rest; it is aggravated by sneezing, laughing, coughing, and lifting; and it is relieved by exercise. General weakness and numbness appear later, and sensitivity to heat and touch diminishes. Sometimes there is a rarely reversible paralysis in one or more areas of the body, and perhaps loss of bladder and bowel control. The child's reflexes and gait are disturbed, and the tumor is often accompanied by scoliosis (curvature of the spine) and torticollis (wry neck, a spasm that causes a head tilt).

Early diagnosis and treatment are essential. Diagnosis is by spinal x-rays and spinal MRI. Some of these tumors can be cured by surgery alone. Radiation is often given, even for patients with spinal metastases. In some cases chemotherapy is employed, depending on the origin and type of the tumor. Prognosis is improved with early diagnosis and treatment. In one study 60% of survivors regained normal function, some needed braces to walk, and a few were confined to bed or a wheelchair. The results were poorer when the spinal tumor was a metastasis from a primary tumor.

Benign or Low-Grade Tumors of the CNS

Many tumors diagnosed in the CNS are called benign, but in the case of a brain or spinal tumor this doesn't necessarily make the mass any less dangerous. The prognosis depends on the location and the response to treatment. A benign mass that is inoperable is still life-threatening because it is taking up valuable space within the skull and squeezing brain tissue, thus interfering with normal function.

Special Problems

CNS tumors are hard to diagnose and treat because of the obscurity and variety of symptoms, many of which mimic other disorders. Early symptoms are not definitive, and children may adapt their behavior or movements to compensate for the changes caused by the tumor. There is potential for long-term neurologic defects caused by the tumor itself or its treatment. Paralysis or blindness may even occur.

If elevated pressure develops in the brain because of fluid collection there, the doctor may limit liquids to prevent additional buildup. It may also be necessary to limit sedation so that the level of consciousness can be assessed to indicate the condition of the patient. If the child is confused, delirious, lethargic, or hard to arouse, a doctor should be consulted.

Seizures are rare, although possible, so those caring for these children should prepare by using bedrails to prevent falls and small firm pillows to avoid smothering. Doctors recommend turning a child who is having a seizure on his side, so that the limp tongue does not block the airway, and waiting it out.

Late Effects

Surgery, radiation, and chemotherapy for brain and CNS tumors can affect school performance, with children who are very young at diagnosis having the greatest risk. Growth issues and learning disabilities may appear soon after surgery or even many years later. Slower learning, problems with math, a drop in IQ, memory difficulties—these and more may be in the future for these children. Parents or guardians have to advocate for testing and special services. Schools in the United States have a legal obligation to provide appropriate services like one-on-one aides, tutors, and physical adaptations (perhaps a keyboard for a child who has difficulty with handwriting). Be sure to get everything in writing. Have an individual education plan (IEP) in place for your child. Insist on expert testing. This could require a lot of time and effort on your part, but it may be the only way to ensure that your child reaches his full potential.

Because brain and CNS tumors are such a common type of childhood malignancy, there is a wealth of information and some good publications available to help families understand the disease. This chapter therefore is only an introduction; check the section on print resources for helpful citations.

Further Resources

READING

Epstein, Fred J., MD, and Elaine Fantle Shimberg. *Gifts of Time*. New York: Morrow, 1993.
   This fascinating and very readable book describes the work of Dr. Epstein, a pioneer in brain tumor surgery in places once thought inoperable—the brain stem and spinal cord. Encouraging and honest, the stories of several patients are moving; Dr. Epstein's connection to the families involved is especially touching. Descriptions of surgical techniques and a few referral suggestions are woven though the chapters.

Plichart, Matthieu, et al, "Parental smoking, maternal alcohol, coffee and tea consumption during pregnancy and childhood malignant central nervous system tumors." *European Journal of Cancer Prevention*, vol. 17 (4) (August 2008), p. 376–383.

Shiminski-Maher, Tania. *Childhood Brain and Spinal Cord Tumors: A Guide for Families, Friends and Caregivers.* Sebastopol, CA: O'Reilly, 2002.

A "Parent-Centered Guide," this authoritative and up-to-date volume not only provides a wealth of detailed information for families but has much anecdotal content that is both instructional and often reassuring.

ORGANIZATIONS / WEB SITES

American Brain Tumor Association (2720 River Road, Suite 146, Des Plaines, IL 60018; 847- 827-9910; 800-886-2282; www.abta.org)

Includes "A Primer of Brain Tumors, 8th edition," free to download. Funds and encourages research, publishes educational materials. Some publications available in Spanish. Pen pal programs.

Association of Online Cancer Resources (www.acor.org)

Has an online discussion group for brain tumor topics.

Childhood Brain Tumor Foundation (20312 Watkins Meadow Drive, Germantown, MD 20876; 301-515-2900; 877-217-4166; www.childhood braintumor.org)

Articles and information on their research-related mission. Has an ombudsman program to help patients and survivors with insurance and other issues.

Children's Brain Tumor Foundation (274 Madison Avenue, Suite 1301, New York NY 10016; 212-448-9494; www.cbtf.org)

Information on hospitalization, home care issues, schooling, etc. Publishes a free "A Resource Guide for Parents of Children with Brain or Spinal Cord Tumors". Also available in Spanish. Support programs. Funds research.

Healing Exchange Brain Trust (www.braintrust.org)

Has an online discussion group.

National Brain Tumor Foundation (www.tbts.org or www.braintumor.org; West Coast office: 323 Geary St., Suite 510, San Francisco, CA 94102; 415-296-0404; 800-934-CURE (934-2873); East Coast office: 124 Watertown St., Suite 2D, Watertown, MA 02472; 617-924-9997; 800-770-8287)

Merged with the Brain Tumor Society, this expanded organization has publications and other resources for adults and children, patients, and caregivers. Publications (some in Spanish), conferences, support network, research funds. Excellent, well-illustrated publications for readers of all levels. "My Name is Buddy—A Book for Children about Brain Tumors" follows a golden retriever through diagnosis and treatment for a brain tumor using a sly humor that will appeal to older readers, too. They have a nifty interactive "tour of the brain" on the Web site.

Pediatric Brain Tumor Consortium (www.ptbc.org)

Supported by the National Institutes of Health and the National Cancer Institute, this group and its foundation gather about a dozen top research centers and experts to study these tumors and improve their therapies.

Pediatric Brain Tumor Foundation (302 Ridgefield Court, Asheville, NC 28806; 828-665-6891; 800-253-6530; www.pbtfus.org)

Seeks causes and cures of childhood brain tumors through medical research, public awareness, early detection and treatment. Informative booklets are available in English and Spanish. Sponsors conferences. Funds research. Scholarships (includes a list of other resources for educational funds).

10

Retinoblastoma

R etinoblastoma is a highly malignant cancer of the retina. The most common primary eye tumor, it accounts for 3% of childhood malignancies. Because of changes in the appearance of the eye, it is often first noticed by parents (unless children are being regularly screened for the tumor because other family members have had it).

Retinoblastoma begins at the rear of the retina, invades the orbit, grows rapidly, and if untreated spreads to the brain via the optic nerve and then elsewhere in the body.

About 30% of the cases are bilateral (in both eyes). Tumors may arise in each eye at different times, with intervals as long as 19 months between the appearance in the first eye and the second. Doctors think this represents independent growth in each eye rather than spread from a single primary tumor. Retinoblastoma also typically appears simultaneously in several spots within the affected eye.

Unilateral cases are usually discovered around the second birthday, while bilateral disease is typically found about a year earlier. A vast majority, 95% of cases, appear before the age of 5. Some parents and supporters are lobbying for legislation that requires routine screening of infants for retinoblastoma at birth, allowing detection at a very early stage, when it is usually curable by surgery alone.

A small portion of these patients, 5% to 15%, have a syndrome called trilateral retinoblastoma. These include children with both the spontaneous and familial or bilateral forms but with an added intracranial tumor. Aggressive therapy offers some promise against this form of the disease, which has a poor prognosis.

Genetics

Some forms of retinoblastoma are known to be inherited, a clear genetic link that has been much studied. This permits some cases to be predicted and therefore diagnosed at a very early age, often shortly after birth, when cure is most possible. At least two genetic mutations have been found that are responsible for this trait, which is passed as a dominant gene (in other words, more likely to be passed on than not). In the inherited form, a child's disease may be bilateral even if the parent's was not.

Brothers and sisters of retinoblastoma patients have a 1% to 3% risk of developing the disease, if the parents have not been affected. If more than one sibling develops retinoblastoma, the chances of others being affected are 50%, even if neither parent has had a tumor, because one of the parents is probably a carrier. Spontaneous cases—without any family history—also seem to be on the rise. Current theory holds that retinoblastoma requires the presence of two or more causative factors to develop. One factor appears to be the genetic predisposition in susceptible families, and the second may be environmental.

Genetic counseling is recommended for those who have survived this tumor, to explore the possibility of it being passed on to offspring. This is advisable even for those who develop retinoblastoma without any family history of the disease. Children of retinoblastoma survivors have a 50% chance of inheriting the gene, and of those 90% develop retinoblastoma. Of all cases, 40% are hereditary, and of those, 40% are bilateral. (Currently, all bilateral disease is considered familial.) In unilateral disease, 10% to 20% of the survivors seem to have hereditary disease, even without a family history. Therefore, their children carry a 7% to 10% risk of developing the tumor. People from families with retinoblastoma who are not affected themselves may still be carriers of the gene. If one of their children is affected, there is a 50% chance that others will be as well.

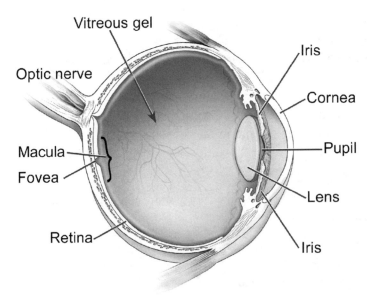

FIGURE 10.1 Diagram of the eye
Courtesy: National Eye Institute, National Institutes of Health.

Incidence

About 300 new cases of retinoblastoma are diagnosed each year in the United States, mainly in infants and young children, with 95% diagnosed before the age of 5. Rates are equal for boys and girls, blacks and whites. Internationally, higher rates of retinoblastoma are found in India, Pakistan, and, to a lesser degree, Latin America.

Signs and Symptoms

Symptoms of retinoblastoma are more specific than those of most other forms of childhood cancer, although in one study of retinoblastoma patients, 15% of the cases had been initially misdiagnosed, half of those as an inflammation of the eye. Delay in getting proper therapy lowers the rate of survival.

Obvious symptoms are changes in the appearance of the eye:

• White pupil
• Cat's eye reflex (whitish spot on the pupil, most easily seen when viewed from the side of the eye)

- Squint
- Later, a pearly glint may appear.
- Eye misalignment, like crossing of the affected eye
- A late sign may be limited or complete loss of vision, indicating large bilateral tumors.
- Sometimes there is glaucoma (raised pressure in the eye and accumulation of fluid in the cornea).
- Red and painful eye, possibly with glaucoma (indicates extensive disease)

Other symptoms are very rare and are related to metastases; they appear later in the course of retinoblastoma:

- Bone pain
- Enlarged liver
- Swollen lymph nodes in the neck
- Headache
- Vomiting

Diagnosis

Diagnosis of retinoblastoma is made through a series of examinations and tests:

- A family history is taken.
- An eye examination is made under general anesthesia using a binocular ophthalmoscope (examination under anesthesia [EUA]).
- Computed tomography (CT) scan (shows anatomy of the eye, optic nerve, and brain)
- Skull x-ray
- Spinal tap (if headache and vomiting are present)
- Bone marrow aspiration (if headache and vomiting are present, to see if any malignant cells are lurking there)
- Magnetic resonance imaging (MRI) (repeated at decreasingly frequent intervals for 3 years to watch for brain tumor development)
- Ultrasound
- Bone scan

Staging

Staging of retinoblastoma is slightly different from that of other childhood cancers. Rather than the extent to which the disease has spread, here doctors note the size, the site, and any extension of the tumor into the eyeball. Size is indicated by optic disc diameters, which compare the mass of the tumor to the diameter of the optic nerve. For example, 2 disc diameters equals twice the size of the nerve, and so on. Tumors are rated from group I (least extensive) to group VI. The presence or absence of tumor outside of the affected eye is another staging factor.

Treatment

The treatment plan for each case of retinoblastoma depends on whether the tumor has spread beyond the eye. Curing retinoblastoma means eradicating the tumor while sparing the child's vision. Patients should be treated in major medical centers by specialists, including an ophthalmologist, experienced in the diagnosis and treatment of this tumor. While every attempt is made to save vision, that must remain secondary to saving the patient's life.

In the case of bilateral disease, each eye is considered separately in terms of surgery and radiation. Often the more affected eye will be removed and the other treated with radiation. Interestingly, in some cases treating both eyes initially sometimes provides greater improvement in the more affected eye. Forms of treatment in retinoblastoma include surgery, perhaps followed by radiation and/or chemotherapy. Current clinical trials are investigating the efficacy of combination chemotherapy drugs to save the eye, peripheral stem cell transplantation, and intra-arterial therapy (infusing drugs into an artery for direct delivery to the eye).

Surgery

If vision has already been lost, the eye is usually removed. The aim of this surgery, which is called enucleation, is to remove the eye without rupture—which is like shelling a nut. As much of the optic nerve is removed as possible, because cancer can spread through the nerve into the brain. Retinoblastoma is not usually discovered in a single eye early enough for useful vision to be saved through radiation rather than removal. This does occur, however, in patients who are carefully monitored because of a family history of the disease.

A special technique used in the treatment of cancer is photocoagulation, a series of treatments that use a powerful beam of light from a xenon arc lamp to destroy small retinal tumors and the blood vessels supplying them. The decision whether to use photocoagulation depends on the site and size of the tumor. Its major use is in treating small tumors that recur after radiation.

Some specialists use powerful laser beams rather than cutting instruments to remove small malignant eye tumors. Watching the beam's progress on a monitor throughout the operation, the doctor first inserts a tiny probe into the eye, then applies the laser beam with split-second timing. Because it cauterizes as it cuts, postoperative bleeding is prevented as well. Lasers are easier to control than xenon arc lamps.

Another technique is cryotherapy, a freeze–thaw method that destroys small or recurrent tumors. The opposite form of treatment is thermotherapy, using heat to destroy cancer cells.

Radiation

Radiation therapy plays several roles in the treatment of retinoblastoma. Because it is a radiosensitive tumor, radiation offers an opportunity to save vision, if sight is still present. However, radiation alone is not effective if there is local involvement, like tumor in the optic nerve that threatens the patient's survival. Some patients lose their sight after radiation, and cataracts may form on the lens, but this is not common. When only one eye is affected, the radiation beam is carefully aimed to avoid damaging the healthy eye.

Radiation treatments require complete immobility for accuracy. Swaddling a young child or infant firmly but comfortably may lull him to sleep, but virtually all small children have to be anesthetized or sedated to allow accurate targeting of radiation. While immobilization devices will hold most of the body in one place, they clearly will not work with the eyes.

A special form of radiotherapy is the implanting of radioactive seeds in small or solitary tumors. This is called brachytherapy.

All patients are examined 4 to 6 weeks after radiation treatments to assess the affects. If treatment has not been completely successful, photocoagulation or cryotherapy may be performed.

The base of the brain, the head, or the spine may be radiated if the central nervous system is involved, and other metastases may be radiated to relieve symptoms. However, specialists are careful to use as little radiation as possible to avoid the development of another malignancy later in life. This is especially important in children with bilateral or inherited retinoblastoma.

Chemotherapy

Drug therapy plays less of a role in the treatment of retinoblastoma than it does in other childhood cancers. In the case of groups IV and V (metastatic) retinoblastoma, a combination of drugs may be used to fight the disease. Carboplatin, etoposide, vincristine, doxorubicin, and cyclophosphamide are among the agents used. For recurrent retinoblastoma, there is a high response rate (85%) to etoposide and carboplatin. Trials are under way to determine if chemotherapy will shrink large tumors, making subsequent cryotherapy more effective.

Researchers have seen promising results using high-dose chemotherapy and autologous stem cell transplant in children with bilateral metastasized retinoblastoma. With this approach they were able to avoid radiation, with its risk of second malignancies. This therapy may preserve some vision for the patient. Intra-arterial delivery of chemotherapy drugs directly into the eye is being investigated.

Metastasis

Retinoblastoma is spread by the blood to the skeleton, spinal fluid, the brain, the lymph nodes, and the liver; rarely are the lungs affected. It first breaks out of the eyeball and grows into orbital tissues and sinuses, and then it metastasizes. It tends, however, to remain a local disease for long periods.

Prognosis

There is a gratifyingly high success rate in the treatment of retinoblastoma, because the tumor is so accessible for early diagnosis and treatment. Prognosis is stage-related, with group I disease classified as very favorable and group V and orbital tumors (group VI) very unfavorable. Over 90% of the patients are cured, with a majority retaining useful vision (defined as 20/20 to 20/200 vision in at least one eye). Even in the case of group V and orbital tumors, a third of the patients live, some with good eyesight. Treating metastatic disease with chemotherapy may increase survival by as much as 18 months to 2 years.

In the familial form, if only one eye is affected at diagnosis, there is a 70% chance of recurrence in the other eye.

Recurrence

A child with the hereditary form of retinoblastoma has an increased risk (5% to 15%) of developing a brain tumor during treatment.

Retinoblastoma that recurs in the orbit has a poor prognosis, although surgery and radiation may be repeated. If the recurrence is in the skull or at a distant spot in the body, a combination of chemotherapy and radiation may have good results. Recurrence is rare after 2 years but may be seen 3 or more years after diagnosis. If the regrowth occurs after radiation treatments, an attempt may be made to save vision through photocoagulation, cryotherapy, or radioactive implants. However, metastasized retinoblastoma is difficult to treat and the prognosis is not good.

Second malignancies may occur up to 50 years later in up to 30% of the bilateral cases and less frequently in patients with unilateral disease; the incidence is significantly higher in patients treated with radiation. Familial patients may develop osteosarcoma (about 1% by age 10), soft tissue sarcoma, or melanoma, commonly in but not limited to patients who had radiation, especially before the first birthday.

Family Precautions

Survivors, their siblings, and other family members should have regular ophthalmoscopic examinations to detect tumors. Children of survivors should also be examined soon after birth and carefully watched for retinoblastoma. Doctors have recently been able to identify the gene that is either missing or nonfunctional in retinoblastoma patients. This is important because doctors may be able to identify children with the faulty gene and screen them. With modern treatments, these tumors can be located and treated when they are very small, giving an excellent chance for cure and retained vision.

Further Resources

READING

Bruner, Sharon Higgins. *Perfect Vision, A Mother's Experience with Childhood Cancer.* Fuquay-Varina, NC: Research Triangle Park, 1996.
  A very readable story of a child with retinoblastoma (daughter of a man who had survived the disease himself). May be difficult to find but uplifting in tone despite the child's eventual death.

ORGANIZATIONS/WEB SITES

Association of Cancer Online Resources (www.acor.org)
  Provides retinoblastoma discussion lists.

Childhood Eye Cancer Trust (The Royal London Hospital, Whitechapel Road, London E1 1BB, UK; 020-7377-5578; www.Chect.org.uk)
  With a British focus, this group has information for adults and children, including appropriate links to other sites.

Eye Cancer Network (115 East 61st St., New York City, NY 10021; 212-832-8170; www.eyecancer.com)
  Educational website with links to excellent illustrations of retinoblastoma (some of which may be a bit graphic for general readers).

11

Soft Tissue Sarcomas

S oft tissue sarcomas are malignant tumors arising from muscle, connective tissue, blood vessels, and fat. They account for about 7% of childhood malignancies, with a few hundred new pediatric cases each year in the United States. The majority are rhabdomyosarcoma, which will be discussed in detail, as will the next most common forms, synovial sarcoma and fibrosarcoma. Others include angiosarcoma, liposarcoma, mesenchymoma, neurofibrosarcoma, synovial sarcoma, and alveolar soft part sarcoma.

With all of these cancers, survival depends on the control of tumor at the primary site, and the prognosis is based on the site of origin, the extent of the disease, and the cell type involved. Some genetic disorders factoring in the development of sarcomas include Li-Fraumeni syndrome, neurofibromatosis type 1, and Beckwith-Wiedemann syndrome.

Rhabdomyosarcoma

Rhabdomyosarcoma, a muscle tumor, is the most common soft tissue sarcoma in children. Its occurrence peaks before the age of 5 and also between 15 and 19. The majority of cases appear in the first decade of life, with a lesser peak in adolescence.

Sites

Rhabdomyosarcoma can occur in any muscle tissue in the body. The most common sites are the head (including the eye socket) and neck (35% to 40%), the genitourinary tract (25%), and the extremities (25%). Tumors in the urinary and genital tracts occur in the bladder, prostate, uterus, vagina, or spermatic cord. Primary tumors are also found in muscles of the limbs, buttocks, and trunk.

Signs and Symptoms

Symptoms depend on the site of the primary tumor. In many cases the initial complaint is a painless lump or swelling. Other possible signs and symptoms include:

- Eye socket: swelling of eyelid, squint, eye bulging, vision problems
- Neck and throat: hoarseness, difficulty swallowing
- Nasal cavity: nasal discharge or blocked nose, inflammation of the sinuses
- Urinary tract: blood in urine, difficulty urinating
- Middle ear or mastoid: pain, discharge from ear canal, mass in ear canal
- Vagina: bloody discharge, tissue like "cluster of grapes" protruding from vagina

Diagnosis

A biopsy is necessary to make the diagnosis. Various types of x-rays and scans are then used to delineate the exact size and location of the primary tumor and determine whether it has spread locally:

- Chest x-ray
- Complete blood count
- X-ray of affected area (to see if there is any local extension)
- Computed tomography (CT) scans (areas of primary tumor and chest)
- Magnetic resonance imaging (MRI)
- Gastrointestinal (GI) series (if abdominal symptoms are present)

- Cystoscopy (if urinary symptoms are present)
- Ophthalmoscopy (if the eye is affected)
- Ultrasound
- Positron emission tomography (PET) scan

Other tests may be carried out to determine whether any metastases are affecting vital organs and to distinguish rhabdomyosarcoma from other tumors:

- CT and MRI for chest tumors; CT for metastases to the lungs
- Bone scan (to see if there is any bone involvement)
- Urinalysis

Staging and Histology

There are several different ways to classify rhabdomyosarcoma—staging, risk groups, favorable or unfavorable sites. The National Cancer Institute has a discussion of these systems on its rhabdomyosarcoma page. For simplicity, the staging system is easiest to understand.

To determine the stage of rhabdomyosarcoma, doctors assess the extent of local and distant disease. The more the cancer has spread, the higher the stage number. Stage (or group) I is still localized, without lymph node involvement, and can be completely removed by surgery. Stage II is local or regional with microscopic tumor residual after surgery. Stage III is regional with a lot of tumor left after surgery. Stage IV is metastatic at the time of diagnosis.

A histologic or microscopic classification of the specific tumor is also made. Specialists study tumor cells to determine whether the malignant cells have developed from immature or relatively mature muscle cells. Some specimens have a variety of cell types and some cannot be distinguished. This histologic subtyping helps determine the prognosis.

The two major histologic types of rhabdomyosarcoma are embryonal (about 80%), which arises from immature cells and is quite responsive to treatment, and alveolar, which usually affects older patients and is more aggressive in growth and spread.

Treatment

Treatment of rhabdomyosarcoma depends on the extent of local disease and whether distant spread has occurred. The aim is to remove the tumor and prevent or eliminate any metastasis while maintaining function of the affected organs or limbs. Therapy consists of a combination of surgery and chemotherapy and sometimes radiation as well.

SURGERY

Until recently, the major treatment of rhabdomyosarcoma was a radical operation to remove the entire affected muscle group along with large amounts of local tissue; sometimes an entire limb was amputated. Today doctors remove local tumors, sparing as much normal tissue as possible. Although the kind of treatment depends on the location of the tumor, the trend today is toward less surgery because rhabdomyosarcoma is responsive to radiation and chemotherapy. This helps preserve the function of the affected limb or organ.

RADIATION

The local area of the mass is radiated after surgery. Tumor in the eye socket is difficult to remove surgically without harming the eye, so radiation is used as the primary treatment with chemotherapy in hopes of saving vision. Metastases to lungs and the liver may receive radiation. Brachytherapy (implanted radioactive seeds) may be used in some genitourinary or head and neck tumors with gratifying results.

CHEMOTHERAPY

Therapy includes combination chemotherapy to attack any residual primary tumor and metastases, whether or not any spread is detectable. Two or three months of chemotherapy may be followed by radiation for several weeks and then further chemotherapy. A number of medications have proven effective against rhabdomyosarcoma.

Patterns of Metastasis and Recurrence

Rhabdomyosarcoma can metastasize to the lungs, lymph nodes, bones, bone marrow, liver, or brain. Local recurrences and metastases may appear up to 5 years after treatment, although most relapses occur in the first 2 years.

Clinical studies have looked at the efficacy of autologous stem cell transplants in some rhabdomyosarcoma patients, but results to date have been disappointing. Still, even patients with recurrent rhab-domyosarcoma may have a 40% chance of survival, depending on the site of the recurrence, the histology of the tumor, and the intensity of the initial therapy.

Prognosis

Children between the ages of 1 and 7 have a better chance of surviving rhabdomyosarcoma. Children under the age of 1 fare especially poorly. The prognosis with rhabdomyosarcoma also depends on the primary site, the extent of disease at diagnosis, and the histologic pattern. Children with orbital tumors (which are obvious and therefore seen early) or bladder tumors and girls with genital cancers have a better prognosis, as do those with primary sites in the head and neck. Conversely, tumors arising in the extremities and chest carry the greatest risk.

The overall prognosis is improving with the advent of better che-motherapy. Recent statistics show 90% survival in stages I and II, 65% in stage III, and 20% in more advanced cases. Overall 71% of patients survive this disease.

Other Soft Tissue Sarcomas

The other group of tumors that fall within the scope of this chapter are non-rhabdomyosarcoma soft tissue sarcomas (NRSTS). They appear slightly more often in boys and blacks, with peaks in infancy and adolescence.

These other forms of soft tissue sarcoma are quite rare. In lieu of staging they are placed into three classes:

- *High risk*: metastatic (treated with chemotherapy, radiation, and possibly surgery, especially for lung metastases)
- *Intermediate risk*: higher-grade, larger tumors that can't be sur-gically removed
- *Low risk*: smaller, removable tumors, even of high grade. Surgery is the first line of treatment, with a goal to remove the whole tumor if possible.

Radiation may be used before or after surgery, with external beam, implanted seeds, intensity-modulated radiation therapy (IMRT), or proton beam therapy. NRSTS in children, especially those under the age of 4, have a better outlook than those in adults.

These tumors tend to be drug-resistant, but chemotherapy is used more often now, especially in tumors that cannot be completely removed by surgery and those that have metastasized. Agents might include doxorubicin and ifosfamide.

Risk factors for these soft tissue sarcomas are:

- Li-Fraumeni syndrome
- Neurofibromatosis type I
- Previously radiated site
- Hereditary retinoblastoma
- Epstein-Barr virus (leiomyosarcoma in patients with AIDS)

Therapy is individualized in each child's case, depending on the size of the tumor, whether and where it has spread, and the histologic grade of the cells involved. There is a great variation of tissue type involved with these sarcomas:

- Liposarcoma (fat cells)
- Angiosarcoma (walls of blood vessels and veins)
- Leiomyosarcoma (smooth muscle)
- Fibrous, adipose (connective tissue)
- Synovial sarcoma
- Fibrosarcoma (fibrous tissue like scars or connective tissue around tendons or nerves)

The prognosis also varies with these rare tumors. Generally speaking, the earlier the tumor is found, the better, with perhaps 90% of patients with favorable factors (tumor grade and resectability) living 5 years after diagnosis. Those who relapse have significantly lower survival rates.

Further Resources

READING

Spunt, Sheri L., et al. Pediatric non-rhabdomyosarcoma soft tissue sarcomas. *The Oncologist* vol. 13 (2008), p. 668–678. Accessed at www.TheOncologist.com, 7/3/2008.
This detailed article reports current research with type-specific information.

ORGANIZATIONS/WEB SITES

Association of Cancer Online Resources (www.acor.org)

Online discussion list called "Rhabdo-kids" for rhabdomyosarcoma patients.

The American Cancer Society (www.cancer.org) and the National Cancer Institute (www.cancer.gov) have up-to-date disease-specific resources for rhabdomyosarcoma.

12

Germ Cell Tumors

G erm cells are the primitive cells that mature into sperm and egg cells. Because of the role they play in reproduction, each one retains the capability to create any kind of tissue or structure in a new human. When these cells become malignant, they can incorporate a bizarre collection of tissue types within a single tumor. Germ cell tumors (GCTs) include teratomas and endodermal sinus tumors. They are characterized as gonadal and extragonadal GCTs.

Teratomas

Teratomas, also called dysembryomas, include a wide variety of malignant and benign tumors present at birth, although they may not be diagnosed for some time. While some teratomas grow large in the prenatal stage, others do not cause symptoms until young adulthood.

Teratomas are groups of cells that appear in the wrong place in the body, such as when bone cells appear in the ovary. They often contain a variety of tissues, such as teeth, kidney tissue, hair, skin, and fat. These tumors arise in many sites, including the brain, testicles, ovaries, base of the skull, palate, mediastinum, and near the base of the spine. A large percentage of teratomas are benign tumors; some of them also become malignant.

Brain teratomas peak in infancy and again between the ages of 10 and 15. The rate of survival is lower for infants.

Ovarian teratomas may be benign cysts. Accounting for 1% of all childhood tumors, they almost always affect only one ovary and seldom appear before puberty. Diagnosis is made at surgery. Tests to determine the extent and nature of ovarian tumors include a blood test to determine levels of alpha-fetoprotein and the hormone beta-hCG. Surgery may cure localized cases; for others, chemotherapy is used. Most survivors have normal puberty and menstrual periods.

Teratomas are frequently sacrococcygeal (that is, located near the base of the spine). Although they are the most common solid tumor diagnosed at birth, they affect about only one baby in perhaps 40,000. In newborns these teratomas are almost always benign, but by the age of 4 months nearly half are malignant with germ cell elements. Most patients are girls. A family history of twins is often seen in these cases. Symptoms include constipation or a swelling at the midline of the body or buttocks. Diagnostic tests include rectal examinations and scans. Surgery, often followed by chemotherapy, may be used to treat malignant tumors.

Diagnosis

Diagnosis of teratomas in general is made by biopsy. A battery of tests determines the extent of disease:

- Chest x-ray (to check for lung metastases)
- Skeletal x-ray (to check for bone metastases)
- Computed tomography (CT) scan
- Magnetic resonance imaging (MRI)

Malignant teratomas produce alpha-fetoprotein and the hormone beta-hCG, so measuring the level of these substances is useful in diagnosis and in assessing response to therapy. If the teratoma had germ cell elements, laboratory tests can detect a recurrence at an early stage:

- Alpha-fetoprotein assay
- Beta-hCG (a hormone)
- Urine and blood (checking for an elevated level of gonadotropin)

Treatment

Treatment of teratomas depends on the degree of malignancy and site of origin. Surgery is the first line of attack against localized disease. Surgery is especially valuable in treating benign and nonmetastasized malignant disease. Chemotherapy may also be used before or after surgery to shrink the tumor. High doses of radiation are risky for children under 2 because of side effects.

Prognosis

Prognosis is difficult to determine for teratomas; some recur locally or metastasize years after initial treatment. In the case of sacrococcygeal tumors, the survival rate is lower for children over the age of 1; overall about a third of the children receiving multidrug chemotherapy achieve long-term remission. With ovarian teratomas, the outlook for benign disease is good, and for malignancies, it is guarded, although improved chemotherapy has brightened the picture recently.

Immature teratomas are treatable 85% of the time with surgery alone, with postoperative observation. Low-grade or benign teratomas are resistant to both radiation therapy and chemotherapy. Recurrences treated with chemotherapy carry an excellent long-term survival potential. Malignant teratomas respond to chemotherapy but radiation is rarely used except in central nervous system tumors.

Gonadal and Extragonadal Germ Cell Tumors

Until the advent of multidrug chemotherapy, the outlook for patients with malignant germ cell tumors was grim, with only 15% to 20% surviving 3 years after surgery and radiation. Fortunately, the picture has brightened dramatically, with 5-year survival rates of 75% to 94%, depending on factors such as age at diagnosis, type of cell involved, stage, and primary site.

Most germ cell tumors are benign, and they rarely appear before the age of 15. They are divided into two types: gonadal (arising in the ovaries or testes) or extragonadal (arising outside the gonads). Extragonadal germ cell tumors constitute only about 2% to 3% of all childhood cancers. In young children most are benign. Malignant extragonadal germ cell tumors appear equally in boys and girls, although the adult form is more common in men than in women by a factor of nine. There are no identified environmental risk factors.

Extragonadal Germ Cell Tumors

Extragonadal means outside the testicles or ovaries; these tumors form from cells that should have matured into sperm or eggs but instead traveled elsewhere in the body, chiefly the brain, abdomen, or mediastinum (area in the chest between the lungs).

In testicular cases, the child is usually diagnosed between the ages of 6 months and 2 years; after that, the prognosis may be poorer. The symptom is a painless mass in one testicle, perhaps discovered while bathing. Surgical removal of the testicle alone cures more than half the patients with localized disease and almost all can be cured with chemotherapy.

Symptoms of other forms are site-related. Those arising in the presacral area (just above the buttocks) usually appear as a mass in the lower abdomen or buttocks. The swelling may cause difficulty walking, urinating, or defecating. Before the age of 6 months, the tumor is often benign, but after that age 65% of tumors are malignant.

Presacral tumors are diagnosed by MRI and CT scans of the chest, seeking to identify the primary site and to locate any metastases. The diagnosis is confirmed by biopsy.

Some of these tumors arise in the brain; while they could be included in the chapter on brain and central nervous system tumors, their origin in embryonic cells places them with germ cell tumors instead. With tumors arising in the pineal area (the middle of the brain near the pineal gland), symptoms are caused by pressure on the brain being squeezed by the foreign growth or by impeding the flow of cerebrospinal fluid. Nausea and vomiting, loss of memory, vision difficulties, or lethargy may be other indications.

Pineal tumors are diagnosed by head CT and MRI, with laboratory tests conducted to look for elevated levels of alpha-fetoprotein or beta-hCG. These tumor markers usually establish the type of tumor, and a rapid drop in levels of the markers during therapy is a good indication that treatments are succeeding. Low levels of tumor markers at diagnosis usually indicate a better prognosis.

Presacral tumors (located above or in front of the hip, the lower abdomen, or the buttocks) are treated with chemotherapy to shrink the tumor, followed by surgery, with a potential for repeating this sequence. Presacral GCTs have a disappointing long-term survival rate of less than 30%, much lower in the presence of metastasized disease. Pineal GCT patients have a much better prognosis: about 80% are long-term survivors.

Another group of extragonadal GCTs is classified as seminoma or nonseminoma. The latter include embryonal carcinoma, malignant teratoma, endodermal sinus tumor, choriocarcinoma, and mixed GCT. More males, usually young adults, are affected by these aggressive tumors. Benign extragonadal GCTs are simply removed surgically.

A subset of these tumors is the endodermal sinus tumor, also known as a yolk sac tumor, which appears in infants. In boys the tumor arises in the testicles and in girls it is vaginal. In either sex it can occur in the abdomen, near the base of the spine, or other sites. In its pediatric form it almost always occurs before the age of 2.

As with most forms of cancer, treatment for these tumors varies according to cell type (histology), stage, primary site, level of tumor markers present at diagnosis, and age of the patient. Therapy consists of a varying combination of surgical removal of the tumor, radiation, and/or chemotherapy, the latter showing excellent results with recent drug regimens. Drugs used include etoposide, cisplatin, bleomycin, and ifosfamide.

Prognosis for extragonadal GCT patients is heartening. Overall, almost all seminoma patients live for the 5 years after diagnosis that to some constitutes a cure. Nonseminoma prognosis is more dependent on risk factors, but over 90% of the lowest-risk patients survive, while nearly half of those with highest risk are survivors.

Gonadal Germ Cell Tumors

These tumors arise in the ovaries or testicles. Therapy depends on the location of the primary, the stage, and the type of tumor. Most patients are treated with surgery, possibly followed by chemotherapy. Clinical studies are under way to determine the optimal course of treatment for these tumors based on risk groups (taking into account location, type of tumor, and spread).

Almost all testicular germ cell tumors arise in boys under the age of 4, although a second peak appears in adolescents usually over the age of 15. Each of these types has distinctive cell types and high survival rates.

Ovarian germ cell tumors appear most often in girls under the age of 15. The treatment varies, again, according to the type of tumor, with the intent of eradicating disease while preserving fertility. The latter, however, is not always possible. Lowest-risk patients have their tumors completely removed by surgery and may not undergo any other therapy, although they are followed closely for some time to spot any recurrence quickly.

Those who still have tumor detectable after surgery may receive platinum-based chemotherapy and, less frequently, radiation.

Some high-risk patients, especially older adolescents and young adults, may be candidates for high-dose chemotherapy followed by peripheral blood stem cell transplant. Pediatric use of this strategy is so far uncertain; it is mainly used in relapsed pediatric patients.

Further Resources

ORGANIZATIONS/WEB SITES

National Cancer Institute's Physician Data Query (www.cancer.gov)

Has especially helpful fact sheets explaining these varied tumors and stages.

13

Testicular Cancer

First, a note of explanation: Most testicular cancers are a form of gonadal germ cell tumor and could have been included in the previous chapter. However, these tumors deserve their own brief chapter because they strike adolescents and young adults and because diagnosis may be delayed due to embarrassment. Awareness is a key to early detection and treatment.

While infants and children do not often develop testicular tumors, the incidence begins to rise after puberty. From the age of about 15 on, boys and their parents should be aware of the signs and symptoms of this cancer. White males have a much higher risk of testicular cancer.

Testicular tumors are almost always malignant, often highly so, with the major symptom a mass in the scrotum. The lump is usually but not always uneven and hard. Any such swelling should be drawn to the doctor's attention right away. Delays in reporting these masses are common, which is unfortunate, especially since this cancer carries such a favorable prognosis when it is treated early.

Risk Factors

Most testicular tumors are in fact diagnosed at an early stage. Some boys carry a higher risk of these tumors because of undescended testicles.

Even surgically correcting that condition may not remove the possibility of developing a malignancy. Still, the procedure does make it easier to examine the testicle for any lumps.

Some boys with Down syndrome develop testicular cancer, as did sons of women who took the hormone DES during pregnancy in earlier years. Males with Klinefelter's syndrome are also at a greater risk of getting testicular cancer.

Symptoms

The major symptom is a mass in the testicle, possibly painful. While there is no evidence that any accident or injury causes these tumors, an accident may draw attention to a lump that is already there. Testicular tumors may also be metastases from leukemia, lymphoma, melanoma, and other cancers.

Diagnosis and Staging

The diagnostic and staging process may include the following:

- Chest x-rays
- Alpha-fetoprotein (AFP) assay and hormonal studies; high levels of AFP, beta-hCG, or lactate dehydrogenase (LDH) can indicate the presence of masses too small to be felt, can help distinguish among the types of testicular tumors, and can alert the patient and physician to watch for subsequent spread
- Lymphangiography
- Ultrasound
- Computed tomography (CT) scans of the abdomen, chest, and pelvis
- Biopsy
- Positron emission tomography (PET) scan
- Magnetic resonance imaging (MRI)

Stage I disease is localized and contained in the testicle. Stage II disease has spread to the lymph nodes in the abdomen. Stage III has spread widely, perhaps to the brain or lungs. The American Cancer Society's Web site has a much more detailed explanation of stages and substages of testicular cancer.

Treatment

Treatment depends on the stage of the disease, the patient's age, and the cell type (60% of cases are slower-growing seminomas and the rest are more aggressive nonseminomas). Sexually mature patients may want to seek counseling on banking sperm, since later fertility can be compromised. With a high cure rate, most patients live to marry and wish to father children. Sperm is damaged by chemotherapy, radiation, and some surgical techniques. Decreased sperm counts may improve naturally over time, with no special risk of congenital problems in subsequent offspring.

The entire testicle is removed for biopsy and identification of the tumor type. In early stages, the operation will be followed by radiation to abdominal lymph nodes if there is evidence of metastases (in the case of seminoma) or possible removal of the lymph nodes (nonseminoma). Sometimes the removal of the encapsulated tumor is all that is needed with stage I disease, although the doctor will carefully observe the patient for any subsequent spread or recurrence.

Chemotherapy may be added if there is residual disease. Drugs involved may be some combination of etoposide, cisplatin, vinblastine, bleomycin, cyclophosphamide, and ifosfamide. Renal function may drop during therapy but will then become and remain stable.

Since most recurrences appear in the first 2 years, patients should be screened for at least that long but optimally for life. Cured patients have a 2% to 5% risk of cancer in the remaining testicle over 25 years. A very small risk of leukemia secondary to treatment has been reported.

The use of autologous stem cell transplant for widespread recurrent testicular cancer is under investigation. Clinical studies are also examining various combinations of surgery and chemotherapy, seeking the most effective mix with the lowest toxicity.

Prognosis

Patients with localized disease at diagnosis have a nearly 100% long-term survival rate. Even those with disease detected beyond the testicle have, with state-of-the-art therapy, survival rates of 80%

or more. Overall, patients diagnosed between the ages of 15 and 19 have a 92% 5-year survival.

Testicular cancer, while fairly rare, is sufficiently common that all males should be taught testicular self-examination, just as females are urged to examine their breasts. The potential embarrassment is far outweighed by the early detection of a highly curable tumor, especially in its early stage.

Further Resources

READING

Armstrong, Lance. *It's Not About the Bike, My Journey Back to Life.*
    Putnam, 2000.
Tour de France winner is diagnosed with testicular cancer, undergoes therapy, and comes back to win the grueling race again. Moving and positive story, well written.

Feder, David, R.D "Testicular cancer." *Cure* vol. 3 (2) (Summer 2004),
    pp. 48–55. Available at www.curetoday.com

ORGANIZATIONS/WEB SITES

Fertile Hope (www.fertilehope.org)
    Web site for those seeking parenthood after cancer treatment. Works with other organizations to publish brochures on cancer-related fertility problems and resources.

Lance Armstrong Foundation (2201 East 6th St., Austin, TX 78702; 512-236-8820; www.livestrong.org)
    This foundation provides many resources to patients and families dealing with various types of malignancies, partly funded by sales of the ubiquitous yellow LiveStrong wristbands.

National Cancer Institute & National Institutes of Health (www.cancer.gov)
    Besides the usual excellent PDQ and other information, the Web site has a fact sheet, "Testicular Cancer: Questions and Answers."

Testicular Cancer Resource Center (www.tcrc.acor.org)
    Has clear explanations of the cancer, treatments, possible side and late effects, and plenty of opportunities to contact others with the disease. Hosted by the Association of Online Cancer Resources, this is a trusted site with a wide range of information and a bit of an attitude with style.

14

Rare Cancers of Childhood

Of the estimated 12,400 newly diagnosed cases of childhood cancer in the United States each year, 10% are forms of tumor so rare that they receive little attention in the media; statistics on incidence and prognosis are often limited. Thus, the cancers included in this chapter were selected somewhat arbitrarily, although an effort has been made to include those representing the different sites that can be affected. Generalizations and useful information on symptoms and diagnosis are provided when possible. The cancers are grouped roughly by the part of the body affected.

Thyroid Cancer

Located in the front of the neck, the thyroid is a gland in the endocrine system that regulates metabolism, the process that transforms food into energy for the body's growth and functioning. Tumors in the thyroid can be adenomas (benign) or carcinomas (malignant). The cancerous form is slow-growing and of lower malignancy, so a diagnosis of thyroid cancer is not quite as frightening as many other cancers.

Although rare (representing 1.5% of childhood cancers), thyroid cancer does occur in adolescents, usually after the age of 15. Radiation of the thymus in infancy and early childhood to treat gland enlargement, acne, or enlarged tonsils is the most important risk factor in the development of this cancer. Used more frequently in the United States than in Europe, this practice stopped some years ago because of the obvious danger it poses. About 6% of the radiated patients develop a low-grade form of cancer from 4 to 24 years later, with the average onset 8.5 years. Most patients are girls. A person at risk because of previous head or neck radiation should be screened at least every 2 years for early signs of thyroid cancer. Another group that may be at risk of developing thyroid carcinoma in the future is Hodgkin disease patients who have received radiation to the neck nodes.

The major symptom is a neck mass, usually painless; in younger patients this is often a swollen lymph node. A nodule in the thyroid can be detected during a careful examination of the area. Hoarseness may occur if the mass presses on the larynx, while pressure on the esophagus may cause difficulty swallowing.

Diagnostic tests may include:

- Ultrasound
- Thyroid scan with radioactive iodine
- Laryngoscopy in the event of hoarseness
- Biopsy
- Computed tomography (CT) scan
- Magnetic resonance imaging (MRI)

There may be no laboratory evidence that the thyroid is not functioning properly.

Treatment of thyroid cancer begins with surgery to remove the mass and perhaps some lymph nodes. Local recurrences and metastases to lymph nodes may also be removed surgically. Tumor still evident at the primary site after surgery and local recurrences may be treated with radioactive iodine. Thyroid cancer patients may also benefit from chemotherapy.

Thyroid cancer metastasizes first to neck lymph nodes and the bones and then to the lungs. Recurrence is quite treatable, even in the presence of lung metastases. Thyroid cancer patients need lifelong synthetic thyroid hormone replacement.

Long survivals are common even when the cancer is widespread. In one study 99.5% of patients were long-term survivors. Metastases even after 20 years are not unknown, but they are treatable.

Renal Cell Carcinoma

Although the vast majority of kidney cancers in children are Wilms tumors, a tiny percentage are renal cell carcinomas (RCC) of the kidney. Cases of this adult-type tumor have been recorded in young patients, especially between the ages of 10 and 19. They may appear in children with hereditary von Hippel-Lindau disease or with tuberous sclerosis. (In adults, tobacco and industrial chemicals seem to play a role.) A type of RCC that runs in families has also been reported. In adults, males are twice as likely to get RCC as females, with the incidence among African-Americans increasing more rapidly than among whites.

Often there are no warning signs, but symptoms might include:

- Blood in the urine
- Abdominal mass
- Pain
- Weight loss
- Nausea and vomiting
- Weakness
- Night sweats
- Elevated blood pressure
- Fever

Special diagnostic tests include voiding cystourethrography (VCUG), renal angiography, MRI, CT scan, and ultrasound. The disease is classified as stage I (local) through IV (distant metastases and recurrence).

Treatment consists of surgical removal of the affected kidney. If the tumor is encapsulated, that may be the only treatment needed. Solitary metastases to the lungs may also be surgically removed. The disease metastasizes to the liver, regional lymph nodes, and bones. RCC is less radiosensitive than Wilms tumors, but radiation is attempted if the disease has spread or is inoperable.

Metastatic RCC is treated with surgery, including removal of affected lymph nodes, with the possible addition of immunotherapy (interferon-alfa and interleukin-2, for example).

Prognosis, as is the case in most cancer, is related to the stage of the disease at diagnosis; complete removal of the tumor is important.

In one study the 5-year survival rate for stage I was 89%. Overall survival rates are improving with current therapy.

Lung and Bronchial Tumors

Primary tumors of the respiratory system are very rare in children, accounting for less than 1% of all pediatric cases. Lung metastases from Wilms tumor, rhabdomyosarcoma, lymphosarcoma, and bone cancers are much more common. Primary lung and bronchial tumors, occasionally benign, are seen more often in adolescents. They may be discovered during routine chest x-rays, and the majority are first misdiagnosed as lung infections.

Symptoms might include:

• Cough
• Chest pain
• Shortness of breath
• Coughing up blood

Diagnosis is achieved through biopsy to distinguish benign from malignant tumors, possibly followed by:

• Bronchoscopy
• Bronchial brushings
• Cellular analysis of mucus from sputum

Bronchial adenomas (or carcinoid tumors) arise in the trachea or large bronchi. The primary treatment of these tumors is surgical removal, followed by radiation and/or chemotherapy only if metastases are present.

Pleuropulmonary blastomas appear in the tissue covering the lungs. Children with these tumors may have a family history of similar cancers. A surgically removed tumor may still recur and spread. Radiation (external beam or phosphorus-32) may be used if the tumor cannot be removed. Chemotherapy with vincristine, cyclophosphamide, dactinomycin, and doxorubicin may also be used.

The child's best chance for survival with these lung and bronchial tumors is through complete surgical resection of the primary tumor. The prognosis is guarded, with too few cases to compile meaningful survival statistics.

Colorectal Cancers

A tiny percentage of colorectal tumors diagnosed each year in the United States affect children. Those pediatric cases include lymphomas (discussed in Chapter 4) and carcinomas. The highest incidence of carcinoma is among males and blacks. Disease is commonly advanced at diagnosis, with metastases already present, and the prognosis is poor.

Colorectal tumors grow on the surface of the bowel and spread into adjacent muscle, or they may break out of the bowel altogether and spread malignant cells throughout the abdomen, to other organs, or elsewhere in the bowel itself.

A history of ulcerative colitis is often associated with colorectal carcinoma, with the risk increasing with each decade after diagnosis. Some colorectal tumors develop in children with an inherited disorder characterized by the growth of many benign polyps in the colon and rectum. In these patients surgery to remove the large bowel, anus, and rectum and to bring the small bowel out on the abdominal wall for removal of body wastes is performed for most patients as a preventive measure.

Symptoms of carcinoma include:

- Abdominal pain
- Vomiting
- Rectal bleeding
- A mass (lump)
- Changes in bowel habits
- Weight loss
- Decreased appetite

Diagnosis is made by:

- Checking the stool for blood
- Liver and kidney function tests
- Colonoscopy to identify any polyps present
- CT scan of the chest
- Bone scans

Many patients have metastases at the time of diagnosis. The disease is treated by surgically removing the tumor and affected portions of the intestinal tract, although this approach is not especially useful in the presence of widespread disease. Radiation or chemotherapy may follow; in the latter case, the drugs used are 5-fluorouracil (5-FU) with leucovorin, possibly irinotecan, or oxaliplatin. Aggressive therapy is essential because the prognosis is so gloomy.

Although children with ostomies have special problems adjusting to wearing bags to collect their body wastes, they can live completely normal lives. Valuable assistance and further information are provided by the United Ostomy Association (see resource section for further information).

Liver Cancer

Liver cancer is rare in the United States, accounting for 1% to 2% of malignancies in all age groups. Worldwide, liver cancer is responsible for about 1% of pediatric cancers. The rate is high, however, in Africa, especially parts of Ethiopia. Metastases to the liver, on the other hand, commonly result from neuroblastoma and Wilms tumor. Primary liver cancers may appear at first to be rhabdomyosarcoma or one of several other malignant tumors. Patients at risk for primary liver cancers are those with Beckwith-Wiedemann syndrome, hemihypertrophy, premature birth, or diagnosis of hepatitis B at a young age. Immunization to hepatitis B may lower the risk of hepatocellular carcinoma.

Two forms of primary liver tumors affect children:

Hepatocarcinoma (Hepatocellular Carcinoma)

Hepatocarcinoma is an adult type of liver cancer that usually appears in American children after the age of 5 (most often between 10 and 19). It has a higher incidence in Japanese children. A third of the cases are associated with cirrhosis. Patients with hepatitis B or C are at higher risk as well. Hepatocarcinoma is not responsive to standard chemotherapy, although new forms being tested show promise. The prognosis for this form of pediatric cancer is poor, with an overall survival rate less than 20%.

Hepatoblastoma

More than half of pediatric primary liver cancers are hepatoblastoma, affecting young children and infants; 90% of patients are under the age of 3 and 60% are less than 1 year old. The incidence of hepatoblastoma is rising; the increased survival of premature babies with very low birth weight is one explanation. While genetic factors may make the child more susceptible to this tumor, it is responsive to chemotherapy. This cancer has a much brighter prognosis, with up to two thirds of the children surviving.

Liver tumors in infants and children differ from those in adults: they tend to be unifocal (arising in one spot), they are more readily removed by surgery, and they may be highly curable.

Symptoms include:

- Abdominal mass or distention, sometimes painful
- Loss of appetite
- Vomiting
- Anemia
- Fever
- Jaundice (in advanced cases)

The diagnosis is made by:

- Biopsy (only if tumor appears inoperable, because it may seed or bleed)
- Bone scan
- Ultrasound (to locate tumor)
- Liver function tests (results may be normal)
- Alpha-fetoprotein assay (may be a tumor marker and useful for diagnosis and prognosis)
- Angiography (to determine whether the tumor is operable)
- Chest CT scan
- Chest x-rays (repeated to check for lung metastases)

Initial treatment of these tumors consists of surgically removing the affected part of the liver. This is possible in only about 60% of hepatoblastoma cases and a third of hepatocarcinoma cases. Surgery is sometimes preceded by a few courses of chemotherapy (doxorubicin/cisplatin) to shrink the tumor. Preoperative radiation may also help prepare an initially inoperable tumor for the surgeon. Infants and children can usually tolerate the removal of up to 80% of the liver because the organ regenerates to its original size within 6 months. Metastases may also be removed surgically. If the liver must be removed and no metastases are present, liver transplants have shown promise.

Because the liver has a low tolerance for radiation and organ regeneration may be threatened, radiation is less useful than in some other types of cancer. Radiation does have some value in combination with chemotherapy to shrink initially inoperable tumors before surgery and for palliation.

Anticancer drugs are more toxic because of impaired liver function. As a result, doctors may have to wait a short time after surgery, when regeneration is well under way, before starting chemotherapy. Chemotherapy is used to destroy any undetected metastases, although there is no real proof that this does or does not prevent recurrence. For children whose tumors cannot be completely removed surgically, drug therapy is especially important. A new form of chemotherapy that is sometimes used on resistant hepatocarcinoma is anti-angiogenesis (chemoembolization chemotherapy), or drugs injected to starve the growing tumor of its blood supply. Other agents that have been employed, especially with hepatocellular carcinoma even when the tumor has been completely resected, include, in various combinations, cisplatin, vincristine, fluorouracil, doxorubicin, and, in advanced cases, ifosfamide.

An especially interesting factor with liver cancer is the clear role played by hepatitis B. According to the Children's Oncology Group, universal immunization against hepatitis B (which showed a decrease in hepatocellular carcinoma in Taiwan) could reduce the incidence of the more challenging liver carcinoma and perhaps even prevent it.

Breast Cancer

Although very rare, children can be diagnosed with malignant breast cancer, whether sarcoma, lymphoma, or carcinoma. About 85% of cases had already metastasized at diagnosis. Surgical removal is the first line of therapy for each type, with chemotherapy and radiation treatment similar to adults with the disease. Long-term survival was better for sarcoma (90%), while over half of the patients with carcinoma survived. One reason for this discrepancy is that sarcoma was more likely to be diagnosed while it was still localized.

Malignant Melanoma

Skin cancers are rare in children because they have not lived long enough to experience the prolonged exposure to the sun and other environmental factors that lead to this disease in adults. One type of skin cancer that does occasionally affect adolescents is malignant melanoma, which may develop from moles or certain benign skin disorders; sometimes it can run in families. Malignant melanoma in youngsters is similar to that in adults in terms of sites, symptoms, spread, and prognosis; incidence peaks in the late teen years.

Suspicious signs on the skin, whether a mole that has changed appearance or a new spot, are identified by the same ABCDE rules that apply to adults. Have a doctor check a spot for:

- Asymmetry (the halves are unlike each other)
- Border (scalloped or uneven)
- Color (varies from one area to another, even white spots)
- Diameter (even smaller than a pencil eraser)
- Evolving (changing in size, color, or other appearance)

Because they sometimes become cancerous during adolescence, some kinds of moles on the soles of the feet, palms, genitals, mucus membranes of the anus or rectum, soft tissue beneath a nail, or on the lower extremities should be removed. Perhaps one mole in 2 million undergoes this cancerous transformation. Changes in size and color of a mole may signal the onset of malignancy that can spread throughout the body. Both sexes are equally affected, with boys' tumors primarily on the trunk, head, or neck and girls' tumors more likely on the extremities. Blacks rarely develop melanoma. With early diagnosis and treatment, complete recovery is possible.

Symptoms include:

- Small groups of blue-black nodules on normal skin
- Changes in color of a mole (red, white, and blue areas)
- Variations in the outline or height of a mole
- A mole that bleeds or forms an ulcer

Diagnosis is by biopsy and examination of the tissue under a microscope. Melanomas are treated by surgical removal of the tumor and possibly of lymph nodes in the area. Skin grafts may be necessary if large portions of tissue must be removed. Radiation is uncommon except to relieve symptoms of painful soft tissue, bone, and brain metastases. Chemotherapy with cisplatin, vinblastine, dacarbazine (DTIC), interleukin-2, and interferon is used with widespread melanoma.

Metastases to regional lymph nodes are common. Late recurrences are known, with some relapses after 5 years.

The prognosis is similar to adult melanoma and stage-related (depending on depth of tumor, thickness, and extent of spread at diagnosis). The deeper the tumor has spread, the less likely the child will survive. A completely resected tumor is highly curable; other prognostic factors are the location of the lesion, the cell type, and the extent of spread in the lymph system. Overall 5-year survival is a heartening 94%.

AIDS/HIV-associated Cancers

The spread of AIDS/HIV around the world has had implications for pediatric oncology as well. As with adults, children with immunodeficiency disease are more likely to have malignancies, too. An article noted that "Children with HIV infection have a high risk of developing cancer... This was the conclusion of a study of 4954 HIV-infected children, of whom 124 developed cancer before, at, or after they developed AIDS. One hundred had non-Hodgkin lymphoma, eight had Kaposi sarcoma, four had leiomyosarcoma, two had Hodgkin disease, and ten had other types of cancer. These rates were much higher than the rate of cancer in healthy children."

Kaposi sarcoma (KS) is a rare cancer appearing as raised skin lesions; while there was some incidence of KS prior to the identification of the AIDS virus, the number of patients has increased, and a finding of KS today is a strong indication of HIV infection even when it has not previously been detected. KS lesions may be treated with radiation, and the malignancies are responsive to some chemotherapy drugs (bleomycin, vincristine, vinblastine, and doxorubicin in various combinations). Similar to other cancers, the prognosis for children with localized disease (in the skin and lymph nodes with little KS seen in the palate) is considered good.

Leiomyosarcoma is a very rare form of soft tissue sarcoma arising in the walls of blood vessels or in smooth muscles of the uterus or abdominal cavity. If the disease is localized, doctors will use chemotherapy and surgery to treat it, although controversy exists regarding which should be used first: chemotherapy to shrink the tumor or surgery to debulk, with chemotherapy mop-up sessions to eradicate any remaining cancer cells. Chemotherapy drugs may include doxorubicin (Adriamycin), ifosfamide, dacarbazine, and/or cyclophosphamide. Clinical tests are under way to determine whether other chemotherapy agents or immunotherapy might be active against this cancer.

Hodgkin disease and other forms of lymphoma are discussed in earlier chapters in this section.

Further Resources

READING

Biggar, Robert J., et al., "Risk of cancer in children with AIDS." *JAMA, Journal of the American Medical Association*, vol. 284 (2) (July 12, 2000), p. 205.

ORGANIZATIONS/WEB SITES

National Cancer Institute (www.cancer.gov)
Has materials on these types of pediatric cancers.

What we can do about Childhood Cancer: The Treatments

15

Introduction to Childhood Cancer Therapy

While cancer in any age group is a life-threatening disease, in recent years there have been greater advances in the treatment of childhood forms than of those that strike adults. For instance, radiation equipment has been refined to target tumors precisely, sparing surrounding tissue to a greater extent than was previously possible.

Chemotherapy has seen much improvement also, both in the number of useful drugs and in the new ways they are given for greater effectiveness. Today each patient usually receives several drugs in combination rather than single ones used in sequence after relapses. Researchers have also discovered a way to use potentially lethal doses of one drug to kill cancer cells (for example, methotrexate) and then to "rescue" the body through use of another (citrovorum, in this case).

Support therapy (beyond the basic surgery, radiation, and chemotherapy) includes transfusions with specific blood components like platelets or white blood cells and new antibiotics to control infections that not long ago were fatal for children with cancer. Patients who have lost all resistance to infections through drugs or through deliberate destruction of the immune system in preparation for a bone marrow transplant can be protected in well-designed hospital rooms.

Surgical techniques have improved as well, so that more tumor can be removed while destroying less of the nearby healthy tissue.

What is a Protocol?

Most patients are placed on treatment programs called protocols. These are combinations of therapy based on medical expertise from across the country and internationally. Some are part of research efforts to find more effective treatments, while others are based on customary clinical practice. Protocols are planned to take advantage of the known action of drugs and radiotherapy plus the known behavior of the specific cancer involved. They are individually tailored and can be altered depending on the patient's response. If the therapy does not work as planned, or if the child cannot tolerate it, a different protocol can be tried. Even if a protocol is experimental, the doctors base it on previous known responses to particular drugs and types of treatment. The participation of so many children in these protocols over the past several decades is one reason the cure rates for pediatric cancer have improved so much.

Treatment Centers and Clinical Trials

A major disappointment for me and for some other parents we met at the clinic was the failure to attempt to trace the cause of our children's illnesses. We felt we should be "grilled" about our lifestyle, habits, environment, genetics—anything to understand why the child developed cancer. When we asked why that was not done, we were told that such a "third degree" might lead to more guilt. I do not think that would have been the case. There must be a reason why Lisa developed such a rare tumor; why not try to find out? Was it an allergy medication or a garden pesticide I used while I was pregnant? Was my husband exposed to some chemical during his Vietnam service? We will never know, because research at that time focused on cure with limited side effects. As well, Lisa's disease was so rare that it would be unreasonable to attempt epidemiologic research for a single case. With advancements in genetics, many families today understand better why their child became ill.

Taking Part in Research

Children with cancer are offered treatment on clinical trials and their response to therapy is included in research reports. These studies identify the most effective treatments. If there are alternative treatments available, the doctor will explain in advance what to expect and what choices there may be. The parents can be assured that the child will receive at least the best therapy available, with the possible addition of a drug or procedure the doctors have good reason to believe will be even more effective.

Care in scattered clinics and hospitals around the country and around the world varies widely, but participation in clinical trials places the youngster under strict protocols followed carefully and reviewed by your doctor's peers from other institutions. As W. Archie Bleyer, MD, who is Clinical Research Professor in Radiation Medicine at Oregon Health and Sciences University, wrote in a letter to the editors of *U.S. News and World Report*, "Owing to clinical trials, tens of thousands more U.S. and Canadian children have been cured than would have been if the progress achieved by these trials had not occurred. Millions of additional patient-years of life have been saved. More than 200,000 U.S. children with cancer have survived their disease and are alive today, 5 to 40 years after their date of diagnosis, and most of them were treated on at least one of our clinical trials... Clinical trials have allowed us to transform what was a highly fatal disease, as recently as the 1970s, into one that is now cured in 75% of affected children."

Parents have a legal right to know if the treatments offered are experimental, and they also have a right to refuse such therapy. The doctors must tell you both verbally and in writing why these treatments are being offered, what they are, their risks, side effects, what tests will be done before and after the treatments, what monitoring procedures will be done, and what expectation there is of improvement. Parents sign an "informed consent" form on behalf of their children.

Informed Consent

Before your child receives any treatments, the doctors will tell you about potential side effects, even if only one patient in a thousand develops the problem. This well-intentioned information can backfire. Parents already in a state of shock over the diagnosis are often terrified about the potential harm these treatments can do to their child. Ask the doctor what effects are likely, and try not to worry about the rare ones.

TABLE 15.1   Questions to Ask Your Doctor About Clinical Trials

---

Article date: 2000/10/05

You may want to ask your medical team detailed questions about clinical trial opportunities; consider beginning with the ones below:

What are my clinical trial options?
- Do members of my health care team participate in clinical trials? If so, what type of trials are they involved in?
- Am I eligible for a nationally sponsored clinical trial?

Who is running this study and what is its purpose?
- What is the study trying to determine? Is the purpose to determine the safest dosage of a new drug or to determine the most effective treatment for breast cancer?
- Who is sponsoring the study? Has it been reviewed by a respected national group, such as the American Cancer Society or the National Cancer Institute? Has it been reviewed by an institutional review board?

How does this trial treatment compare to other treatments?
- What results could I reasonably expect from the trial treatment? In initial stages of the trial, how has the effectiveness of the trial treatment compared to the effectiveness of treatments currently used on my type of cancer?

How would this clinical trial affect me?
- How would my cancer most likely progress or change if I joined this study? What treatment plan would I pursue if I didn't join the study?
- How would being in the study affect my daily life? Would I be able to continue work? Would I feel like pursuing social activities?
- Would I have to be hospitalized? How often and for how long?
- What kinds of additional tests, such as blood tests or biopsies, would I undergo for the specific purpose of the study? Do any of these have side effects or risks that are of particular concern to me?
- How long would my active participation in the study last?

- What are the potential short-term and long-term side effects of the treatments being tested? Are any of them likely to be permanent or life threatening? Would I be allowed to take medications to alleviate side effects such as nausea? Would I be able to continue other medicines?
- If I seemed to be harmed during the research program, would I be entitled to care for problems related to the treatment?

How and where would my response to the trial treatment be evaluated?
- Where would I be treated and evaluated? Would I have to travel? How frequently?
- How would I know if the treatment was working properly or if I was responding? How would I determine whether I should receive a different treatment plan from the one being studied?

Who would look out for my care?
- What type of follow-up care would I receive after the study is completed?
- How much would my personal physician be involved in my care?
- Who would be professionally responsible for my health care while I am in the trial?

How would I pay for this trial treatment?
- Would the treatment involve additional expense? Would any or all of the costs be covered? If not, are there other sources I can turn to for financial help?
- Do you know of any organizations that could help me convince my insurance company or health plan to cover the costs?

The American Cancer Society is the nationwide community-based voluntary health organization dedicated to eliminating cancer as a major health problem by preventing cancer, saving lives, and diminishing suffering from cancer, through research, education, advocacy, and service. Used with Permission

My husband and I vividly remember sitting with the doctor day after day as he told us about the therapy and what side effects to expect. It is better to digest this information over a period of time. Ask the doctor to write down unfamiliar terms and names so you can learn to recognize them. You might want to tape record these conferences for later referral. Some families ask a friend or relative to go with them to these meetings, perhaps to take notes.

The standard here is "informed consent." Current medical practice requires that consent be obtained without coercion or undue influence, nor may those who consent be required to waive their legal rights concerning any liability for negligence. A great deal of understandable information about this process is available through the National Cancer Institute, either from the toll-free number 1-800-4-CANCER or online (www.cancer.gov). The NCI's Web site contains a wealth of material on clinical trials.

What is the child's role in this process? Patients under the age of 18 must have a parent or guardian sign the consent form. Another issue is the child's assent to the treatments. According to the NCI's Cancer Trials Web site, experts have "established age 7 as a reasonable minimum age for involving children in some kind of assent process. It is felt that most children this age can understand information tailored for their knowledge and development level." Many parents, though, ask that consent not be obtained from the youngest children because they fear the children are not ready to hear all the details of treatment. The NCI Web site has a wealth of information on the assent process and ways to involve the child in treatment planning.

The Health Care Team

The best medical care for children requires a multidisciplinary approach with a team of experts working together. There will be dozens of trained specialists helping to treat your child, including some people you'll never see. Depending on the type of malignancy your child has, the team may include:

The doctors

- Your family pediatrician
- An oncologist or hematologist (the latter may treat even patients who do not have leukemia, because chemotherapy is usually given in the blood)
- Pediatric surgeon (or subspecialty surgeon like urologist, neurosurgeon, or orthopedist)
- Anesthesiologist

- Pathologist (studies tumor tissue under a microscope)
- Radiologist (uses x-rays and radioactive materials to diagnose disease)
- Radiotherapists (plan and administer radiation therapy)
- Microbiologist (studies infectious disease in the laboratory)
- Endocrinologist (experts on glands and hormones)
- Neurologist (nervous system specialist)
- Nephrologist (kidney specialist)
- Cardiologist (heart specialist)
- Geneticist (studies heredity)
- Ophthalmologist (eye specialist)
- Psychiatrist
- Interns and residents (the house officers and hospital staff in training under the specialists at teaching hospitals)

Other medical staff

- Nurses and nurse clinicians/nurse practitioners (nurses are now educated on several levels to take on increasingly skilled duties in patient care)
- Nurses' aides
- X-ray technicians
- Laboratory technicians
- Respiratory therapists
- Nuclear medicine technologists (administer tests involving injection of radioactive substances)
- Physical therapists
- Pharmacists
- Occupational therapists

Your social support network

- Home health aide
- Social workers
- Clergy
- Child life worker (specially trained person who is an advocate for the child's comfort and care)
- Speech therapist (especially with brain tumors)
- Play therapist (helps child deal with the illness through play that entertains, educates, and aids in expression; the child life worker may perform this role as well)

- Art or music therapist
- Teacher or tutor
- Hospice team (if the illness is terminal)
- Parents
- Siblings, grandparents, other extended family
- Friends

Do not forget the most important member of the treatment team: the child/patient.

It seems appropriate to note here the important role of the pathologist in treating children with cancer, for he is usually an invisible member of the team. This specialist studies the tissues taken in biopsy, both with the naked eye and under the microscope, to determine whether the suspicious mass or cells are malignant or benign. If it is malignant, he determines whether it is of low grade (slowest-growing) or high grade, based on the percentage of cells that look almost normal and how many are in the process of dividing at a time. Several grades may be represented in a single tumor. The pathologist assesses how far the tumor has spread in the area where it arose and elsewhere in the body: is it just in one place, or has it invaded nearby organs, lymph nodes, or distant areas of the body? (This is called "staging.") He also determines whether the tumor has been completely removed.

No patient, no matter how complicated the case, has all these health professionals involved in his diagnosis and treatment, nor is any patient cared for by all involved specialists at one time. The infectious disease specialist, for example, may be called in to help with a troublesome infection.

Where Should Your Child be Treated?

With most childhood cancers, your first chance at curing the disease is your best. The failure of initial therapy is a very serious problem. Once in a while a local doctor will treat the child until relapse, then refer him to a major center, where treatment options are narrower than would have been the case at the outset. Even diagnostic studies like the biopsy should be carried out at the center where the child will be treated. These early procedures should be performed by specialists who can handle whatever they find.

The Cancer Center

Studies have shown that patients who receive at least part of their care at medical centers staffed by experienced pediatric specialists have an improved chance at long-term survival. Although not every town and city has such a hospital, there are dozens scattered across the United States and in foreign countries. It may be necessary to travel for some distance to get this care, but the atmosphere and top-notch, up-to-the-minute treatment are worth the effort. (See Appendix A for a list of these hospitals.)

The American Academy of Pediatrics, in its "Guidelines for the pediatric cancer center and role of such centers in diagnosis and treatment," states that

> children with cancer should be treated and followed at pediatric cancer centers by board-certified pediatric cancer specialists. These centers have the most appropriately trained support personnel and equipment to effectively treat children with cancer. The child's pediatrician, however, should continue to serve a supportive role during cancer treatment.

The article cites membership in the Children's Oncology Group as an indication that the hospital has specific equipment, staff, specialized personnel, and "access to increasingly complex equipment and facilities...critical to success in diagnosis, treatment, and long-term follow-up."

It takes a special knack to deal with children, as every parent has learned, often the hard way. Since not all doctors have this knack, it is important that these centers are staffed by pediatric specialists, trained and equipped to deal with rare and catastrophic illnesses in youngsters and adolescents. A parent need not fear referral to these hospitals. In our experience they offer a support network that is simply unavailable at community institutions. If the clinic is some distance from home, there are houses and apartments, many funded by the McDonald's Corporation and parent groups, where families can stay for minimal cost during treatment. At these houses and these clinics, the psychological support, the warmth and compassion, and the friendships formed with others in the same boat are invaluable in dealing with your child's disease.

"Patient- and family-centered care is an innovative approach to the planning, delivery, and evaluation of health care that is grounded in mutually beneficial partnerships among health care patients, families, and providers. Patient- and family-centered care applies to patients of all ages, and it may be practiced in any health-care setting." With these words the Institute for Family-Centered Care sets a high bar for an approach to medical care that includes the family (as defined by the patient—family may be by blood, legal, or emotional ties). See the contact information at the end of this chapter to find out more on this gold standard of care.

Role of the Pediatrician or Family Doctor

This does *not* mean that your local pediatrician or family doctor is not important; far from it! He has discovered that your child has or may have a serious problem, and he also knows that these centers regularly treat patients with these rare diseases, whereas a general pediatrician may see only a handful of them in a lifetime. Particularly with the rapid advances in modern medicine, it is unreasonable to expect every doctor to keep up on every development in cancer, cardiology, orthopedics, and all the other medical disciplines.

Your local pediatrician remains an important member of the treatment team. He keeps track of normal pediatric care; fields questions on child development like teething and nutrition; receives (or should receive) regular reports from the center on the child's treatment and progress; maintains records on immunizations and gives any that are permitted, depending on the child's treatments (some are too risky); and provides regular care for the patient's brothers and sisters, too. The pediatrician treats problems that can be handled at the local office or at the community hospital and recognizes which should be drawn to the attention of the cancer specialists. When the child has finished treatments, you will have made a strong investment in the future—a relationship with your local doctor strengthened through crisis.

If you live far from a major pediatric cancer center, it can sometimes be arranged to evaluate the child at the referral center, stabilize his condition, begin treatment, and perhaps operate. The center specialists will prescribe therapy and determine what can be carried out at a local hospital near your home. They will then, if appropriate, provide chemotherapy drugs and special medications like controlled painkillers to be administered there. The community hospital might be used in the event of minor setbacks, but major problems and regular checkups are carried out at the center. Working together in this way, the special center and the local medical community can treat the patient with the least possible disruption of everyday life.

How is Cancer Managed Today?

Once the child's disease has been diagnosed and the extent or stage is known, the treatment team gets together to decide who will do what, and when. The theory of management of cancer, put very basically, is:

1. The surgeon removes the tumor, if possible. (This applies only to solid tumors, not leukemia.) Sometimes the surgery is intended to debulk, or remove as much of the tumor as possible.
2. Radiation cleans up remaining cancer cells in the area where the tumor was found.
3. Chemotherapy kills off even invisible clumps of cells that have migrated elsewhere.

This all depends on the type of tumor, its location, stage, and numerous other factors like the child's general state of health and age. Some patients don't receive every form of therapy, and for others the order is altered. This section will examine in some detail the treatments used against these cancers, but it will not cover specific doses and protocols; that is a matter for the professionals.

Should you get a Second Opinion?

Because pediatric cancer usually requires immediate treatment on an emergency basis, families often have only a short period to obtain a second opinion before therapy begins. However, if you have serious doubts about the diagnosis or proposed therapy, or if you just want another team to evaluate the proposed care, any good doctor will help you find another specialist to consult as quickly as possible. It is your right to have a second doctor or team of physicians examine your child to confirm or question the diagnosis and treatment plan. Except in the case of emergencies, some insurance companies recommend or require this course of action, either as protection for the patient or to ensure they are not being asked to pay for unnecessary treatments. Insurance companies pay for this second evaluation most of the time.

In going to another doctor, you should take along your records (including copies of imaging and pathology slides) from the first doctor so your child doesn't have to repeat any tests. The second specialist may, on the other hand, perform different tests. The first doctor or clinic may send your slides and records, perhaps electronically, to the physician providing a second opinion, write a letter, or fax or phone the test results to the consultant, or may have you take the records along to your appointment. They might be accessible through the computer, too. (If time is short, taking them along with you is advisable; errors or delays in transporting the records occur all too often.) Whatever method is used to transfer the information, check ahead of time to make sure it is all organized and available. If it has not arrived, you may have wasted a trip. The safest method is to hand-carry everything yourself.

If you as a parent want still a third opinion, you may have to pay for it yourself or have a battle with the insurance company. If two or three specialists disagree on the diagnosis or treatment, it may be difficult to determine whom to believe and trust. This is a real problem because there is often more than one "right" way to treat a disease. If, on the other hand, several doctors agree on a diagnosis you don't want to accept, you may be fleeing from reality. But perhaps your parental gut instinct is accurate, too.

Pediatric cancer specialists generally agree with the Mayo Clinic's Dr. Gerald Gilchrist, who writes, "A solid honest physician or surgeon should welcome a request for a second opinion—if his position is confirmed, it's a feather in his cap—if not then he's learned something!"

If for some reason your doctor cannot or will not refer you elsewhere, you might find the names of appropriate physicians through your state or local medical society, directories at the library, your insurance company, or physicians' professional organizations like the American Association of Pediatric Hematology/Oncology or the National Cancer Institute. (See Web sites and addresses listed in Appendix B.) If you are looking for a surgeon, try to find one who is a *pediatric* specialist in cancer surgery for the particular area of the body involved in your child's case.

Because almost all of our daughter's operations and the initiation of treatment for her tumor were handled as emergencies, we didn't give any thought to getting a second opinion. We were referred to a major center in a city an hour's drive from our home, where fortunately we both trusted and liked the doctors involved in her care. But the inevitable happened: she was scheduled for follow-up surgery a few weeks ahead of time, and it dawned on me to wonder if, as a good parent, I should seek another opinion on this operation (it was her fourth or fifth) for her sake. Personally, I didn't want our daughter treated at any other hospital by any other surgeon.

I first broached the idea with the clinic secretary, a wonderful woman who has become a good friend. She, and then the nurse clinician, also a friend, supported the idea as my right and offered to discuss it with the oncologist. Before I had them do that, however, and with a what-have-I-gotten-myself-into sinking feeling, I phoned our pediatrician.

My sense of relief at her reassurance was enormous. She began by agreeing that she regularly suggests in her practice that parents seek second opinions on their children's care. In this case, however, she saw no reason to do so. I remember her words clearly.

"Normally I don't give two hoots about a surgeon's ego," she said, "but in this case [the doctor] has a lot invested in your daughter." She continued by reminding me that my daughter has an unusual anatomy because of previous surgery, and that this surgeon knows that anatomy intimately because he created it. (Even a quarter of a century later, she wanted him to be present for her kidney transplant, but he had retired.) In addition, the man has a national reputation and it was possible that some other surgeon might egotistically make a different treatment suggestion just to second-guess the prominent physician. I was relieved and happy to drop the whole matter of the second opinion, secure in the knowledge that having Lisa treated by the doctor I knew and trusted without an outside evaluation was not only best for me but also best for her.

Other parents in other situations will no doubt decide differently.

Further Resources

READING

"Be an active member of your health care team," U. S. Department of Health and Human Services, Food and Drug Administration. Available at www.fda.gov/cder/consumerinfo/active_member.htm

Bleyer, W. Archie. Clinical trails debate. *U. S. News and World Report* (November 29, 1999), p. 6

Chan, Helen S. L. *Understanding Cancer Therapies.* Jackson, MS: University Press of Mississippi, 2007.
Replete with explanations and tables of information, for adult readers.

Finn, Robert. *Cancer Clinical Trials—Experimental Treatments and How They Can Help.* Sebastopol, CA: O'Reilly, 1999.
Primarily for adult patients, a brief section covers clinical trials for pediatric patients. Trials are very common with childhood cancer patients. Includes an interesting discussion on gaining the child's assent to trial participation (age 7 and up). Comprehensive discussion of trials, how to find them, what to expect, when to get help (including financial issues).

Getz, Ken, and Deborah Borfitz. *Informed Consent: The Consumer's Guide to Volunteering for Clinical Trials.* Boston: CenterWatch, 2003.
The downside of clinical trials, the risks and benefits to participants. The thoughtful chapter "Vulnerable Populations" has a discussion of pediatric patients in clinical trials and poses important questions for parents or guardians to ask of clinicians.

Gilchirst, Gerald. Private Correspondence. February 1985

Giller, Cole A., MD, PhD. "Speaking out: lessons learned—as the patient, as the doctor." *Cure* vol. 5, (4) (Fall 2006), p. 80. Also available at www. curetoday.com

Leukemia and Lymphoma Society. *Understanding Clinical Trials for Blood Cancers.* White Plains, NY: The Society, n.d. Also available online at www.LLS.org
This clearly written booklet is packed with information and resources for all cancer patients, not just those with leukemia or lymphoma.

Mohrman, Margaret E., MD. *Attending Children: A Doctor's Education.* Washington, DC: Georgetown University Press, 2005.
Interesting and readable look at the other side of the desk.

"Policy statement: Guidelines for Pediatric Cancer Centers reaffirmed", *Pediatrics*, vol. 123 (1) (January 2009), p. 188. Also online at www.aap.org.

ORGANIZATIONS/WEB SITES

Cancer Trials (a service of the National Cancer Institute; www.cancer.gov/clinicaltrials)
Provides patients, family members, health care professionals, and members of the public with easy access to information on clinical trials for a wide range of diseases and conditions. This site currently contains approximately

5500 clinical studies, with heavy U.S. emphasis but somewhat international in scope. A "Children's Assent" section is especially informative.

CancerNet Treatment (www.cancer.gov/cancertopics/youngpeople.html)
See the full text of "Young People with Cancer: A Handbook for Parents." National Cancer Institute introduction to hospitalization, therapy side effects, etc. Very comprehensive Web site.

Candlelighters Childhood Cancer Foundation (www.candlelighters.org)
Several excellent articles on informed consent and pediatric childhood cancer trials have appeared in the Candlelighters newsletter and are accessible through their Web site.

Cure Our Children Foundation: "Checking on and Selecting Your Doctor and Hospital" (www.cureourchildren.org/doctors.htm)
This private Web site has excellent advice on choosing a doctor and offers an amazing array of links to Internet resources that check state and other certifications for hospitals as well as medical personnel.

Foundation for the Children's Oncology Group (www.nccf.org/childhoodcancer/clinicaltrial.asp)
"What is a Clinical Trial, From Lab to Bedside" is a careful explanation of the need for and the benefits of clinical trials in pediatric cancer.

Institute for Family-Centered Care (www.familycenteredcare.org)
This organization promulgates core concepts for the care of patients of any age.

16

Surgery

Surgery is the oldest and still most widely used treatment for cancer patients with solid tumors (as opposed to leukemia). Removing the primary tumor sometimes makes even widespread cancer treatable by chemotherapy. Still, surgery plays its most important role in the early stages of disease, when a great percentage of patients can be successfully treated.

Infants and children respond well to surgery and recover more quickly than their parents usually expect. The doctor will therefore remove as much tumor as possible. Rehabilitation can come later, but if too little tissue is removed, a relapse might occur, necessitating even more surgery.

Expert care of the child from the first day is vital, for even the biopsy technique can have an effect on subsequent therapy. If an inexperienced doctor takes tissue samples improperly, subsequent surgery may be made more difficult. The role of the surgeon therefore begins before the biopsy is performed and continues through diagnosis, patient evaluation, surgery (perhaps more than once), and rehabilitation. In many situations the staging is based on the surgeon's observations and degree of success in removing tumor tissue. He or she is not a team member for just a few hours but also follows the patient long after the operation is over.

Cancer surgeons sometimes disagree about the amount of tumor that must be removed to best benefit the patient. Thus, surgical decisions will vary somewhat from doctor to doctor, with each one taking into consideration factors such as other therapies that are available to destroy remaining disease and the effects of surgery on normal tissues and organs.

Unfortunately, not all tumors are operable, depending on their size and site. With local extension and distant spread, surgery is less effective. During the operation the surgeons may discover that the cancer has spread more widely than they had previously thought. In that case, the team may leave the tumor as it is, or they may remove as much as possible (called debulking). After some chemotherapy or radiation has shrunk the tumor, surgery may again be attempted.

When to operate is a matter of individual judgment, but timing is important:

- **Emergency** surgery is needed at once.
- **Urgent** surgery must be performed as soon as all tests are completed and the results analyzed. This may take up to a few days.
- **Planned** surgery is needed within weeks or months.
- **Elective** surgery is not essential, but the patient would be better off having it.
- **Optional** surgery may be performed for cosmetic or psychological reasons rather than medical ones.

Factors that influence the surgical decision include the age of the patient, his physical and mental condition, and the stage of the disease at it appears from diagnostic tests. Angiography might help the doctor examine the tumor's blood supply, and scans might show the extent of the disease. The patient's kidney function is assessed through laboratory tests and medical imaging. Fluid balance is checked, especially when there is vomiting or diarrhea, and if the child has been bleeding, a transfusion of platelets will improve clotting.

Recent techniques have improved precision and decreased postoperative complications, and better anesthesia, new intensive care procedures, and superior nutritional support have played significant roles in increased survivals. Nor is surgery the "stand-alone" technique that it was in the past. Modern therapies often include radiation or chemotherapy *during* the surgery, when specialists can treat the tumor bed with drugs or radiation sources to enhance the tumor's removal and sweep up any stray cancer cells while sparing normal tissue. Rarely, during surgery the doctors might also implant radiation seeds or other sources, or install a tube or other device for "after loading" radiation implants at a later date.

Categories of Surgery

There are five categories of surgery: diagnostic/staging, specific, supportive, preventive, and rehabilitative.

Staging and Diagnosis

The staging operation may be performed at a distance from the apparent tumor to gauge how far the malignancy has spread. In some patients, the abdomen is examined for signs of disease, even though the primary symptom may be elsewhere in the body. In other cases surgeons may perform exploratory surgery, which involves looking at the area of a suspected tumor, checking its size, and determining whether there are visible metastases. Information gained from this operation will help determine the approach to be used in subsequent surgery aimed at removing the tumor completely.

With today's high-tech tests like magnetic resonance imaging (MRI), some staging and other surgery may be completely avoided, since the images can reveal enough information that the doctors don't need a direct look.

A biopsy may be done by taking a sample of the tumor tissue for examination under the microscope to identify its type. The pathologist may be in the operating room to make sure the biopsy specimen taken is clear and usable. The surgical team will decide whether further surgery is of value, taking into consideration any physical scars or disfigurement that might result and weighing that against the effectiveness of other available therapies. If the tumor is accessible, intact, and encapsulated, the team may omit the biopsy and take the whole tumor out. Sometimes biopsy is avoided because cutting into the mass might allow tumor cells to escape and spread or "seed" elsewhere in the body.

Specific

Specific surgery is the main operation, an attempt to cure the disease. This aims to remove all tumor and leave the patient with full body functions. The surgeon removes the primary tumor with surrounding tissue to prevent a local recurrence, taking care to avoid contaminating the body with cancer cells. The lymph channels and nodes in the area may also be removed because they are often the route through which cancer cells disperse throughout the body. Specific surgery may include operations to remove masses that recur locally where there is no evidence of metastasis, or surgery after radiation has failed. Isolated single colonies of tumor in such locations as the lungs may be removed surgically, especially with osteogenic sarcoma, Wilms tumor, Ewing tumor, and rhabdomyosarcoma. During these operations the team may place metal clips in the body to identify the biopsy site and to help target future radiation treatment.

Supportive

Supportive, or palliative, surgery is used when the tumor has spread so much that removal alone will not cure it but may help relieve its symptoms. Palliative surgery can ease pain that is unresponsive to narcotics by severing the pain-transmitting nerves (called a cordotomy) in a patient expected to live for some months. Blockages, even scar tissue from surgery, may be removed if doing so will ease pain and discomfort. Complications such as abscesses, abdominal pain from the tumor or infection, intestinal bleeding, and tumor-related bone fractures may be treated through palliative surgery. Hormone sources that may stimulate growth are sometimes taken out. This is not done very often in children, and then almost always in those without hope of cure, so there is little concern about long-term effects. Any of these measures may increase the child's comfort and life span significantly.

Preventive

In preventive surgery, certain polyps and moles or even whole organs (like the colon) are removed that, if left, have a reasonable likelihood of becoming malignant.

Rehabilitative

Rehabilitative surgery helps restore the function of vital organs damaged by cancer or treatments. This includes plastic surgery reconstructions and operations to reverse colostomies where possible.

Preparation for Surgery

Preparing the child for surgery takes place in stages and begins with the preparation of the parents. They should know the mechanics of the child's trip to the operating room, what procedures will be used in the hospital room, how long the child will be in the holding area before surgery, who takes him there and who will stay with him, and how far the parents can accompany him. How the parents are "prepped" and how they react has a direct bearing on how the child copes both before and after surgery. Well-informed parents are better able to cope and can give a truly informed consent to a procedure, so ask questions until you are satisfied you know what will happen. You are entitled to clear answers that you understand, and you should know about problems that may arise and what alternatives may be available. You should know what might happen if the surgery is not performed, and you should be given some idea of what pain your child will experience, how long it will last, and what can be done about it.

The doctor, nurse, and parents, possibly in combination with a social worker, a member of the clergy, or another patient who has had the same operation, may take part in preparing the child. Explain in simple, age-appropriate language what is going to happen and the probable results. With younger children, it may be wise to wait until the day of the surgery to talk about the operation. Stay with your child as much as you possibly can, within reason.

I remember a child of about 6 who was scheduled for brain surgery. His mother was understandably upset and became hysterical. In order not to upset the boy, she left the hospital and did not return until after the operation. She was gone from evening until the following noon. The child was calm and the nurse kept him occupied, but I wondered whether someone could not have been found among the family to sit with him for the hours when he was awake. But perhaps others would criticize me, for while I stayed late on nights before surgery and reappeared at dawn, I did go home for a few hours' sleep. I was not at my daughter's side all night then, although many parents are. Several times when she was older and was hospitalized for surgery or a serious medical condition, I did stay with her day and night.

In telling the child what is going to happen, be honest or he may later feel betrayed. Try to hear and relieve your child's fears if possible, clear up any misunderstandings, reassure him when you can, and explain why this must be done. Ask the hospital staff if the youngster can visit the operating room and the recovery room ahead of time; this is sometimes allowed. If crutches or a wheelchair will be used after the operation, let him try them out ahead of time. The child will also be carefully measured for any prosthesis at this time. Make sure the child understands that none of this is happening because he has been "bad." Emphasize what will happen after the operation rather than the procedure itself.

Explain what preparations have to be made. Tell the child that an intravenous line may be started to make sure his body has enough fluid (if he doesn't have a central line or similar device). Warn the child that no food or drink may be allowed right before surgery or even for a few days. He may be given a light meal or Jell-O and clear soup the night before. If the operation is scheduled for the morning, he probably won't be permitted anything at all after midnight, but the nurse may wake him up for a drink as that deadline approaches. The nurse will put a note on the bed saying "NPO," an abbreviation for a Latin phrase meaning "nothing by mouth," and a young child, if up and walking around, may have such a note pinned to his pajamas, too, to make sure aides and play therapists know. This precaution is to prevent the child from vomiting under anesthesia and choking. Eating a crayon or Play-Doh in the activity room carries the same danger as breakfasting on bacon and eggs.

Not getting breakfast can be pretty stressful, especially for a child too young to understand why he can't eat. So take a walk if you must; get the child out of the sight and smell of food before the trays appear. If you have a private room, close the door and distract him.

Studies have shown that children can be distracted even in a preoperative or waiting room area by handheld video games. Many adults prepare for surgery using mind-body techniques like relaxation and visualization. See the chapter on complementary and alternative medicine (Chapter 21) for resources that might be helpful.

If the operation will require opening the intestines, a clean-out before the operation may be required. The repeated enemas, laxatives, and clear liquid diet are upsetting for the child. The intent is to clean out as many germs as possible to prevent them from escaping into the body during surgery, because they could cause some nasty infections. There isn't much you can do to relieve the procedures themselves, but you can help your child not think about it between sessions. New books, records, and tapes from the library might help. The playroom might have some toys the child can play with in his room; if not, borrow some from friends or neighbors. This is not the time to worry about spoiling your child—that will come later!

Surgical Complications and Their Prevention

Surgeons are careful not to cut through or handle the tumor more than necessary, and they tie off adjacent blood vessels and lymph channels early in the surgery to prevent malignant cells from escaping. They carefully remove the tumor and all tissues that may have cancer cells, avoiding contamination of healthy tissue with surgical instruments or even stitches.

New Surgical Techniques

Recent developments in pediatric surgery include fine-tuning techniques for optimal outcome and the widening use of new methods like laparoscopy and laser surgery. In skilled hands, these procedures preserve organ function, lower risks, provide greater precision, and perhaps spare limbs.

Laparoscopy

Laparoscopy is a forerunner in the "minimally invasive" area of surgery. With special instruments guided by computer images, specialists can perform operations using very small incisions and tiny, high-tech equipment. A fiber-optic cable (lighted instrument with a camera) can be inserted to the site of the tumor, showing doctors on a screen where to excise the tumor, while computerized robots allow more precise techniques than those that surgeons can perform on their own.

With these techniques, there is less blood loss during surgery and faster recovery, with smaller wounds. In major centers like Massachusetts General Hospital, an operating room right out of the future is filled with voice-activated equipment, special cameras, scopes, fiber-optic cables, robotic camera holders, and digitally enhanced equipment. Surgical robots make three-dimensional ultrasound images for real-time imaging. Information from this equipment is disseminated not only to those in the operating room and to observers nearby, but also online digitally or through a webcam for teaching purposes.

Laser Surgery

Advances in laser surgery have also helped treat pediatric cancer patients. Lasers use a very narrow, intense, and carefully controlled beam of light to treat some tumors. Unlike light from familiar bulbs, this beam can cut through steel. Some laser therapy is aimed at relieving or palliating symptoms like bleeding or an obstruction, while in other instances it will shrink or destroy tumors with heat. This precise surgical work also requires very expensive equipment used by highly trained specialists. As an adjunct, the heat sterilizes the site and reduces infection, seals blood vessels, and shortens recovery time. Some types of laser surgery are handled as outpatient procedures. This technique is useful with retinoblastoma and has potential for cancers of the skin, head, neck, and brain, among others.

Cryosurgery

Cryosurgery destroys tumors by freezing them with argon gas or liquid nitrogen at nearly minus 200 degrees Centigrade. A small incision is made and a hollow probe is inserted into the tumor, where the liquid gas is injected. The dead tumor cells are broken down and reabsorbed harmlessly into the body. This is used for skin, mouth, and other surface cancers and, more recently, with bone tumors. In the case of internal tumors, ultrasound or MRI is used to guide the probe to cancer cells while avoiding as much damage as possible to normal tissues. Cryosurgery may be done at the same time as standard surgery or through the skin. Frozen tissue thaws and is absorbed by the body or is dissolved and sloughed off as scabs (external). Cryosurgery is used for some small retinoblastoma tumors and in Kaposi sarcoma (AIDS-related cancer) for localized skin tumors.

Side effects depend on the location of the tumor but may include scarring, swelling, hair loss, pigmentation loss, and possibly bone fracture. With the small incision, there is less pain, less bleeding, shorter hospital stays, and lower costs. Sometimes cryosurgery can be performed with local anesthesia and can be repeated. It is sometimes effective where other surgical techniques have failed or cannot be used. Long-term effectiveness is as yet unknown, and the National Cancer Institute suggests that some insurance carriers may balk at the expense.

Transplantation

Organ transplantation is certainly not new, but improvements in both preparation for the procedure and aftercare have moved most of these life-saving operations from the realm of the experimental into the mainstream of medicine. Newer drugs are more effective against rejection. Children with hepatoblastomas that can't be completely resected benefit from living donor liver transplants. Transplants are rarely the first therapy used with cancer patients. Replacing major organs has no impact on the metastatic process, which continues through escaped cells, and the problems of transplants in cancer patients are enormous. The major exception to this rule is the transplantation of bone marrow and stem cells, used increasingly for leukemia and other pediatric cancers. These procedures are common enough now to earn their own chapter (Chapter 19).

Surgical Procedures

During surgery, the doctors watch for loss of blood, fluctuations in blood pressure, pulse, urine output, and body temperature. When they are through, the incision is closed with stitches and with paper tape strips. You may be surprised how insubstantial they look! These strips are removed in a few days, but the wound is easy to see.

Regular adhesive tape causes tape burns, which the paper strips avoid. The wound is also more accessible for cleansing.

"Second-Look" Operations

Operations to take another look to determine how effective treatments have been are not as common today as they used to be. High-tech imaging by MRI, computed tomography (CT) scans, ultrasound, and the like provide much of the same information without the invasion that surgery requires. A second look might be considered if the tumor was initially inoperable but subsequent radiation or chemotherapy seems to have improved its status. In cases like these, the operation is performed within 6 weeks to 3 months after radiation treatments are completed, before scars form. Second-look operations are at any rate not useful in the presence of metastases.

Anesthesia and Sedation

The anesthesiologist is a physician who examines the patient, prescribes the drugs and technique to be used before and during surgery, and administers or directs the administration of the anesthesia. In the United States, an anesthetist is a specially trained nurse who administers the anesthesia.

Anesthesia medications are safer now and can be used for longer periods. This means that more radical and complex operations can be carried out. The anesthesiologist visits the patient and parents before the operation, usually the day before. He does a physical examination, takes the patient's history, and checks whether the youngster is allergic to any drugs. If the child has a cold, the operation may be postponed to be safe. If all systems are go, there are four types of anesthesia that might be used:

1. **General anesthesia** is given by intravenous injection or is inhaled through a mask or a tube inserted into the windpipe from the mouth. It renders the patient unconscious.
2. **Spinal anesthesia** is given by a needle injected into the spinal canal to deaden sensation in only parts of the body. The patient may be awake for surgery. Depending on the drug used, a spinal anesthetic may take longer to wear off. These epidural anesthetics can cause a severe headache; a blood patch will relieve this pain, which Lisa said was like a bad migraine.

3. **Local anesthesia** is injected into the tissue at the incision site for superficial minor procedures, such as drilling teeth or some biopsies.

4. **Regional anesthesia** is injected into the nerves that transmit pain from the area of the body to be operated on.

Anesthesia drugs do not paralyze the patient, so he may also be given a muscle relaxant to make inserting tubes into the trachea (and similar procedures) easier.

Our experiences with anesthesia and sedation were mixed. At our daughter's initial surgery the doctors used a rectal medication to "knock her out" before she was taken to the operating room. Holding a child who has been anesthetized is frightening, for there is a loss of muscle tone unlike that of a sleeping child. Beware, and protect yourself and your clothing from urine and feces!

Sometimes children have reactions opposite to those expected from some sedation. On one occasion when Lisa was about 2, a sedative was used before a delicate test. Perhaps the dose was wrong. At any rate, she because hyperactive, belligerent, hostile, and hysterical. It was terrifying to watch, and she had to be restrained to keep from hurting herself. An antidote helped, but there were repeated episodes of the violence over a couple of hours, and afterwards she slept for 14 hours. She never had the test. Once, on the other hand, before an outpatient cystoscopy, Lisa was so calm that no medication was needed before she went into the operating room.

Postoperative Care

Where your child is taken after surgery depends on several factors, not least of which is the site and extent of the operation. Most patients go to the recovery room or a holding area near the operating suite, where they stay until they regain consciousness. In some circumstances they may be kept there for several days, although that is not common. In our experience, however, it is always longer than you expect and longer than you think you can bear. In the recovery room the vital signs are checked and the dressings are examined for bleeding or other discharge. There is usually an intravenous line still in place, which may be kept in for days; if it is dislodged from the vein, it may have to be restarted elsewhere. If the child is in pain, medication is given to relieve it (or to prevent it). Dressings may be checked to make sure they aren't too tight. Once, our daughter's catheter was held by a stitch that was pulling, causing her pain. That was correctable.

Nausea and vomiting is common after anesthesia. Studies at Yale have shown that acupuncture may be as effective for postoperative nausea and vomiting as intravenous medications.

After brain surgery and in certain other circumstances, the child is transferred to a pediatric intensive care unit (ICU or PICU). In the ICU the patient may be disoriented because of the constant noise, lights, lack of sleep, sedation, confusion, and monitors. There are a lot of instruments, which can be frightening, and the other patients may be alarming as well. We shared the ICU with a young boy who had just had both legs amputated after being struck by a train; such trauma is common in these units. Your presence gives your child someone familiar to focus on.

Ask ahead of time where the child will go after surgery. Our daughter was taken to an ICU because her major surgery was per-formed on an emergency basis on a Saturday—for years after, one house officer remembered her because of that!—and on weekends, the recovery room may not be open. The transfer is standard proce-dure, but we weren't told that, and we were devastated to hear she was there instead of on the regular pediatric floor.

Sometimes respiratory therapy—deep breathing and coughing—begins as soon as the patient regains consciousness to avoid pneumo-nia and lung collapse, although these complications are much less common in children than adults. The therapist or nurse may want to teach the child the procedure before the operation, when it is less frightening. The patient may be turned over often after surgery to aid in circulation, to help the lungs recover, and to help the heart by moving, even passively, the limbs. There may be nausea and vomiting after general anesthesia, yet the child may be thirsty because of the preoperative medication given to dry mucous secretions during sur-gery. If the child can't keep fluids down, try some ice chips or let him suck on a lollipop.

Regardless of where your child is taken, it will be devastating to see him lying pale with tubes and monitors hooked to various parts of the body, disoriented or in pain, especially if he seemed healthy before the surgery. In the ICU the child may also have electrodes attached to the chest for an electrocardiogram (ECG), a respirator, and perhaps a tube that is kept in the windpipe for days. With all this gear, it is hard, perhaps impossible, to pick up your small child or to hug your older one. But do talk to the child, touch him, make sure he knows you are there. Do this even if he is unconscious; the child will know.

Return of Body Function

Your child's body will slowly return to normal. After the operation the nurses will check the pulse, blood pressure, breathing rate, temperature, urine output, the contents of the various drainage tubes, general level of consciousness, and appearance. There may be a nasogastric (NG) tube through the nose and down into the stomach. This irritates the nose and throat, but makes it easier for the digestive system to heal.

If a Foley catheter is in place (a tube through the urethra into the bladder held in place by a small balloon) for the period right after surgery, there may be a loss of sensation when it is removed. To avoid the embarrassment of an older child wetting himself, urge the child to go to the bathroom frequently until the sensation returns. If a toilet-trained child does have postsurgical "accidents," reassure him that it is not his fault.

If your child has abdominal surgery, the doctor will check his abdomen with a stethoscope, listening to rumblings that signal that the bowels are working again. Another sign is passing of gas. This happens after 1 or 2 days, and until it does, there will be no hamburgers or spaghetti, maybe nothing at all or just sips of water, then Popsicles and clear juices. When the digestive system is working again, good nutrition does aid in healing. This could be a problem with a finicky eater. Check with your doctor to see if the child can have things you bring from home like yogurt, fruit, or canned soups that you know are his favorites.

Meanwhile, most patients are out of bed the first day or two after the operation, sometimes even the same evening. Parents may hold their infants then, too.

Antibiotics may not be used routinely unless there are signs of infection like an elevated white blood cell count or a fever. They are more likely to be employed if the bowel, urinary tract, gallbladder, or liver have been opened. If so, they may be started before the operation and continued until several days later.

The pain medications that are used depend on the age of the patient, his condition, and the extent of the surgery. The child may fear getting a "shot" (although indwelling catheters eliminate this) and not ask for pain relief. After an amputation, phantom limb pain and a feeling that the limb is twisted into an awkward position may continue for some time, perhaps for years.

Rehabilitation

With modern reconstructive surgery and rehabilitation techniques, surgeons can remove limbs and even some whole organs and the patient can still lead a relatively normal life. Right after the operation the child will begin to walk, exercise, and help in his own care. After 72 hours he will be walking with crutches and beginning physical therapy. If a limb has been amputated, after 2.5 to 3 months, when the stump and body weight have stabilized, the patient will be fitted for a prosthesis using measurements of the original limb taken before surgery. Functional, natural-looking artificial limbs come in a variety of new man-made materials and make it possible for an amputee to return to normal activity with minimal embarrassment and discomfort.

If the primary tumor was in the genital or urinary organs, surgery may leave the patient with a stoma (an artificial opening in the abdomen through which urine or feces are secreted). This may be temporary, until sensitive tissues have healed, or permanent, but the child, after some special training, can resume normal activity. I learned that two uncles, a friend, and a beloved nurse all wore bags to collect urine and I never knew. These people swim, make love, have babies, and are just like the rest of us. The Internet has made it possible for "ostomates" to make contact with one another for support.

Successful rehabilitation depends on positive support from the parents and the hospital team. You must encourage the child, particularly when things are going badly, because he no doubt sees himself as "different." Rehabilitation in general is discussed in more detail in Chapter 22.

Other Therapies

Other therapies will ordinarily be used as well. If there is to be chemotherapy and radiation, they will be continued or resumed as soon as possible, probably when the child is taking liquids orally and keeping them down.

Further Resources

ORGANIZATIONS/WEB SITES

United Ostomy Association of America, Inc. (P.O. Box 66, Fairview, TN 37062; 800-826-0826; www.uoaa.org)

Has support groups in many locations. Publications and online information. Many links, including several child-related.

17

Radiation

About half of all children with cancer receive radiation therapy. It is most often used in the early stages of treatment with chemotherapy. After the primary tumor has been partially removed by surgery, radiation effectively cleans up tumor cells that may have been left behind.

Radiation therapy, also called irradiation or x-ray therapy, combines neatly with surgery, for it "gets" the residual local cells that the operation misses, while surgery can debulk a large tumor that radiation could not cure.

How it works

Radiation is a form of energy, which in cancer therapy is either produced by the breakdown of unstable elements called radioactive isotopes or generated by machines. Some isotopes, like the rare element radium, are found in nature, and others, like cobalt-60, are man-made. X-rays are created by machines, while gamma rays result from the breakdown of radioactive isotopes. Radiation changes the internal structure of cells regardless of the form of beam used. Some types of radiation therapy use waves like ultraviolet or x-rays, while others bombard the cell with atomic particles (electrons or neutrons). It takes several "hits" of radiation to kill a cell.

Radiation therapy destroys cells by eliminating their ability to divide. Cells differ in their reaction to radiation ("radiosensitivity"). Since cancer cells are growing and dividing more rapidly than normal cells, they are more vulnerable to radiation "hits." Normal tissue in general recovers faster than cancer cells. Cancer cells that are not usually destroyed by radiation at a dose that is safe for nearby normal cells are called radioresistant. The radiosensitivity of tumor cells tends to parallel that of the tissue from which they arise. For example, lymph tissue is radiosensitive and breast tissue is not, so lymphomas are more affected by radiation than breast tumors. Most children's cancers that arise from rapidly dividing "embryonal" cells are radiosensitive. Another variable is the degree of malignancy—the less malignant a cell, the less responsive it is to radiation. Some parts of the body, including the lining of the digestive tract, hair follicles, reproductive organs, and bone marrow, have many especially fast-growing cells. Radiation's effects on these normal cells leads to side effects above and beyond the killing of tumor cells.

All tissues and tumors are susceptible to radiation to some extent, but it may vary from tumor to tumor within the same type and even within the same mass at different moments. For example, cells at a resting phase in their reproductive cycle are less sensitive to the treatments. Speaking very broadly, radiation is used for brain tumors, sarcomas, and more advanced stages of neuroblastoma, Wilms tumor, and perhaps non-Hodgkin lymphoma.

Because of serious side effects, it is necessary to avoid radiating large portions of the lungs, kidneys, and intestines. Testicles and ovaries are carefully shielded as appropriate to avoid infertility. Radiology procedures should be performed only when necessary, using the smallest amount of radiation that will provide good image quality. Besides therapeutic use, radiation is also often a step in biopsy and in placing central lines or chest or drainage tubes. Each treatment or test must be carefully planned to limit exposure, which can lead to serious side effects.

A Brief History

Wilhelm Roentgen discovered x-rays in 1895, and they were first used to treat cancer in 1899. That patient lived for at least another

25 years. By the 1950s, radiation played a large role in treating not only cancer but some benign diseases as well. Its use to cure acne and similar problems was halted when it was discovered that some of the patients later developed a malignancy in the region of the original therapy.

Supervoltage radiation became widely available in the 1950s, providing deeply penetrating, high-energy radiation from cobalt machines, linear accelerators, and betatrons. This radiation destroyed tumors that were buried beneath layers of normal tissue, and it reduced the damage to the skin. Early treatments were unpredictable and occasionally dangerous, but modern equipment has minimized many of these problems.

Why Radiation?

There are clear benefits in treating a child with radiation. Depending on the child's age, the area to be treated, and the dose, no mutilation results if the therapy is properly planned. Radiation therapy doesn't hurt, individual treatments are not time-consuming (although they may be given daily for weeks or months), and they may salvage body functions that surgery would destroy. They usually require little or no hospitalization and, unlike surgery, there is no risk of spreading the tumor during the treatments.

On the other hand, radiation is not without its disadvantages. The equipment and skilled therapists needed may not be available near the child's home. Normal cells will be damaged. Particularly in small children and infants, the growth patterns of bones and other tissues can be altered, and there is a possibility in a small but significant proportion of cases that a second cancer may appear some years later. If the pelvic area is radiated, sterility may result. These risks have to be weighed against the benefits when therapy is planned.

New equipment has reduced some of the side effects and enhanced the effectiveness of radiation. Today maximum doses can be given to various depths of body tissue with less concern for skin damage. The survival rates of patients with some radiosensitive forms of tumor have increased by leaps and bounds with these improvements and with the advent of combination therapy (adjunctive chemotherapy).

Overall, new techniques allow more precise targeting and therefore more potency—both very good news for our children.

Special Applications

The usual purpose of radiation therapy is to control local and regional disease. There are specialized uses as well. In leukemia and certain other cancers, cells have a tendency to hide in the central nervous system out of reach of chemotherapy distributed by the bloodstream. Then, just when the patient seems cured, the malignant cells reappear, thus spoiling the remission and perhaps the child's chances for cure. Radiation to the brain and spinal cord has been used as a treatment for certain patients who have evidence of leukemia in those areas at the time of diagnosis or as a preventive measure. Because of serious side effects in learning, thinking and other mental skills, central nervous system radiation is not used as commonly today. Instead, drugs are injected into the spinal fluid; cognitive effects are less severe with this therapy.

With Hodgkin disease, custom-made shields protect the heart and the lungs. These treatments may be given in conjunction with chemotherapy, and doses of each have to be carefully monitored to avoid more extreme, or "enhanced," side effects when the two are combined.

Total body radiation is also used sometimes to "turn off" the patient's own immune system and to eradicate all traces of leukemia before a bone marrow or stem cell transplant.

Sometimes radiation is delivered during surgery; the surgeons remove as much tumor as possible and move critical organs out of the way, and then a radioactive beam can target remaining cancer cells. This is called intraoperative electron beam radiation.

Where is Radiation Performed?

The availability of sophisticated equipment and skilled personnel is a major consideration in planning a patient's radiotherapy. The dosage and the timing of the treatments are critical. It takes expertise to calculate the exact doses that will control the tumor without causing overwhelming future problems. If chemotherapy will be part of the regimen, it may be necessary to alter the dose because some drugs (dactinomycin and doxorubicin [Adriamycin] in particular) enhance the effects, good and bad, of the radiation. Since most pediatric cancer centers have the latest equipment, and experienced radiotherapists can plan an individually tailored program that includes several forms of treatment, experts recommend that children be treated there.

Who Performs Radiation?

The doctor who plans the timing and the length, site, aim, and dose of the radiation treatments is called a radiation oncologist, therapeutic radiologist, radiation therapist, or radiotherapist—all names for the same specialist. The treatments themselves are administered by a trained radiation therapy technologist or technician. A physicist helps plan the individual child's therapy using computers to calculate the densities of the various body tissues and to plot the pathway the radiation beam should take, the volume of tissue to be treated, and the dose that will be delivered to the tumor and normal tissues. These specialists are members of the patient's whole team, along with the oncologist and nurses. At pediatric centers, these staff members have special pediatrics training in addition to their general qualifications.

Equipment

The type of radiation given and the equipment involved depend on what's available at the center where the child is to be treated, the site of the tumor, and the need to protect adjacent tissue. With modern x-ray therapy the target area can be carefully restricted, which causes less damage to normal cells. With sophisticated machines and careful treatment planning, tumors the size of a match head in the lungs, brain, abdomen, and other internal areas of the body can be pinpointed with accuracy by a beam of radiation. The patient may be rotated or the equipment may be repositioned to alternate the direction of the beam, approaching the tumor from different angles.

Thus the skin and other tissues overlying it receive less radiation, while the tumor is hit with a maximum dosage.

Types of Radiation

External beam, or **teletherapy**, projects radiation to the tumor site from a machine in a carefully targeted stream. The isotope that is most frequently used is cobalt-60. These isotopes emit rays all the time, unlike an x-ray machine, which can be turned off. The machines are constructed to focus a beam of radiation during treatment. At other times the isotopes are shielded and pose no danger.

Proton accelerators more accurately target cancer cells when compared to conventional x-rays that go through other tissues, losing potency in the process. They reach deep-seated tumors. This new equipment rotates the machinery rather than the patient to alter the beam's direction and uses imaging techniques like magnetic resonance imaging (MRI) and positron emission tomography (PET) to pinpoint the site with great accuracy. Although not used widely, proton beam therapy has promise for pediatric patients, whose small size demands precision; results have already been seen in pediatric head and neck tumors.

Low-dose involved field radiation therapy (LD-IFRT) is sometimes used after chemotherapy to wipe out residual disease, for example in Hodgkin disease. This therapy replaces the wide-field radiation used in earlier years, which had unacceptable side and after-effects.

Conformal radiation involves "shooting" the tumor from several directions at one time for a three-dimensional image. This spares normal tissue.

Specialists use **radiosurgery** to send a large one-time dose of radiation to a tiny, carefully targeted place in the brain. The equipment used for this procedure (stereotactic radiosurgery) is a gamma knife, or a special linear accelerator. The dose is much larger than usual and the target is much smaller, so the patient's head must be completely immobilized with a custom head frame.

Brachytherapy uses radioactive implants (seeds, wires, or needles) that are inserted directly into the tumor. They provide highly localized, constant radiation therapy. Radioisotope solids may be placed on the skin or inserted in body cavities. The implants are put in place while the patient is under general anesthesia and removed after a few days or up to a week or so later. Techniques have been developed to implant tubes during surgery, and then, after the tubes are in place, to insert the radioactive substance. This "after-loading" is much safer for the surgeons and other staff. Brachytherapy may be occasionally used in rhabdomyosarcoma, Ewing sarcoma, and retinoblastoma patients, among others. Sometimes radioactive seeds are implanted that give off radiation for about 2 weeks, and then become inert and remain harmlessly in place. Radioactive isotopes that are commonly used include radium, cobalt, gold, iodine, iridium, cesium, and, in trials, a radioactive form of phosphorous, P-32. Radioactive isotopes may be injected intravenously, either for diagnostic purposes (scanning) or as treatment. The isotopes seek out and concentrate in the tumor, and then are visible on a screen. When used in larger doses for therapy, they help destroy it.

Dose Factors

Dose prescription is a tricky matter, requiring the skills of a specialist. Dosages are determined by identifying the therapeutic ratio, or the relationship between the radiation sensitivity of cancer cells and of normal cells, so that the number of tumor cells killed will be maximized and unacceptable side effects minimized. The dose is expressed in numbers of rads, a shorthand term for "radiation absorbed dose." The size of the mass, the body site, the age and sex of the child, the child's general condition, the radiosensitivity of the tumor cells, the tumor's growth rate and pattern (is it infiltrating normal tissue?), whether or not cure is the intention, the side effects after treatment begins—all are taken into consideration when determining radiation dosage.

If cure is the aim, the highest possible dose tolerable to the adjacent tissue is given. Damage to the liver, lungs, brain, spine, heart, kidneys, bone marrow, and intestines is limited when possible, but effects on less important organs may be considered acceptable. Possible consequences might include sterility, or damage to the salivary glands, leading to dry mouth. The radiation oncologist discusses all this with the patient and the family before therapy begins.

The dose also depends on how tolerant the organ being treated is to radiation. In some instances this varies with the age of the patient.

The younger the patient, the more carefully the dose must be calculated and administered.

An important consideration is what other treatments are being used on the same patient. Here again the team approach is important. If chemotherapy is being given at the same time, the dose may have to be reduced as much as 20% to alleviate side effects like suppression of bone marrow, nausea, and vomiting. Radiation doses may vary over the course of treatment; often there is a rest period between courses.

Split-course regimens of radiation are especially useful when the patient will also receive chemotherapy. Because the drugs intensify the side effects as well as the desired effects of radiation, the child may need to rest between treatments until the reactions subside.

Schedules

In radiation therapy the total dose is divided into multiple applications called fractions, a process called fractionation. Therapy is commonly given on a daily basis, perhaps five times a week, over several weeks until the total dose is delivered. Blood counts are checked regularly to monitor any effects on the bone marrow, particularly if chemotherapy is being given at the same time or if a wide area of the body is receiving radiation.

Large tumors, even those considered inoperable, are sometimes shrunk by radiation, improving the possibility of totally removing them surgically. Area lymph nodes can be treated, too. After the radiation treatments, a rest of up to 4 weeks allows the body to recuperate and the therapy to take maximum effect.

Postoperative radiation treatments are used to clean up local tumor cells that may have been missed during surgery. Some metastases may also be radiated. Palliative radiation is used to relieve symptoms of the tumor, such as pain or blockage of a vital organ, but it is not expected to affect a cure. Brain masses and painful bone metastases are often the targets of palliative radiation. Palliative radiation takes time, effort, and money and can thus impose an additional burden on the patient and the family. By slowing the cancer growth, however, these treatments can make life more pleasant for the time the patient has remaining. That time can be greatly extended by the palliation.

Preparing the Patient

If the child has surgery before radiation begins, the surgeon may take that opportunity to place metal clips near the tumor that will show up on x-rays. The clips delineate the extent of the tumor and help the radiation therapist design the treatment fields. They are harmless and are simply left in place when therapy is over. They will not set off airport metal detectors or cause any other problems.

There are some steps you can take before the radiation treatments begin to help your child accept them. First and foremost, you should be well informed about the side effects, what alternative treatments are available, and what the prognosis will be if the radiation is not given. This will enable you to give informed consent to the procedures. Shields of lead or tungsten are used to protect tissues and organs near the tumor, like the lungs and kidneys, during radiation treatment. These shields, or blocks, will be custom-made according to the shape of the radiation field and should be comfortable and well fitting. A machine called a simulator, which is identical to the radiotherapy machine but without the radioactive elements, is used to plan the fields and the shape of the blocks. Lead blocks several inches thick are custom-designed with a hole for the beam to pass through while nearby vital organs are shielded. These shields are mounted on thick clear panels that slide onto the machine like a photographic lens. These preparations involve a lot of measurements but no pain or discomfort.

The child may wear cast-like, custom-made immobilization devices. If so he may look like a hockey goalie or a baseball catcher. The ovaries may be repositioned during surgery to keep them out of the beam of radiation. Computed tomography (CT) or MRI scans may be used to locate and size the tumor specifically, thus helping to target the treatments.

Take the child to the clinic for a visit before the treatments are to begin. Try to make the visit fun by showing the child that he will be "on TV." Help the child understand that although the machines are large and may appear frightening, the treatments are not painful. He will hear clicking and buzzing as the machines are operated. The child may be afraid because he will be left in the room when the actual therapy is given, but reassure him that the therapist will be in sight in the adjacent room and will talk with him through an intercom or watch him on a TV monitor. Child life specialists and occupational therapists "play" with the child and show what will happen during treatments. This experience helps young patients feel more comfortable with the therapy and may reduce the need for anesthesia.

Because it is essential that the target be hit precisely, the youngster must be immobile; those over the age of 3 will hold still when they realize it doesn't hurt. Sedation will be used judiciously for any child who is unable to keep still and in treating tumors such as retinoblastoma (because of course no restraint can hold the child's eye still). Many centers prefer to use a short-acting general anesthetic rather than relying on sedation when delivery of the radiation to a restricted area is critical. It will be easier if you can arrange for the treatments to take place at about the same time each day. The radiation department will try to schedule your child's treatments for his best time of day. For most youngsters, this is morning: I've never met a child who was at his best at 4:30 pm, known around our house as The Poison Hour.

The doctors and technicians get to know the child and the parents on early visits to defuse the drama. The clinic can also provide special services if needed—a translator, for example, if the patient's family doesn't speak native English. Children (and adults, for that matter) fear the unknown, and a small amount of preparation time can eliminate that fear.

You are probably daunted by the prospect of daily trips to the hospital over a period of several weeks. Fortunately, most radiation treatments take less time than most chemotherapy visits. The child is ordinarily in and out within half an hour, including waiting time. The departments begin to see patients early in the morning, so some can make appointments before work or school and others after. If any equipment fails, however, the waiting period will be longer, so be prepared. Dressing the child in loose, easily removed clothing will expedite any changes required for the treatments. Any metal jewelry that the child wears must be removed for each treatment if it is in the target zone, but it can be put right back on afterward. Few areas around the world are spared extreme weather of one sort or another, so ask the doctor ahead of time what to do if travel is affected by a storm.

A Typical Radiation Visit

Most radiation appointments are very brief, since the therapy itself only takes a few minutes, although the need for anesthesia or sedation will stretch your visits. The first few visits, however, when therapy is planned, are an exception to this and may take half a day. During a routine visit the child may have to stop first at the laboratory for blood tests to monitor the blood counts. The technician then calls the patient and the parent from the waiting room and positions the child on the table precisely, using immobilization devices if necessary.

The parent and the technician step out into a control area, where they can see and talk with the child. After a quick and painless treatment, the child and the parent are safely reunited and may go about their daily business.

Care of the Radiation Patient

First and foremost, the child needs reassurance. The child may think that his personal possessions have become radioactive; this is not so. Playmates and classmates may have to be told that he is not dangerous.

The child's diet is important. He needs foods with high calorie content and high protein content for energy and to rebuild tissues. He may prefer small, frequent meals and snacks. If the child is having trouble eating regular food, a blender, food processor, or baby food grinder may solve the problem while allowing him to eat family food. Drinking lots of liquids and resting before meals may help, too. In the meantime, your doctor may want to control nausea with medication, although this is avoided in young children if at all possible. Behavior modification techniques may help, too. (See the chapter on alternative and complementary medicine, Chapter 21, for suggestions.) If in the second or third week your child develops diarrhea or constipation, medication and a change in diet can improve the situation. Sometimes therapy has to be stopped temporarily until the diarrhea is controlled.

Skin care is very important. If your child's skin has dyed marks on it to target the treatments, do not wash them off. These marks outline the treatment port to ensure that the same area is treated each time.

Avoid excess sun without sunscreen on the radiation field for a year. Temperature changes on the site of radiation, such as those induced by heating pads and ice bags, should also be avoided. Keep the skin clean, dry, and clear of infection. Do not use anything but a mild soap for 2 weeks after the treatments without checking with your doctor. This includes ointments, lotions, powders, deodorants, and perfumes, which may contain metals that would increase skin reactions. Bathe the child normally but don't scrub. Do not let him wear tight-fitting clothes, and don't use adhesive tape on the radiated area, because irritation could result. If the skin is itchy, a mild steroid cream can be prescribed. For dry mouth and sore throat, topical anesthetics and mouthwash will help. Ask the doctor what types to use. Except as noted, continue the precautions for 4 to 6 weeks after the treatments are over.

If the mouth is in the radiation field, your child may have an increase in tooth decay due to decreased saliva flow. Ask about fluoride treatments to prevent unnecessary problems. If the child has braces on his teeth, they may have to be removed for the duration of the radiation therapy. Your doctor will explain these precautions in detail. Many radiation oncologists request a dental consultation before beginning therapy to that area.

The number of white blood cells, which fight infection, may fall, depending on the dose and field size. If so, they begin to return to normal about 3 weeks after the treatments stop. During the period of radiation therapy, blood counts will be taken often to see if a transfusion is needed for anemia or if the child should be watched especially carefully for signs of infection. If the white blood count or platelet count drops very low, the treatments may have to be interrupted until it rises somewhat.

Side Effects

Before therapy begins, the doctor will also discuss the side effects that your child may develop. Some are short term and some will last over a period of time. Nobody will experience all these effects, or even many of them, and some patients don't have any at all. The severity and kind of side effects will depend on the site under treatment, the dose, the amount of tissue treated, the child's age, and how the dose is fractionated. These effects occur because the radiation hits not only the cancer cells but others that are also growing and dividing rapidly. The affected tissue may be adjacent to the target zone or in a part of the body well removed from the target zone.

Some of the early side effects are:

- Hair loss (only in the radiation target zone, not generalized as in chemotherapy. It is temporary, and regrowth begins in 2 months or so.)
- Depressed bone marrow and blood counts
- Nausea and vomiting (especially in wide-field radiation or if the head or abdomen is in the target area)
- Diarrhea
- Fatigue (if the central nervous system has been radiated. This may last for a week or two and may even begin several weeks after therapy is completed. This fatigue may be accompanied by dizziness, irritability, a decrease in appetite, vision problems, and a fever. Tell your doctor about these symptoms.)
- Ear infection and dizziness (if the ear is in the target zone; hearing loss is rare at the doses given to children)
- Sore throat and sore or dry mouth (if the head and neck are radiated)
- Mucositis (inflammation of mucous membranes in the target area, which may become infected)
- Inflammation of the esophagus, eye, or tongue (if these tissues are radiated; intravenous fluids and a nasogastric tube can be used until the adverse reaction subsides)
- Skin burns (including dry patches, moist patches, and blistering), beginning a week or so after treatment begins. In more serious cases, surface scars or layers of fibrous tissue may form under the surface. Ask your doctor about a salve to soothe this.
- Enhanced side effects if radiation is given in combination with chemotherapy. Doxorubicin with radiation, for example, may increase the risk of damage to heart tissue.
- Radiation-induced inflammation of the lungs
- Inflammation of the cornea, iris, and conjunctiva of the eye
- Stomach ulcers
- Depressed bone marrow and blood counts

Late effects may not appear for some time, maybe years after the treatments have ended. These include:

- Alteration of growth patterns, especially in the youngest patients. With modern combined therapies, more children are surviving for a long time and therefore more late consequences are being found. A radiated limb may not grow as long or to the same diameter as the other. If muscle is scarred by radiation, the effect may be like a bowstring and cause curving of bones to which the muscle is attached.
- Damage to the pituitary gland if it is radiated, which can lead to short stature. Hormonal replacement therapy can counteract the problem.
- Cataracts and inflammation of the eye covering and possibly suppression of tears. These occur in only a few cases, when the eye has been radiated. The cataracts develop slowly, are sometimes correctable with contact lenses, and can be removed by surgery.
- Joint stiffness and impaired function if the joint is in the treatment field (physical therapy helps)
- Lung fibrosis (if the lungs are in the target zone)
- Injury to bladder, bones, kidneys (if they are in the treatment field)
- Sterility. Failure to menstruate and to develop secondary sexual characteristics may result from radiation to the pelvis or abdomen before puberty. Some of this can be avoided by repositioning the organs in question during surgery. Data will be collected as our children become long-term survivors to see what effects these therapies have on subsequent generations. So far, there appears to be no additional risk to our grandchildren in most cases.
- Bone fragility
- Tooth cavities or decreased saliva (if the nose and throat are treated)
- Kidney damage
- Smaller breast growth and problems breastfeeding if the chest is radiated (less likely with newer equipment)
- Heart muscle damage (if the chest is radiated)

- Delay of appearance of teeth (if the jaw is radiated)
- Second malignancies (a small percentage of patients develop a second cancer, with several years' latency before that happens)

This list looks pretty formidable, but remember that no child will experience all or even most of these side effects. Remember, too, that your child may have a reduced chance for survival if the therapy is not given. The risks are acceptable when that is taken into consideration.

Future Developments

Researchers are working on substances to make cancer cells more radiosensitive, thus allowing a lower and more efficient radiation dose. Other drugs that increase the effect of radiation on tumors are being tried experimentally, and radioprotective compounds that minimize the side effects are also being developed.

The drug C225 (cetuximab, a monoclonal antibody) enhances the effects of radiation: the radiation damages the cell and the C225 antibody stops a growth factor that the cell needs to reproduce.

Proton beam therapy is super-accurate, damaging cancer cells with little injury to adjacent tissue. However, it is unlikely that this extremely expensive therapy will be generally available for some time. Protons, neutrons, and pi-mesons are some of the subatomic particles currently under study.

Intensity-modulated radiation therapy allows higher doses of radiation to reach tumors without affecting surrounding tissues.

A child receiving radiation therapy will have to be followed lifelong to make sure the original cancer does not return and to detect any late consequences. In this way information can also be compiled to help future patients.

Further Resources

READING

Kornmehl, Carol L., MD. *The Best News about Radiation Therapy: How to Cope and Survive*. Howell, NJ: Academic Radiation/Oncology Press, 2003.

Not specific to pediatric patients. Photographs of radiation equipment are especially useful, including positioning and blocking devices. A lot of information about placement and immobilization techniques.

ORGANIZATIONS/WEB SITES

"Radiation Therapy and You—A guide to self-help during cancer treatment." National Cancer Institute. Available at www.cancer.gov.

18

Chemotherapy

Chemotherapy, or the treatment of disease with drugs, has brought about a revolution in the fight against cancer, particularly in children. Because surgery and radiation treatments are limited to specific body sites, they do not affect any tumor cells that are not directly removed or radiated. Since drugs are circulated throughout the body, chemotherapy is the primary treatment for leukemia and lymphoma, known to be widespread at diagnosis; "chemo" is the treatment for solid tumors that are assumed to have spread (metastasized).

Most tumors are not detectable by even the most sophisticated means until they contain about billions of cells. Most primary tumors are much larger when diagnosed. After surgical removal, if even one cancer cell of the primary tumor were left behind after treatment, it could grow to become a new tumor, metastasize, and kill the patient. By the time most tumors are discovered, there is a good likelihood that at least a few of those cells are elsewhere in the body, having been carried away from the tumor by the bloodstream or through the lymph system. Even if these metastases can't be detected, doctors assume they are present and go on the offensive against them. Using chemotherapy to find and destroy these cells is called adjuvant, or adjunctive, chemotherapy.

Currently, doctors have in their arsenal several dozen drugs that kill cancer cells. To use these powerful drugs safely, the physician

TABLE 18.1 Chemotherapy Drugs

Name of drug & alternate names	Description & route	Side effects	Frequency of effects	Diseases
Actinomycin-D Dactinomycin Cosmegan	Clear yellow liquid, IV	Nausea and vomiting Bone marrow depression Mouth sores Loss of appetite Diarrhea	Common	Lymphomas Retinoblastoma Wilms tumor Sarcomas Liver cancer
		Hair loss Acne Skin burns or ulcers Liver effects Fever, malaise Causes tissue burns if it infiltrates	Less common	Teratomas Germ cell tumors Testicular tumor Rhabdomyosarcoma Ewing tumor ANLL Kaposi sarcoma Osteosarcoma
Adriamycin Doxorubicin Rubex	Clear red liquid, IV	Nausea and vomiting Pink urine (not blood) Bone marrow depression Hair loss Sore mouth	Common	ANLL, ALL Lymphomas Neuroblastoma Wilms tumor Bone tumors Soft tissue sarcomas

Drug	Description	Side effects	Frequency	Cancers treated
		Heart damage Fever Loss of appetite Changed taste or smell Diarrhea Sun sensitivity	Less common	Thyroid cancer Kaposi sarcoma Testicular tumors Rhabdomyosarcoma
ara-C Cytosar Cytosine Cytarabine	Clear colorless liquid IV, spinal injection, subcutaneous arabinoside	Nausea and vomiting Loss of appetite Tingling, numb hands or feet Taste, smell changes Sore throat or mouth Bone marrow depression	Common	ANLL, AML Chronic leukemia Lymphomas Brain tumors
		Conjunctivitis Headache Diarrhea	Less common	
		Lowered fertility	Late effect	
BCNU BICNU Carmustine	Clear colorless liquid, IV	Burning along vein of injection Bone marrow depression (3–4 weeks later) Nausea and vomiting Dizziness Nerve damage	Common	Lymphomas Bone tumors Brain tumors Melanoma

(continued)

TABLE 18.1 Chemotherapy Drugs (*contiuned*)

Name of drug & alternate names	Description & route	Side effects	Frequency of effects	Diseases
		Renal failure Liver damage Shortness of breath	Less common	
Bleomycin Blenoxane Bleo	Clear, colorless liquid; IV, intramuscular, subcutaneous	Fever Mouth ulcers Shortness of breath Sun sensitivity	Common	Lymphomas Testicular tumors Kaposi sarcoma Kidney cancer
		Nausea and vomiting Loss of appetite and weight Hair loss Skin lesions Allergic reactions Liver, kidney damage	Less common	

Drug	Route	Side effects	Frequency	Uses
Busulfan Myleran	Oral, IV	Hair loss Bone marrow depression Skin rash Raised heartbeat and blood pressure Dry mouth Diarrhea	Common	CML, ANLL BMT preparation
		Seizures Nausea and vomiting	Less common	
		Lung and kidney damage potential with high dose Decreased female fertility	Late effect	
Carboplatin Paraplatin	IV	Bone marrow depression	Common	Leukemias Head and neck tumors
		Tingling and numbness of hands and feet Nausea and vomiting Hearing loss Mouth sores Hair loss Rash, dry skin Liver changes Kidney effects	Less common	Testicular tumors Brain tumors

(continued)

TABLE 18.1 Chemotherapy Drugs (*continued*)

Name of drug & alternate names	Description & route	Side effects	Frequency of effects	Diseases
CCNU Lomustine Ceenu	Oral (capsules on an empty stomach)	Nausea and vomiting Bone marrow depression (delayed)	Common	Hodgkin disease Non-Hodgkin lymphoma Brain tumors
		Kidney, lung, liver damage Loss of appetite Dizziness, weakness Hair loss Mouth sores Blurred vision	Less common	Melanoma
Chlorambucil Leukeran	Oral (tablet)	Bone marrow depression Loss of appetite Rash Hair loss Liver effects Seizures	Common	Lymphomas Clear cell adenocarcinoma (kidney) Testicular tumors

		Side effects		Uses
Cisplatin(um) Platinol AQ CDPP	Clear colorless liquid; injection IV	Less common	Nausea and vomiting Cough, shortness of breath Diarrhea	
		Common	Bone marrow depression Loss of appetite Taste and smell effects Kidney function effects Ringing in the ears Nausea and vomiting	Common: Brain tumors Lymphomas Leukemias Testicular tumors Head & neck tumors Melanoma
		Less common	Diarrhea Allergic reactions Blurred vision Muscle cramps	Less common: Osteosarcoma Neuroblastoma Germ cell tumors
		Late effects	Hearing loss (bilateral and irreversible) Kidney damage	
Cytoxan Cyclophosphamide CTX, CPM Neosar	Clear, colorless liquid; pills	Common	Bone marrow depression Nausea and vomiting Loss of appetite Hair loss	Common: ALL, AML Lymphomas Neuroblastoma Wilms tumor
		Less common	Irritation of bladder,	Less common: Bone tumor

(continued)

TABLE 18.1 Chemotherapy Drugs (*continued*)

Name of drug & alternate names	Description & route	Side effects	Frequency of effects	Diseases
		blood in urine Sore mouth Diarrhea Taste & smell changes Fluid retention Shortness of breath Heart damage Blurred vision Liver effects		Retinoblastoma Sarcomas Rhabdomyosarcoma Teratomas Head & neck tumors Testicular tumors
		Bladder cancer, other second malignancies (rare) Leukemia Lowered fertility Lung disease (with high dose)	Late effects	

Drug	How given	Common	Less common	Late effects	Used to treat
Dacarbazine DTIC, Imidazole Carboxamide	IV	Bone marrow depression, Nausea and vomiting, Loss of appetite, Taste & smell changes, Flu-like symptoms	Liver changes, Sun sensitivity, Blurred vision		Melanoma, Soft tissue sarcoma, Neuroblastoma, Hodgkin disease, Osteosarcoma
Daunomycin Rubidomycin DMN Daunorubicin Cerubidine	Clear red liquid	Pink urine (not blood), Bone marrow depression, Hair loss, Loss of appetite, Diarrhea	Mouth ulcers, Nausea and vomiting, Fever, Heart damage, Liver damage, Sun sensitivity, Tissue burns if the IV infiltrates	Heart damage, Second malignancy	ALL, ANLL, Lymphomas, Neuroblastoma, Wilms tumor, Bone tumors, Kaposi sarcoma

(continued)

TABLE 18.1 Chemotherapy Drugs (*continued*)

Name of drug & alternate names	Description & route	Side effects	Frequency of effects	Diseases
Flavopiridol (clinical tests)				ALL Glioma Soft tissue sarcoma
5-Fluorouracil 5-FU Adrucil	Clear, colorless liquid; IV Topical cream	Nausea and vomiting Bone marrow depression Sun sensitivity Loss of appetite	Common	Bone tumors Cancers of the colon and rectum Liver cancer
		Diarrhea Mouth ulcers Hair loss Skin rash Liver damage Conjunctivitis, excess tears Dizziness, confusion	Less common	Head & neck tumors

Drug	Route	Common	Less common	Uses
Gemcitabine Gemzar (pediatric clinical trials)	IV	Bone marrow depression Diarrhea Nausea and vomiting Flu-like symptoms Skin rash and itching Loss of appetite	Hair loss Kidney, liver effects Mouth sores Fluid retention Tingling or numb hands or feet	Solid tumors Leukemia (resistant)
Idarubicin Idamycin	IV	Bone marrow depression Hair loss Mouth sores Diarrhea Nausea and vomiting Loss of appetite Liver effects Skin irritation Orange urine		AML, CML, ALL, ANLL

(continued)

TABLE 18.1 Chemotherapy Drugs (*continued*)

Name of drug & alternate names	Description & route	Side effects	Frequency of effects	Diseases
		Heart damage Sun sensitivity Burns at injection site	Less common	
Ifosfamide IFEX	Clear liquid, IV	Bone marrow depression Hair loss Bleeding from bladder (mesna prevents) Nausea and vomiting Loss of appetite	Common	Germ cell tumors Testicular tumors Lymphomas Bone tumors Brain tumors Soft tissue sarcomas
		Diarrhea Dizziness, confusion, headache Liver effects Seizures	Less common	ALL, ANLL
L-asparaginase L-asp, Elspar	Thick, colorless IM, IV, subcutaneous	Allergic reaction Fever, loss of energy	Common	Chronic leukemias Lymphomas

Name	How Given	Side Effects	Frequency	Used to Treat
(continued from previous page)		Body aches; Liver, pancreas effects; Lethargy, confusion; Bone marrow depression; Nausea, vomiting; Kidney function effects	Less common	Soft tissue sarcoma; ALL
Melphalan; Alkeran; L-Pam	IV, oral	Diarrhea; Bone marrow depression; Nausea and vomiting	Common	Hodgkin disease; Testicular cancer; Melanoma
		Hair loss; Itching, rash; Shortness of breath, cough; Mouth sores	Less common	Preparation for BMT
6-Mercaptopurine; 6-MP; Purinethol; Lukerin; Mercaleukin; Puri-Nethol	Oral, IV	Bone marrow depression	Common	Acute leukemias; Non-Hodgkin
		Loss of appetite; Nausea and vomiting; Diarrhea; Fever; Jaundice; Mouth sores; Skin rashes; Liver damage (reversible)	Less common	Lymphoma; *May be used in lower dose with allopurinol to ease urinary side effects*

(continued)

TABLE 18.1 Chemotherapy Drugs (*continued*)

Name of drug & alternate names	Description & route	Side effects	Frequency of effects	Diseases
Methotrexate Amethopterin MTX *Avoid alcohol, tetracyclines, A vitamins, chloramphenicol, folic acid, aspirin*	Oral Clear yellow liquid (IV) IM Intrathecal	Mouth ulcers Bone marrow depression Nausea and vomiting Loss of appetite Hair loss	Common	Leukemias Lymphomas Bone tumors Brain tumors Kidney tumors
		Diarrhea Light sensitivity Nerve damage (high dose) Kidney failure (high dose) Lung damage Seizures Liver damage Brain damage (high dose, intrathecal)	Less common	(adenocarcinoma) Liver cancer
Methotrexate with leucovorin calcium rescue (citrovorum factor)	High-dose MTX with rescue IV, oral	Rash Nausea and vomiting Allergic reaction	Common	Osteosarcoma Non-Hodgkin lymphoma Resistant cancers

Drug	Appearance	Common side effects	Less common side effects	Uses
Mitomycin Mitomycin C Mutamycin	Purple liquid IV	Nausea and vomiting Bone marrow depression Hair loss Loss of appetite Mouth sores Blue-green urine Skin irritation (at radiation site)	Skin burns, ulcers Sun sensitivity Cough, shortness of breath Tingling hands, feet Dizziness	CML Head and neck tumors
Nitrogen mustard Mustargen Mechlorethamine HN_3	Clear yellow liquid IV	Nausea and vomiting Bone marrow depression Diarrhea Mouth sores Decreased appetite Taste, smell changes Hair loss		Lymphomas Neuroblastoma

(continued)

TABLE 18.1 Chemotherapy Drugs (*continued*)

Name of drug & alternate names	Description & route	Side effects	Frequency of effects	Diseases
		Skin rash	Less common	
		Burns if IV infiltrates		
		Dizziness, tingling hands or feet		
		Second malignancy (high dose)		
Pergaspargase PEG-1 Oncaspar	IV, IM	Similar to L-asparaginase		*Modified form of l-asparaginase, used in ALL patients too sensitive to the original drug*
Plicamycin Mithramycin Mithracin	IV	Bone marrow depression	Common	Testicular cancer
		Nausea and vomiting		Chronic leukemia
		Loss of appetite		
		Taste, smell changes (metallic taste)		
		Diarrhea		
		Mouth sores		
		Liver changes		

Generic and brand names	How given	Common side effects	Less common side effects	Used to treat
			Skin burns or sores Hair loss Skin changes (thickening, blushing)	
Prednisone *Must be tapered slowly if taken more than 7–10 days. Take with meals, avoid aspirin.*	Oral	Weight gain Increased appetite Rounded face Acne Bone pain	Suppression of fever or other signs of infection Mood swings Diabetes Thinning of bones Muscle weakness High blood pressure	ALL, ANLL Non-Hodgkin lymphoma Hodgkin disease
Procarbazine Matulane Natulan *Avoid cheese, bananas; many common drugs interact with this agent.*	Oral capsule	Nausea and vomiting Bone marrow depression	Diarrhea or constipation Dry mouth Fever/chills Skin rash	Non-Hodgkin lymphoma Hodgkin disease Brain tumors Melanoma

(continued)

TABLE 18.1 Chemotherapy Drugs (*contiuned*)

Name of drug & alternate names	Description & route	Side effects	Frequency of effects	Diseases
		Headache, dizziness		
		Loss of appetite		
		Sun sensitivity		
		Hair loss		
Rituxan Rituximab *Monoclonal antibody. Premedicate with acetaminophen or Benadryl for allergic reaction.*	IV	Fever, chills Skin rash (allergy) Shortness of breath Fluid retention	Common	Lymphomas
		Nausea and vomiting Fatigue Low blood pressure Dizziness Muscle, joint pain	Less common	

Taxol Paclitaxel	IV Colorless liquid	Bone marrow depression Hair loss Mouth sores Diarrhea Tingling hands, feet Rash, allergic reaction Muscle aches Blood pressure, heart rate changes Decreased appetite	Common	Head and neck tumors Testicular cancer Melanoma Relapsed leukemia and other cancers
		Nail changes Nausea and vomiting Skin burns	Less common	
Teniposide Vumon	IV	Bone marrow depression Diarrhea Mouth sores Hair loss	Common	Relapsed, resistant ALL
		Lowered blood pressure Nausea and vomiting Severe allergic reaction	Less common	

(continued)

TABLE 18.1 Chemotherapy Drugs (*continued*)

Name of drug & alternate names	Description & route	Side effects	Frequency of effects	Diseases
6-Thioguanine 6-TG	Oral tablet	Bone marrow depression Nausea and vomiting	Common	Leukemias Lymphomas
		Fever Mouth sores Liver effects Decreased appetite Stomach pain Diarrhea Blood in urine	Less common	
Thiotepa	IV Intrathecal Intracavity (bladder)	Nausea and vomiting Decreased appetite Bone marrow depression Hair loss Bladder effects	Common	Brain tumors Lymphomas Preparation for BMT
		Dizziness Skin rash Fever Allergic reaction	Less common	

Drug	Description	Side Effects		Used to Treat	
		Common	Less common	Common	Less common
Vinblastine Velban	Clear liquid IV	Bone marrow depression Numbness, tingling Constipation	Nausea and vomiting Loss of appetite Hair loss Mouth sores Diarrhea Burns at injection site Bowel paralysis Urinary retention	Lymphomas Bone tumors Head and neck tumors	Melanoma Neuroblastoma Kaposi sarcoma
Vincristine Oncovin VCR	Clear, colorless liquid IV	Constipation Loss of reflexes Muscle weakness Tingling in hands, feet Hair loss	Loss of appetite Seizures Skin burns if IV infiltrates Nausea, vomiting Diarrhea Bone marrow depression Mouth ulcers	Leukemias Lymphomas Neuroblastoma Wilms tumor Bone tumors	Retinoblastoma Sarcoma Liver cancer Melanoma Brain tumors Rhabdomyosarcoma Germ cell tumors Kaposi sarcoma

(continued)

TABLE 18.1 Chemotherapy Drugs (continued)

Name of drug & alternate names	Description & route	Side effects	Frequency of effects	Diseases
VP-16 Etoposide Ve-Pesid	Clear liquid IV Oral capsules	Bone marrow depression Lowered blood pressure Mouth sores Diarrhea	Common	Leukemias Lymphomas Brain tumors Neuroblastoma
		Loss of appetite Skin irritation (at radiation sites) Taste, smell changes Tingling, numbness Flu-like symptoms Nausea, vomiting Allergic reaction	Less common	Kaposi sarcoma Testicular (resistant) Ewing sarcoma

Adapted from an earlier edition of Young People with Cancer after work by Sondra R. Tabor, RN, MN, Amie Karen Cancer Center, UCLA, Los Angeles, CA

Note: BMT is bone marrow transplant; CML is chronic myelogenous leukemia; ALL is acute lymphoblastic leukemia; AML is acute myeloid leukemia; ANLL is acute non-lymphocytic leukemia

Murr's poem

Chemo

The first day, in the crowded waiting room
I study others but except for one—
A woman whose bald head declares the truth—
I can't tell who is also there for meds
Or who, like me, has come to add the love.

A large TV, set low against the wall,
Provides some background noise; just morning talk.
And magazines placed near each chair and couch
Show heads of state from several years ago.
They're meant, I think, to stop time passing by
For those whose lives may slowly seep away.

At last, a nurse comes out and calls our name.
Gray lounge chairs edge the square room's outside walls.
Each chair draped with a handmade cotton quilt
A gift, a nurse says, made by a patient's aunt.
I can't help wondering if they were made
In gratitude or as memorial?

Next to each chair a silver pole is set
To hold clear pouches of those potent drugs
Whose dispensation, almost like a rite
Proceeds according to accepted steps.
First dose: an anti-nausea medicine
And next, two drugs prepared to wage cell wars,
Their stealth attack just drip by quiet drip.

—Muriel Dubois (whose husband battled lung cancer)

must be experienced in using them and must have access to a sophisticated hospital laboratory to measure their effect and watch for side effects. Treatments, even if they are carried out at a community hospital, should be supervised by specialists from the cancer center.

Chemotherapy drugs are usually introduced into the bloodstream through pills or an intravenous (IV) infusion. Chemo infusion pumps deliver greater accuracy than regular IVs. The blood carries them to almost every nook and cranny of the body where microscopic tumors can hide. There, through several different methods of action, they stop the cancer cells from growing and dividing. These treatments are the best hope for children with most forms of widely metastasized cancers and, indeed, are essential for virtually all patients.

A Brief History of Chemotherapy

Modern drug therapy for cancer began partly as a result of a poison gas explosion during World War II, when researchers noticed that victims of mustard gas had suffered injury to their bone marrow and lymphatic systems. This was useful to know in treating cancers like leukemia, in which the white blood cells, which are manufactured in the bone marrow and lymph system, multiply out of control. Nitrogen mustard, a chemotherapy drug still used today (but only rarely), is an outgrowth of subsequent research. Then in the late 1940s, Dr. Sidney Farber (after whom a cancer center in Boston is named) first used methotrexate, another type of drug, in a patient with leukemia.

Initially these medications were tried in patients with terminal disease who had nothing to lose. While they all died, some did show improvement. Eventually the drugs were given to patients with earlier stages of cancer who had some hope of surviving. More recently the use of a combination of drugs has led to major improvements in long-term remissions, curing many children with cancer.

The National Cancer Institute (NCI), a U.S. government agency, coordinates an international search for new substances that might be effective against tumors. Thousands of new materials are studied each year, and a few show enough promise to justify laboratory trials in rodents and larger animals. Only 0.1% are ever used in human patients on even an experimental basis.

Scientists are working on drugs to control the side effects of the cancer and the treatment side effects, aiming for substances that are much more precise and less toxic than current medicines. Other investigatory drugs play a role in genetics, either by blocking (or repairing) cancer-causing genetic abnormalities or by enhancing tumor suppressor genes.

Goals of Chemotherapy

Doctors hope that chemotherapy drugs will help their patients by seeking and destroying tumor cells hiding throughout the body. Chemotherapy agents attack cells that are growing and dividing, including certain normal cells as well as cancer cells. Therefore, tissues of the body that depend on rapidly multiplying cells are also affected by the medications—particularly hair follicles, the bone marrow, and the digestive system. There is a fine line between killing all the cancer cells and causing too many detrimental side effects. The major reason these drugs work is that although they harm both normal and cancer cells, the normal ones have a capacity for repair, while cancer cells, which are defective, are less able to do so.

To understand the action of the chemotherapy drugs, it is useful to take a quick look at the life cycle of the normal cell. Simply put, the cell takes in nutrients, incorporates them into essential compounds, and divides into two daughter cells that go on to repeat the process. (Or, the cell is born, eats, grows, matures, reproduces [divides], and dies, and the process is repeated, just like the human body on a tiny scale.) The "brain" of the cell is the nucleus. It contains chromosomes with DNA (deoxyribonucleic acid), the substance that holds the genetic key to all living things. A cell undergoes malignant change because the DNA has become faulty, perhaps through an environmental factor like cigarette smoke or radiation (although these specific factors are rare in children). In a malignant cell, the faulty genetic message gets passed on to its daughter cells, just as normal DNA is passed on to the daughter cells of a normal cell.

Combination Chemotherapy

Cancer cells can become resistant to individual drugs. In the early days of cancer chemotherapy, doctors gave patients a single drug for as long as it was effective. When there was a relapse, they switched to a new medication. This process was repeated until they ran out of drugs and the patient died. Today specialists use several drugs at the same time early in the treatment. This strategy has been the major factor in all subsequent successful treatment programs. Drug combinations are planned to take advantage of agents that have different methods of action or that work on different schedules.

Remission and After

Treatment for some forms of cancer, leukemia in particular, takes place in the following stages:

1. **Remission induction**. Several drugs are given in varying combinations to kill all detectable cancer cells.
2. **Consolidation**. After the child is in remission, additional agents or boosters (larger doses of the same drugs) may be used.
3. **Maintenance**. Chemotherapy is continued for varying lengths of time, depending on the disease itself, to get rid of "the last cancer cell."
4. **Relapse**. If the child relapses, the cycle is repeated with different drugs. While the prognosis is less favorable after a relapse, there is still hope of additional remissions and long-term survival, particularly if the child is not receiving therapy at the time the cancer reappears. Switching to a different combination of drugs may still achieve a successful treatment outcome.

Schedules, Doses, and Lengths of Treatment

Most pediatric cancer patients are treated by a planned course of therapy called a protocol. Chapter 15 has detailed information about protocols and clinical trials.

The drugs are often given over a series of visits followed by a few days or weeks of rest. Each series of doses is called a course. Chemotherapy treatments are carefully monitored by the team of specialists through blood tests and physical examinations. The major early side effect of most of the individual drugs and combinations is to lower the white blood count, the chief cells that fight infection. The count is thus checked before giving these medications. If it drops so low that there is danger of serious infection, there may be a pause in therapy while the body recuperates. Because many of the drugs are either activated or eliminated from the body by the kidneys or the liver, doctors also watch the functions of these organs carefully.

In the initial stages of chemotherapy, blood counts are taken before each course is started and several times over the next couple of weeks. The doctors are trying to find out when the nadir, or low point of blood counts, occurs in the individual patient. They are also watching for trouble, like an especially low platelet count. After a while, when doses have been adjusted and the doctors know how the child will react, some of the blood tests will be eliminated.

These interim tests may be carried out at your community hospital if that is more convenient. Be sure, in that case, that the results reach your clinic doctors quickly. If the community hospital needs written orders before they can perform the tests, perhaps they would be willing to keep a standard order on file or perhaps your doctor will give you a few laboratory slips to keep on hand.

You should have a small notebook that you always keep with you. This is the place to note the names and phone numbers, fax numbers, e-mail addresses, and other contact information for the cancer center and the community hospital, pediatrician, and anyone else you might need to reach in a hurry when you are distracted by a sick child. More suggestions for this pocket-sized essential book are noted in later chapters about supporting your child and handling finances.

Individual doses are based on the child's size, including height, weight, and body surface area. This is why he is measured at the beginning of every course of chemotherapy. Regular blood tests and physical examinations assure the doctors that the kidneys and liver are working properly. The child may also have frequent x-rays of the primary tumor site and places like the lungs where the particular type of cancer is known to metastasize. Urine will provide information on how well the child's organ systems in general are functioning, and in some cases either urinalysis or blood tests will be performed looking for tumor markers. These biochemical tattletales sometimes show that a cancer is recurring before it can be found on x-rays.

Most chemotherapy patients receive a lot of their medication by intravenous injection. This can be a real problem, not only because the drugs are so potent and potentially dangerous but also because young patients have tiny veins. Starting IVs day after day is painful for children, is extremely stressful for parents to watch, and requires patience and skill. As therapy continues, it becomes more difficult to find "good" veins. Some doctors and nurses are better at this than others. It helps if the same person starts the IV each time because he or she will know which veins are more reliable in your child. If the veins aren't cooperating, try putting warm compresses on the area to see if the blood vessels dilate. Lightly slapping or tapping a vein might also cause it to dilate in response. Hold the arm below the level of the heart. If the person starting the IV is having trouble and becoming frustrated, you might quietly suggest taking a break or ask tactfully that someone else start the IV. When she was in treatment, Lisa's veins were so notoriously difficult to "hit" that sometimes the paramedics (who are trained to start IVs in the most difficult circumstances like at accident sites) were called in.

Luckily, much of the IV drama has been defused through the use of skin creams that numb the area to cut down on discomfort. Many children also have indwelling catheters that reduce or eliminate the need for starting IVs on a regular basis. See Chapters 22 and 25 for more information on these welcome improvements.

Side Effects

The therapeutic index is the margin between an effective dose of drugs and a lethal one. In cancer chemotherapy, this is a very fine line. The side effects can be many and serious. It is hard to see your child so sick, but try to remember that if these drugs were not available, he would have a poorer chance for survival.

You probably cannot help being discouraged as you look at the drug table and note the side effects that are possible from these potent drugs. Remember that nobody gets all or even most of them. Almost all side effects are reversible when the therapy stops or even when the child's body becomes accustomed to the therapy. As we'll see, there are ways to avoid or minimize some side effects.

- Nausea and vomiting are common side effects of many chemotherapy drugs. Pills, suppositories, and injections or IV infusions may ease the symptoms; they are most effective when given before the chemotherapy begins, although response varies from patient to patient. Some children are given sedation and sleep through the nausea.
- Some of the chemotherapy drugs can cause constipation, which may be relieved by a change in diet or gentle laxatives.

- Diarrhea may last 2 to 4 days.
- Children receiving prednisone may experience heartburn or bleeding from the stomach or duodenum. Medicines can help prevent this side effect.
- A change in the way food tastes is not uncommon. Meat may taste unpleasant, other foods metallic and bitter. Sucking on a sour candy ball while the medicine is given may help.
- Mouth ulcers are a common side effect with some chemotherapy agents. If these are painful, your child may not eat enough food to keep up his strength. Mild painkillers and mouthwash can be prescribed to ease the pain. Remember, teeth cleaning is vital to avoid cavities, but try having the child use a sponge, a soft-bristled toothbrush, or a cotton swab. Have your child avoid very hot and very cold food and drinks, spicy and highly acidic food, and, of course, smoking and alcohol.
- The weight gain and elevated blood pressure that prednisone often causes through increased appetite and fluid retention may be somewhat controlled if your child avoids fatty and salty foods. Ask your pediatrician or the hospital dietitian for lists of foods to avoid; celery and potato chips, for example, have high sodium content. Otherwise there is little you can do about the weight gain.
- Hair loss is a common side effect of chemotherapy. Some patients lose only part of their hair, and some lose it all—more than once, and not just the hair on their heads but their beards, eyebrows, eyelashes, armpit hair, pubic hair, and leg hair can also be lost. My daughter lost all her hair twice, every single strand, but by the time she had been off chemotherapy for a couple of years, she had hair nearly to her waist. Another girl we know, an adolescent, lost her hair three times but has a lovely full head of hair today. This too shall pass. Upsetting as this surely is, particularly to teenagers, who have such sensitivity about their bodies, it is more important to get the disease under control and keep it there. Wigs are tax-deductible, but some hospitals provide them free of charge. If not, your insurance may cover a wig if your doctor writes a prescription for it. If you are going to get a wig, shop before the hair falls out for the best match in color and style. The hospital will have

a listing of shops that make children's hairpieces. Organizations that provide donated real-hair wigs to sick children are listed in Appendix B. Hair loss may be minimized by either cutting it short or keeping it in a braid or other style that minimizes brushing and combing.

- Low blood counts are very common with chemotherapy. The bone marrow, where blood cells are manufactured, has very fast-growing cells, which are more susceptible to the chemotherapy drugs. If the white count is low, there is a risk of infection; watch for fever, sores, or cracks in the skin, especially near the anus and in skin folds. A child who is tired, pale, and short of breath may be anemic, with a low red blood count. Bruising is an indication of a low platelet count. The clinic staff can combat all of these with transfusions of red blood cells and platelets. Do not use aspirin during therapy unless your primary doctor specifically orders it.
- Bladder irritation is a problem with some of the drugs. Giving the therapy early in the morning and forcing fluids for the remainder of the day helps. Popsicles are helpful here. We used a lot of apple juice because it was easier for Lisa to handle when she was nauseated, and also because it was less unpleasant to clean up when she did vomit. Blood in the urine or difficulty urinating is a symptom the doctor should know about right away. This may persist for several weeks or more. Redness in the urine for up to 2 weeks after the administration of doxorubicin (Adriamycin) and daunomycin probably isn't blood and is no cause for alarm, but report it anyway.
- Weakness, loss of coordination, loss of balance, and clumsiness may temporarily be seen. Guard against falls.
- Nerve damage can cause temporary tingling, burning, prickling, or numbness.
- Allergic reactions, some of them severe, may occur with a couple of the drugs. Because of this, initial doses may be given to the child on an inpatient basis. Otherwise, he is watched closely over a period of time in the outpatient clinic. Sometimes the needle is left in the vein for a while so an antidote can be given quickly if necessary.
- Liver damage is monitored with periodic blood tests.
- Kidney damage is evaluated by urinalysis.

- Skin burns at the site of the injection may occur with some of the medications if the needle comes out of the vein. If this occurs, the doctor or nurse may give a cortisone shot to minimize the burn. An ice pack and pain medication will help. If redness appears after you get home at the site where the medication was given, call the doctor.
- Skin rashes, which may itch and peel, should also be reported to the doctor.
- Sensitivity to the sun is a problem, particularly for patients receiving methotrexate. Sunglasses, protective clothing, and suntan lotions with a high sun protection factor (SPF) are sensible precautions.
- Heart damage, even congestive heart failure (a serious problem that results when the heart cannot pump as much blood as the body needs), can occur with Adriamycin. This is dose-related and cumulative, so the doctor will keep a careful record of the amount of this drug that your child has received. Daunorubicin has this effect as well, and it may occur at a lower dose in children who have had chest radiation. Symptoms to watch for and report to the doctor are difficulty breathing (at first, even after mild exercise, and then even when resting), wheezing, coughing spells, urinating more frequently at night, swollen legs, and eventually pallor or turning blue.
- Reproductive system effects may be noted in adolescents. Low sperm counts may result. This may be permanent or the count may increase as time passes after therapy is complete. Ask your medical team about possibly freezing your son's sperm for future use. Girls may have irregular periods, or they may stop menstruating completely for a time, but their periods may resume when therapy is finished. Researchers have harvested viable eggs from girls as young as 5 years old. In sexually active teenage girls, conception is unlikely during chemotherapy, but it is possible and must be avoided due to the risks to the fetus.

Special Treatments

Methotrexate is sometimes given in huge, normally toxic, doses, and then an antidote, citrovorum, is given after a period of time ranging from a few hours to a few days to stop methotrexate's action on normal cells and rescue the body from the lethal side effects. This is done sometimes in patients with leukemia, osteogenic sarcoma, and non-Hodgkin lymphoma. The therapy is not without risks: brain damage, liver damage, kidney damage, or even death may rarely result.

As was discussed in the leukemia and brain tumor chapters of Section I, killing tumor cells in the central nervous system can be difficult because of the biochemical shield that protects the brain, the blood–brain barrier. To bypass this, methotrexate may be injected directly into the fluid surrounding the spine and brain. Ara-C or hydrocortisone may also be given in this manner. Some other drugs like BCNU pass the barrier naturally, if given intravenously.

Palliation

As with surgery and radiation, chemotherapy may also be given as a palliative measure to relieve symptoms or temporarily control the growth of a tumor that may not be curable. The patient's life is prolonged as the tumor is controlled. Palliative management is discussed in greater detail in Chapter 22.

Other Treatments

Chemotherapy given in conjunction with radiation can enhance the beneficial effects of the treatments, but it can also enhance the toxic side effects. Actinomycin-D does the latter. Radiation may enhance the side effects of bleomycin on the lung if the drug is given either previously or concurrently.

Chemotherapy drugs also interact with other medications, which can cause problems. This is why your doctor needs to know everything your child is taking, including cold medications and other over-the-counter preparations and herbs.

Experimental Chemotherapy

Research on chemotherapy takes several directions. Some studies, for example, are investigating drugs that work only on exposure to light.

Others are using high drug doses to flood affected body cavities (regional perfusion). An implantable drug transfusion pump (ITP) is being tested on some patients. Yet another study is testing chemotherapy in an inhaled form for pediatric patients with lung metastases from bone cancer.

Researchers constantly search for new chemotherapy drugs that won't have serious side effects. They hope to learn, too, of antidotes that will counteract current drug toxicities, the way citrovorum works against methotrexate. No one expects to find a single drug or even a combination of drugs that will cure all types of cancer, because the disease occurs in many forms. Researchers are also trying to find out why some children become resistant to the drugs before every last cancer cell is wiped out, causing relapse and possibly death. Over a quarter of a million substances have been tried out so far in the search for effective drugs to combat cancer. Only a tiny percentage has proven effective against human malignancies.

New drugs are always under investigation. Such studies usually are limited to major medical centers because of the relatively large patient population and the capacity for rigidly controlled testing. These clinical trials are carried out in three stages. Phase I trials seek to establish the maximum dose that can be tolerated and the optimal schedule for a drug used on humans, although laboratory studies on animals have usually given researchers a solid starting point. Phase II trials study the antitumor response rate and side effects. Phase III trials are usually randomized studies to learn the real value of a new therapy or agent in comparison with other drugs, schedules, or doses.

Recordkeeping

Unfortunately, pediatric patients are harmed every day through medical errors. As reported in the *Journal of the American Medical Association* (*JAMA*), about 6% of prescriptions themselves contain errors. In addition, staff can make mistakes in administering the medications. These "adverse drug events" are more harmful to children because their immune systems are more fragile than those of adults. Parents and other caregivers who keep a close eye on the drugs given to their children are one line of defense. Computers are another. Using programs that double-check dosages and print out the prescription (avoiding the sometimes illegible doctor's handwriting) is another important step.

Hospitals that have computerized medical records provide laptops for staff to carry to the bedside and a wireless network for access to the institution's system. Several people can access the records at one time (on a need-to-know basis) and records are kept up to the minute, including patient data like vital signs as well as the care plan and treatments. Benefits of this system also include the ability to amend records, trace staff who are responsible for errors, alleviate paper shuffling and storage, and eliminate the need to repeat information over and over. At discharge the whole record can be printed for the patient. Computers also make it virtually impossible to falsify records. Vigilance is still essential to avoid medical errors. When pharmacists are included in patient rounds, errors can be reduced significantly.

Further Resources

READING

"Chemotherapy and you, a guide to self-help during cancer treatment."
   National Cancer Institute, revised 2007.
   Available online at www.cancer.gov/cancertopics/chemotherapy-and-you with additional information in the PDQ section. Handy one-size-fits-all guide to therapy, side effects, financial information, etc. Not specific to pediatric patients.

Fischer, David S., et al. *The Cancer Chemotherapy Handbook*. Philadelphia: Mosby, 2003 (6th edition).

Kaushel, Rainu, et al, "Medication errors and adverse drug events in pediatric inpatients." *JAMA The Journal of the American Medical Association*, vol. 285 (April 25, 2001), p. 2114–2120.

Krisher, Trudy. *Kathy's Hats: A Story of Hope*. Dayton, Ohio: Marianist Press, 1990.
   A picture book for young children, this story tells about the author's daughter Kathy, who had radiation and chemotherapy for Ewing sarcoma and had to contend with hair loss.

Templeton, Sarah-Kate, "Doctors freeze eggs of girls, 5". *The Sunday Times (London)*, July 1, 2007. Accessed online at www.timesonline.co.uk on July 25, 2008

Understanding Drug Therapy and Managing Side Effects. Leukemia and
   Lymphoma Society, 2007.
   Detailed information on specific drugs, especially helpful in advising
which side effects need medical attention. Also available at www.LLS.org.

ORGANIZATIONS/WEB SITES

Cleveland Clinic (www.chemocare.com)
   This Web site features champion ice skater Scott Hamilton, a testicular
cancer survivor. Care during chemotherapy and beyond. A comprehensive
site with information on drugs, side effects, and adjunctive therapies.

Medscape Drug Info Database (www.rxlist.com)
   Geared to professionals, this searchable online pharmacology site has
information on specific drugs, side effects, and warnings and advice.

Kemo Shark from Kidscope (www.kidscope.org/Kemo)
   Written for the children of cancer patients rather than pediatric patients,
the principles are still applicable.

National Cancer Institute (www.cancer.gov)
   Much up-to-date drug information written for the layperson.

Wigs for Kids (21330 Center Ridge Road, Suite 26, Rocky River, OH 44116;
440-333-4433; www.wigsforkids.org)
   Provides wigs kids can wear during activities like sports.

19

Bone Marrow and Peripheral Blood Stem Cell Transplants

B one marrow transplant (BMT), which was relatively new at the time of the first edition of *Children with Cancer* (1986), is no longer considered experimental. Since it has improved survival rates for leukemia patients, it is now available for more children (and adults) with other malignancies. This procedure involves giving potentially deadly doses of chemotherapy drugs and radiation, which ideally wipe out all remaining disease cells in the body. However, such intense therapy damages, and perhaps destroys, the bone marrow's ability to repopulate the body with new blood cells. It can take many weeks or months for the child's marrow to regenerate the blood cells. A marrow or stem cell transplant can shorten that period of weakened or nonexistent immunity to a couple of weeks. In these cases, the chemotherapy and high-dose radiation wipe out the disease and the transplant is a form of rescue.

Peripheral blood stem cell transplantation (PBSCT or just SCT) is a less invasive procedure that is replacing BMT in many cases. In some countries SCT has replaced BMT entirely, while other countries are conducting studies comparing the two methods in terms of patient outcome, incidence of graft-versus-host disease, time to engraftment, and donor comfort and the need for hospitalization.

New blood cells are formed in the marrow, a spongy material found in the hollows of the long bones. Thus, the first indications of disease may be seen in the marrow even before symptoms appear as a result of irregular blood counts in the peripheral blood, when the body is not getting enough oxygen, for example.

There are two major sources of transplant cells. An allogeneic transplant uses a donor's cells, while an autologous transplant uses the patient's own cells.

In an allogeneic BMT (donor to patient), healthy marrow is drawn from a carefully chosen donor and is given to the patient through an intravenous needle, much like a blood transfusion. With an autologous transplant (patient to self), the patient is the donor. Sometimes cells are drawn during remission and frozen should they be needed in case of relapse. Transplant material can be safely frozen for years.

With SCT the donor receives drugs to stimulate the growth of stem cells, which are then harvested through apheresis, a process that can be performed in a dialysis center.

Another potential source of stem cells for transplantation is banked umbilical cord blood. Some families preserve their cord blood in case it is needed in the future, although such precautions have rarely proven necessary. Cord blood that is donated to a bank for general use stands a much higher chance of being used. Since the number of cells from one umbilical cord is too small to help most patients, several may be combined. The number of antigens that need to match from unrelated donors in a cord blood transplant is generally less than from other donors.

Who are BMT/SCT Candidates?

In the past, doctors performed bone marrow transplants only on patients with end-stage disease, as a last effort to save a life. The results, not surprisingly, were poor. Today the procedure is often carried out when the patient is still reasonably strong and has a good chance for survival.

Doctors are still learning which patients are likely to benefit from this highly specialized procedure and which probably will not. Earlier, it was used exclusively for cancer patients with acute nonlymphocytic leukemia (ANLL or AML), which often does not respond well to chemotherapy. Patients in first remission for AML are often candidates for transplant, and tests have shown that the procedure is effective. Today it is sometimes done when there is a suitable donor in acute lymphoblastic leukemia (ALL) patients who relapse, since the child's chances for long-term survival are reduced if the first remission fails. Success is more likely if the patient receives the marrow while in remission, although a transplant may be performed during relapse in certain cases if necessary.

Children with various forms of leukemia are often candidates for BMT or SCT. Those with non-Hodgkin lymphoma in various forms (such as Burkitt lymphoma) and Hodgkin disease are rarely considered for these transplants if their cancer recurs. Some types of sarcoma, neuroblastoma, and testicular cancer have responded also. Clinical trials are investigating the use of these therapies for some brain tumors, Ewing tumor (therapy-resistant or relapsed), retinoblastoma (metastasized), and Wilms tumor (widespread, therapy-resistant malignancies).

Today patients with ALL are rated as high, moderate, or low risk. Those at high or moderate risk may be chosen for a BMT if they relapse while on maintenance chemotherapy. An appropriate donor must be available for an allogeneic (donor-to-patient) transplant. Autologous (patient-to-self) transplants are discussed later in this chapter.

Factors that are taken into account in choosing which patients will have transplants are the following:

- Is a compatible donor available (allogeneic transplant)? An identical twin (syngeneic transplant) may be ideal, but other close family members may be a good match.
- Has the child received central nervous system radiation? Children who have not have a better chance.
- What age is the patient? Younger patients do better than adults and so may be chosen first; optimal candidates are under 20.

Several factors can threaten the transplant's potential success:

- A recent serious infection
- Other underlying disease weakening the patient
- Severe psychological problems
- Damage to vital organs from the malignancy

Choosing a Transplant Center

There are hundreds of transplant centers in the United States, Canada, and abroad. The staff work together through national organizations to optimize the transplant process. Each center has slightly different procedures and protocols, and if time and logistics permit, families should visit the center before making a final choice. These institutions have differing requirements and if one might not accept your child, another will. Be sure to ask how experienced the center is with your child's specific diagnosis and situation. Ask about survival rates. Make sure the staff is experienced in working with pediatric transplant patients. Larger units generally have better outcome rates because of experience. Centers also vary in the level of isolation, in pretransplant preparation procedures, and in other ways.

Types of Transplants

BMT is being used less frequently today, replaced by SCT. A non-myeloablative or mini-transplant is an even newer option. Preparation for this procedure is easier on the patient, since the goal is not to destroy the patient's marrow completely before the transplant. These patients receive significantly lower doses of chemotherapy prior to transplant. Again, sicker and older patients can be candidates for these mini-transplants.

Matching Donors and Patients

Matching donors and patients is a very complicated task. Briefly, each person has a human leukocyte associated (HLA) antigen identified as proteins found on the surfaces of his cells. These HLA antigens are typed by special blood tests ("tissue typing"). A perfect HLA match is 6 of 6 antigens. An acceptable HLA match may be 4/6, 5/6, or 6/6.

The interaction of the graft (donor) and host (recipient) cells after the transplant is determined by how close the match is. Two possible results are "host-versus-graft effect" (rejection of the transplanted cells) and "graft-versus-host disease" (GVHD) (the donor cells attack the recipient's body). These reactions range from mild (barely noticeable) to severe (life-threatening). A little bit of GVHD may be a good thing, but a lot is dangerous.

To vastly simplify the explanation, think of the cells as teams wearing uniforms. If the recipient is a Red Sox player, the donor should also be from the Red Sox, although sometimes a Yankee will work, too (like the All-Star game when the rivals play together). After the transplant the Red Sox recipient accepts the foreign Yankees donor cells like a traded outfielder. The host-versus-graft reaction is not a problem. On the other hand, if the Yankees donor and the Red Sox recipient engage in a bench-clearing-brawl-like GVHD, the transplant is compromised.

While millions of people have registered with donor banks, finding a match for racially mixed patients is especially difficult, and on top of all that, gender matches are more successful. It is also harder to find donor matches for racial minority patients.

Choosing a Donor

Because identical twins have the same blood and tissue type, a twin is the perfect match, although not necessarily a good donor. With rare exceptions, only siblings can have completely compatible blood. Parents and other relatives are not as well matched but may be used as donors at some centers.

There is a 25% chance that any sibling will be a good donor match. Curiously, although tissue typing is an exact science, patient and donor need not have the same blood type. Centers perform BMTs in which the donor and the patient have different blood types. Special preparations and precautions are required, and when the procedure is over, the recipient has a new blood type—that of the donor.

Doctors at the Massachusetts General Hospital are testing dual simultaneous transplants, in which a donor gives bone marrow and an organ (a kidney, for example). Once the donor's marrow engrafts, the recipient's body will not recognize the organ as foreign. Then the patient will not have to take lifelong anti-rejection medications, as others must.

If the donor is a child, careful preparation and follow-up are necessary so the child understands what is happening. The child may feel responsible for the patient's future health, or he may feel that something he said or did is causing the illness. Some children feel they are being sacrificed for their sibling's sake, and others think they are being punished for their jealousy over the attention being lavished on the sick sibling. It is especially important to reassure the donor child that having a good tissue match for the transplant does not mean that he, too, will get leukemia. The child should know that, should the transplant fail, it is not his fault. In discussing this with the child, parents and professionals should listen to the child carefully for any false impressions he may have.

Depending on his age, the patient should be involved in the transplant decision, as should a child who has been identified as a donor. Encourage questions, and answer them honestly. If the child doesn't ask questions, don't assume he is okay with the idea and understands what will happen. Give the child plenty of chances to talk about the transplant.

Dangers to the Donor

The only physical dangers of BMT to the donor lie in any blood loss and in the use of anesthesia, which always carries some risk. However, in this case the donor is not deeply anesthetized or "out" for a long period, so the risk is minimal. PBSCT donors don't require anesthesia, so the risk is smaller.

Legal Ramifications

BMTs and SCTs have legal ramifications when the donor and the recipient are minors. Some states consider it a conflict of interest for the same parents to give permission for both the donor and the recipient to take part in the procedure. In these circumstances, a guardian is appointed by the court for the potential donor and a hearing is held to decide if the transplant should take place. Institutions usually develop their own internal review procedures to protect the interests of donor and recipient.

Preparation

As explained earlier, there are several potential sources of stem cells for transplants. The bone marrow is the body's nursery, where these cells grow and mature into different kinds of blood cells. While the bone marrow is much richer in stem cells, there are always some in the circulating blood. Another possibility is umbilical cord blood after a baby's birth. Families with a child with cancer or another blood disorder may wish to "bank" the cord blood of a newborn sibling. The process is expensive, so it is not routine after every birth. Other families may donate their cord blood for eventual use by a sick child. See the resource list at the end of this chapter for contact information for a cord blood bank. (The stem cells referred to here, incidentally, are not the same as the fetal stem cells used in research, which is so controversial in the United States.)

Getting ready for a SCT is different from preparation for a bone marrow procedure. Some drugs stimulate the formation and release from the marrow of stem cells. The screened donor is given these "growth factor" drugs that target certain types of primitive blood cells. These drugs are formulated to stimulate specific cells to proliferate. Neupogen, for example, is a granulocyte colony-stimulating factor (G-CSF).

After a few days of taking growth factor drugs, the donor (which in the case of an autologous transplant is also the patient) undergoes apheresis. The donor's blood passes through a centrifuge that spins out the stem cells and then returns the rest of the blood to the donor. The machine looks a lot like the equipment used for kidney hemodialysis, which uses the same blood cleansing principle. This process takes place over several days. The donor is connected to the machine for a few hours each day but is not hospitalized for the procedure. In fact, collecting stem cells in this manner is much easier on the donor, since it does not require hospitalization, anesthesia, or as much discomfort as a marrow donation. Until about the age of 10, child donors can only give bone marrow, although children as young as 2 or 3 may donate peripheral blood stem cells.

During apheresis, the donor may feel lightheaded, chilled, or slightly uncomfortable. The growth factor drugs may cause muscle aches and pains, headaches, or sleep disruption, but these symptoms disappear a few days after the last dose.

To avoid rejection of the transplant, the patient's own immune system is first "turned off," usually through high doses of the chemotherapy drugs like cyclophosphamide (Cytoxan), ara-C, or methotrexate. Total body radiation is effective in killing the recipient's marrow and is still used as a transplant preparation in some cases despite serious risk factors. This suspension of the immune system is essential to prevent the body from destroying the alien donor cells, but it is also dangerous, for it renders the patient helpless against any illnesses and infections. The drugs and smaller radiation doses, besides destroying the body's own immunity, should also kill off any malignant cells hiding within the body.

The recipient is hospitalized, probably in some form of isolation. Lots of fluids are required to keep the kidneys flushed to avoid damage from the drugs. Preparatory doses and regimens vary slightly from center to center, but today the radiation is usually given in split daily doses over a few days rather than as one huge total body jolt, causing fewer adverse effects on normal tissues.

In an autologous transplant, the patient in remission donates some of his own marrow, which is treated to kill any cancer cells by various means, and then is frozen. Should the patient relapse, a second remission is induced and the marrow is transplanted back. The chances for success are better if the relapse doesn't occur for at least 3 months after the marrow is drawn, because then it is more likely to be "clean," or free of leukemic cells. Autologous bone marrow transplants avoid complications such as GVHD.

The Procedure

The actual BMT procedure, in contrast to the preparation and aftermath, is quite simple. After a physical examination and tests to ensure he is healthy, the donor is taken to the operating room and usually given general anesthesia. Needles are inserted into the hip bone, marrow is withdrawn, and the needle is repositioned elsewhere in the bone to repeat the process. The bone is "punched" dozens of times to obtain enough marrow, depending on the size of the recipient.

After filtering it to remove bone fragments and fat cells, the marrow is injected into the recipient's vein like a blood transfusion. The transplanted cells then migrate to the centers of the bones, where, if all goes well, they will "take" (engraft) and begin in 2 to 3 weeks to manufacture a new supply of blood cells for the child.

With SCT, the stem cells collected from the donor through apheresis are injected into the donor, again like a blood transfusion, and the same engrafting process begins.

The Aftermath

The bone marrow donor, who may feel some pain in the hips after the proceedings, is discharged from the hospital a day or so later. Pain medications will relieve any brief discomfort, and any scars will be minimal.

The SCT donor has continued with his normal daily life all along.

The patient is usually kept in some sort of isolation for a time and is watched for signs of rejection of the transplanted marrow or symptoms of infection and other illnesses. His immune system will gradually improve in its ability to fight infection, but he may be at greater risk of illness for 6 months to a year or longer. Preventive antibiotics are useful here.

Isolation, with its potential emotional ramifications, has been found sometimes to be more debilitating for the patient and family than the protection against side effects it might provide. New trends are toward private rooms and adjacent clean areas, with visitors allowed. Rooms with special air flow and filtration systems play a role in keeping away dangerous germs. (These are similar to the HEPA vacuums and other equipment used by asthmatics, for example.)

Precautions like masks and gloves are essential; toys and games, videos, and other objects have to be disinfected. Visitors are carefully screened; those with colds or other illnesses, those with recent exposure to communicable diseases like chickenpox, or those who have recently received live immunizations are understandably barred from close contact with the recovering patient.

Also, the growth factor drugs that were given to the donor before collection of the cells may be given to the patient afterward to stimulate recovery. Besides Neupogen to stimulate granulocyte production to fight infection, another growth factor is Epogen, which stimulates the production of red blood cells. This is a little like using a different fertilizer for roses than for tomatoes.

Reactions

Sometimes the recipient's body recognizes the donated marrow as foreign and rejects it. In many patients the opposite happens—the donated marrow attacks the recipient. This GVHD ranges in severity from mild (maybe even beneficial) to potentially fatal. Developing in the second to fourth week after the transplant, symptoms include a skin rash or blisters; diarrhea; loss of some liver function, with yellow jaundice; and depressed bone marrow. The lungs and joints may be affected, or the child may develop mouth ulcers, infections, or nausea. GVHD is not a risk with autologous transplant. Some patients also develop a graft-versus-leukemia reaction, where the new marrow recognizes and attacks residual leukemia cells in the recipient, another beneficial reaction.

There are other potential hurdles after a transplant. Many bone marrow transplant patients who survive more than 6 months fall ill with herpes zoster, or shingles, a painful disease caused by the same virus as chickenpox. A small percentage die. The drug acyclovir has had good results against this illness.

Some BMT recipients develop cytomegalovirus (CMV), which arises from viruses common in some age groups. CMV outbreaks regularly occur in nursery schools and day care centers, for example. Recipients are also at risk of possibly fatal pneumonias.

Even if the marrow engrafts (or "takes hold") and begins to produce new blood cells, the patient may relapse with leukemia in the new bone marrow. The leukemia cells are not from the donor's marrow, but represent disease that was not wiped out by the drugs and radiation before the transplant.

The child will have to repeat all immunizations—killed vaccines 1 year later and live vaccines 2 years later. With donor transplants, there is an increased risk of infertility for both boys and girls; older patients may want to bank eggs (experimental) or sperm (standard therapy).

The Results

According to SEER (Surveillance, Epidemiology, and End Results cancer statistics gathered by the U.S. government and posted online), results of these transplants have been gratifying. With AML/ANLL, there is at least a 70% success rate in some children. If the patient is not in remission at the time of the transplant, whether he has an allogeneic/unrelated donor transplant or an autologous one, the chance for a cure is at best 30%. ALL patients (who are usually transplanted if they do not respond to therapy or if they relapse) have similarly hopeful results. With CML, transplantation has a success rate of 80% to 90%. With Hodgkin disease and non-Hodgkin lymphoma, in patients who have either relapsed or not responded to chemotherapy, there is a 30% to 40% possibility of cure.

Costs

A BMT is enormously expensive because of intensive nursing care, a potential 2-month hospital stay, and a host of regular laboratory tests. A transplant can cost $250,000. There have actually been some decreases in the costs due to mini-transplants and speedier recovery times from SCT because more outpatient care is possible. Insurance plans like Blue Cross/Blue Shield, Medicaid, or Major Medical may pay the medical costs for covered patients. However, the cost of several months of nonmedical expenses like travel, parking, meals, and living expenses if the center is not close to the patient's home (and it is not likely to be) can be prohibitive. In Canada, transplants are covered by the national health plan, but incidental expenses like travel may not be. Some financial assistance may be available through the Leukemia and Lymphoma Society.

The family's insurance and other financial resources will be checked to determine that the funds are available for the medical costs. Some insurance companies, however, do set coverage limits, and public assistance programs may balk at such an expense. Should a family need financial help, resources are listed in Appendix B for help with fundraising.

The hospital social worker may be able to help parents apply for grants from the American Cancer Society or the Leukemia and Lymphoma Society and to find decent alternative housing for their stay. Some clinics have special dormitories for the families of the patients, and others may have a Ronald McDonald house or an American Cancer Society Hope Lodge nearby. Appendix B lists organizations that arrange free transportation in some circumstances.

Whatever your housing and travel arrangements are, keep careful records and receipts of all out-of-pocket expenses and check with an accountant at tax time; most costs should be deductible if they relate directly to medical care.

Some outpatient housing facilities have special residences (including some Ronald McDonald houses with special isolation suites) where children can recover from their transplants. Other centers may have arrangements with nearby hotels or apartment complexes. The child is not necessarily kept in strict isolation for several weeks after the procedure, but in other centers the isolation rule is upheld. If children can recover near but not in the hospital, more transplant patients will be able to use BMT facilities.

BMT/SCT is a medical specialty that is performed in a growing number of centers in the United States. Because these hospitals have only a few beds at most, the waiting list for admission can be long. Some patients are placed on waiting lists at more than one center so they can take advantage of the first available bed and therefore the earliest possible transplant.

The Future of BMT/SCT

As with other therapies, researchers are constantly seeking ways to improve these treatments to provide the best chance of a cure while lessening the side effects. Trials are under way to determine the optimal doses of radiation and chemotherapy for the conditioning phase of the procedure. A mini-transplant may be used after standard doses of chemotherapy for patients who are too ill to receive the full dose of radiation and drugs that are customarily used. Researchers are also trying to improve procedures to modify bone marrow cells from mismatched donors, allowing transplants that were once impossible. Some centers are trying cyclic transplants, giving the conditioning regimen, then transplanted cells, then a recovery period, with the cycle repeated, depending on the protocol. This latter is more common with central nervous system tumors.

Further Resources

READING

Crowe, Karen. *Me and My Marrow, A Kid's Guide to Bone Marrow Transplants.* Funded by Fujisawa Healthcare, Inc. (now Astellas Pharma US, Inc.).

This booklet talks about the preparation for the process and the transplant itself and has lots of ideas for keeping busy while in isolation and getting back to your regular life. Available at www.meandmymarrow.com.

ORGANIZATIONS / WEB SITES

Association for Online Cancer Resources (www.acor.org)
ACOR has a discussion group online, BMT Talk.

American Bone Marrow Donor Registry (P.O. Box 8841, 2733 North St., Mandeville, LA 70448; 985-626-1749; 800-745-2452; www.abmdr.org)

Blood and Bone Marrow Transplantation (www.cancerindex.org)
A rich index with dozens of links to BMT and PBSCT sites in the United States and abroad.

Blood and Marrow Transplant Information Network (2301 Skokie Valley Rd., Suite 104, Highland Park, IL 60035; 888-597-7674; www.bmtinfonet.org)
Online newsletter. Education and support for families and patients. Lists of transplant centers on their website. Lots of helpful resources.

Caitlin Raymond International Registry (CRIR), University of Massachusetts Medical Center (55 Lake Avenue N., Worcester, MA 01655; 508-334-8969; 800-726-2824; 800-7-DONATE [for donors]; 800-7-AMATCH [for patients]; www.CRIR.org)
Coordinates searches internationally for BMT, SCT, and placental cord blood donors, with affiliates in 43 countries.

CancerBacup (www.cancerbacup.org.uk)
A United Kingdom organization "helping people live with cancer." Good information on bone marrow and stem cell transplants.

Children's Organ Transplant Association (2501 West Cota Drive, Bloomington, IN 47403; 800-366-2682; www.cota.org)
This national nonprofit organization helps children and young adults with fundraising for transplant-related expenses. Matching funds program. Must be U.S. citizen.

Cord Blood Registry (1200 Bayhill Drive, 3d Floor, San Bruno, CA 94066; 888-932-6568; www.cordblood.com)
One company banking umbilical cord blood cells.

Leukemia and Lymphoma Society (1311 Mamaroneck Avenue, White Plains, NY 10605; 800-955-4572; 914-949-5213; www.lls.org)
The Stem Cell Transplant Coloring Book is a road map through the process for younger children. Also many helpful and detailed booklets available on BMT and SCT.

National Bone Marrow Transplant Link (20411 West Twelve Mile Road, Suite 108, Southfield, MI 48076; 248-358-1886; 800-LINK-BMT/800-546-5268; www.nbmtlink.org)

Information resources and peer support programs. Extensive online information regarding the process, handling finances, and much more. A lot of help for caregivers sets this organization above many others. Excellent, thorough, and understandable. One publication with a lot of helpful tips and explanations, available online, is *A Resource Guide for Bone Marrow/Stem Cell Transplant: Friends Helping Friends*, to order or download from the Web site; also available in French Their *Survivor's Guide for Bone Marrow/Stem Cell Transplant* is another knowledgeable and practical guidebook available on their Web site or by mail.

National Cancer Institute (www.cancer.gov)

"Fact Sheet: Bone Marrow Transplantation and Peripheral Blood Stem Cell Transplantation: Questions and Answers" provides reliable and up-to-date information in a readable format.

National Marrow Donor Program (3001 Broadway St. NE, Suite 100, Minneapolis, MN 55413; 612-627-5800; 800-627-7692 [for donors]; 888-999-6743 [patient advocacy]; www.marrow.org)

Donor information. Patient advocacy. Federally funded. Computerized list of potential unrelated marrow donors. "Mapping the Maze: a Personal Financial Guide" is an especially helpful online publication.

National Transplant Assistance Fund (150 North Radnor Chester Road, Suite F-120, Radnor, PA 19087; 800-642-8399; www.ntafund.org)

Helps raise funds for transplant and catastrophic injury patients.

Starlight Foundation (www.bonemarrow.starlightprograms.org)

This organization has a great, clear explanation of bone marrow in a game-like video program for late elementary students and up (and pretty good for parents, too!).

World Marrow Donor Assn. (www.worldmarrow.org)

An international site based in the Netherlands with a registry of over 5 million potential donors, plus educational, research, and grant information. An umbrella organization for registries.

20

New and Experimental Treatments

Basic research attempts to determine exactly what cancer is—what happens to cause normal cells to multiply out of control and how to arrest and reverse that process without causing devastating side effects. As our understanding of this process increases, we are taking major steps towards finding a cure and, ultimately, preventing cancer before it starts.

Investigations are also under way seeking better diagnostic tools to identify tumors at the earliest possible stages. Researchers hope to develop easy and inexpensive tests to locate malignancies when they are most curable and to find more tumor markers that reveal the presence of cancer even before symptoms appear. More accurate methods of staging help doctors pick the best combination of treatments and the precise timing for optimal results. Locating chemotherapy agents with fewer and less debilitating side effects, with the most effective dose timetables, is an ongoing search.

Researchers are heartened, and rightly so, by advances in treating children with cancer, but they are still in the laboratories looking for more improvements. The ultimate aim of current research is to turn cancer from a life-threatening to a chronic disease, to keep patients alive for decades using drugs with no side effects. That day is not yet here.

While pediatric progress is remarkable, some are frustrated because the pharmaceutical companies don't automatically test each new drug specifically for pediatric use. The U.S. federal government has mandated pediatric studies in the past, but the "Pediatric Rule" was suspended by the U.S. Food and Drug Administration after pressure from the drug industry. Parent activists lobbied to ensure that all agents that are tested for adults are also investigated for the much smaller pediatric population, so the Pediatric Rule is again in force. The Candlelighters Childhood Cancer Foundation has been one source of information on this legislation. *Cure* magazine reports on the legal and technical advances. (See Appendix B for contact information.)

The federal Caroline Pryce Walker Conquer Childhood Cancer Act, passed in the summer of 2008, increases funding for pediatric cancer research by $30 million per year for 5 years, beginning in 2009. The act also provides funds for family and patient education, access to therapy, and creates a national childhood cancer database to identify trends in children's cancer rates.

Much but not all of the investigation revolves around new chemotherapy drugs and new ways to administer them. Other areas of research include immunotherapy, hyperthermia, angiogenesis, cancer vaccines, and photodynamic therapy.

Immunotherapy

Patients with known deficiencies of the immune system have an increased rate of cancer of various types, so it appears that the immune system helps determine whether or not a person gets cancer. Researchers now know that in some cases genetics is also a deciding factor.

Let's take a look at how a healthy immune system works. Antibodies are proteins a person's body manufactures to attack and neutralize foreign proteins, called antigens, which are found on the surface of virus or bacteria cells. Simply put, antibodies are the native good guys, who recognize and attack the invading bad guy antigens. (Again, think of the immune system as a sports team; their uniforms identify who's on which side.) Antibodies are produced by cells in the bone marrow and lymph nodes.

Macrophages are large white blood cells found in the liver, spleen, and circulating blood; they gobble up old red blood cells, making room for young replacements. Researchers are looking for ways to recruit the macrophages as allies by activating them with other drugs so that they consume cancer cells instead. Macrophages can remove the cells, but first they have to recognize them. Studies are searching for ways to use macrophages to clean up malignant cells that remain after chemotherapy, radiation, and/or surgery.

Other cancer researchers are trying to find ways to use the body's own immune system to destroy an invading cancer. This treatment is called immunotherapy. It is experimental and is not usually used alone but in combination with chemotherapy and radiation in an attempt to wipe out any remaining tumor cells.

Researchers theorize that tumor cells have unique antigens that the body should recognize as foreign (the other team). If the immune system is healthy, the tumor cells will be destroyed. Therefore, immunotherapy seeks to stimulate the body's defense mechanisms with foreign particles to wipe out the immunotherapy "germs" and the cancer cells as well.

Scientists at Wake Forest University in North Carolina are beginning human testing of a therapy that has been effective in eradicating cancer in mice, using white blood cells (granulocytes) from donors whose immune systems show high levels of cancer-fighting activity. The research is based on the discovery of "cancer-resistant" mice, whose white blood cells have proven highly successful in treating mice with advanced cancer.

One form of immunotherapy takes leukemia or other cancer cells from the child, treats them with radiation and drugs, and injects them back into the body. Vaccines against diseases like measles work this way. Antigens from the disease are created that remain in the body and attack the appropriate antigen whenever it appears again because the person has been exposed to measles viruses, to use the same example.

Agents of immunotherapy are also called biological response modifiers; some of the better known are interferon, interleukin, monoclonal antibodies, "vaccines," and colony- (or cell-) stimulating factors. These substances may prevent the spread of cancer or metastasis; many of them enhance the body's repair mechanisms, fixing normal cells hit by radiation or other therapies; and others may slow the growth of the cancer.

Cancer vaccines, though, differ from the familiar ones in a major way. While "shots" against childhood diseases and smallpox aim to prevent the disease, cancer vaccines would instead cure the disease after it has developed. These vaccines would be most effective against metastases, goes the theory. A vaccine used with melanoma, called Melacine, has been shown to extend survival in patients with advanced disease, yet with fewer side effects. Tests with small population groups have been promising, but large-scale clinical trials are needed.

Monoclonal antibodies have had a lot of press coverage and have raised hopes for some patients. Scientists create these special disease-fighting entities by tacking an antibody-producing cell (which is usually short-lived) onto a cancer cell (which usually lives a long time, at least in a laboratory mouse). The new, altered cell produces antibodies indefinitely, reproducing (cloning) repeatedly. With radioactive tags, the monoclonal antibodies may detect or diagnose cancer and assess the effectiveness of treatments, or perhaps sweep the body free of cancer cells after conventional therapies have had time to work. Rituxan is a monoclonal antibody shown to have some positive effect on recurrent or chemotherapy-resistant B-cell non-Hodgkin disease. Trials are under way with other lymphomas, leukemias, brain tumors, and other cancers.

What about interferon, the drug some in the media elevated to miracle status a while ago? Several varieties have been identified to date that have proven effective against virus infections. These proteins are made naturally by the body when stimulated by a virus or are cultivated in the laboratory. The three groups of interferon are alpha, beta, and gamma. These substances seem to interfere with the growth of the tumor rather than killing it outright (hence, "interferon"). Gamma interferon seems most potent in human trials. They are used in cancers of the kidney and bladder, melanoma, some lymphomas and leukemias (but not ALL), and Kaposi sarcoma.

Interleukins are several forms of colony-stimulating factors that encourage bone marrow cells to divide and differentiate into various kinds of blood cells. Some are used with donors in preparation for bone marrow or peripheral stem cell transplants. They are being tested in brain tumors, some forms of leukemia, some lymphomas, and melanoma. While some patient deaths due to side effects were seen in early tests, smaller doses are preventing them now.

Potential side effects of biological response modifiers include a rash, swelling at the injection site, flu-like symptoms, fatigue, serious allergic reactions, fever, and muscle aches.

Hyperthermia

Hyperthermia uses heat to treat disease. While it is an experimental tool in fighting cancer, the theory is far from new. Records show that the ancient Greeks, and perhaps even earlier civilizations, employed it. Hippocrates used red-hot irons on tumors in 400 BC.

The value of applying heat to cancer in hopes of eradicating it was suggested by a lucky happenstance. Some cancer patients who recovered from an infection with a high fever were found to be free of their malignancy as well, sometimes temporarily and sometimes permanently. Researchers are trying to figure out how to apply this knowledge to therapy.

Recent laboratory studies using cells from patients with neuroblastoma, Ewing tumor, germ cell tumors, and osteosarcoma show that hyperthermia has an enhanced effect on some chemotherapy drugs (called "thermochemotherapy").

Hyperthermia (exposing body tissues to temperatures as high as 106 degrees Fahrenheit) appears to be effective against cancer for several reasons. First, the growing tumor crowds the blood vessels that supply it, causing poor circulation. Because of this, the heat is held within the tumor longer than in nearby healthy tissues, increasing the tumor kill. Second, tumor cells die at a slightly lower temperature than normal cells, so the temperature can be carefully calculated to spare nonmalignant cells. Third, heat may stimulate the body's immune system, unlike chemotherapy and radiation, which suppress it. Heat also damages the cancer cell's ability to repair itself and enhances some chemotherapy.

Applying controlled heat beneath the body's surface is the most challenging aspect of the treatment, because the degree and the intensity of the heat, as well as accurate targeting, are important. The temperature and the length of heat exposure must also be carefully calculated for effectiveness.

Hyperthermia may be used for local tumors, on a body region (for example, a limb), or the whole body. In the case of local or regional therapy, radiofrequency long waves and microwaves heat the tumor or region to temperatures lethal to the malignant cells but tolerated by normal cells. Whole body hyperthermia is used against metastasis via special blankets or thermal chambers. Side effects can include pain and blistering at the treated site.

Angiogenesis Inhibitors

Pioneered by Dr. Judah Folkman at Children's Hospital in Boston, the discovery of angiogenesis inhibitors is one of the most watched of the newer cancer therapies. After receiving a great deal of media coverage early on, this therapy generated a huge demand for a treatment that was not at all close to patient trials.

Angiogenesis is the development of a blood supply by tissue. Cancer tumors thrive because they create their own network of blood vessels to "feed" them with nutrients and oxygen. If that blood supply were cut off, the tumor would starve to death. Trials are under way using anti-angiogenesis drugs like bevacizumab (Avastin) and cetuximab (Erbitux). Results have been mixed but promising.

In theory, this route gets around the obstacle that diverse cancer cell types pose. One cancer drug may hit, for example, a lymphoma but not a rhabdomyosarcoma. With anti-angiogenesis, the cell itself is only affected because the blood supply, presumably similar for all solid tumors, is "hit." The attacked blood vessels don't develop a resistance to the drugs.

Trials to starve tumors by anti-angiogenesis drugs have been started against leukemias, lymphomas, brain tumors, and Kaposi sarcoma. These substances can't be used with patients who need blood supply growth support, like those receiving colony-stimulating factors to stimulate peripheral stem cell growth prior to a transplant. Colony-stimulating factors are special drugs that help the body build the supply of blood cells before the procedure. Some early patients had strokes, lung bleeding, and other serious side effects, but as a rule, with current dosages, side effects have not been so severe. The theory is intriguing and will no doubt be in the news and of great interest as human trial results are generated.

Medical Robots

Modern imaging methods are becoming more precise and miniaturized, allowing doctors to "look" at areas of the body formerly invisible. A three-dimensional miniature endoscope is about the diameter of a human hair. Animal testing is under way with hopes for pediatric use in the future.

Photodynamic Therapy

Also called PDT, photoradiation therapy, phototherapy, or photo-chemotherapy, this cancer treatment under investigation uses the discovery that some chemicals can kill certain cells when they are exposed to a special form of light. Those chemicals are delivered to the cells by way of fiber-optics. To date the greatest use appears to be in lung and esophageal cancer as well as some surface skin cancer, because the path has to be so close to the tumor (about 1 inch). Bronchial tubes are used to deliver the drugs and light directly to the lungs or esophagus. After the therapy the patient will be light-sensitive for several weeks and must wear protective clothing out of doors. Side effects include (depending on the site) skin blistering, difficulty swallowing, coughing, or shortness of breath. Investigations are under way to find methods of delivering photodynamic therapy to deeper tissues. In the future PDT may play a role in treating brain tumors and other malignancies. Information on this and other exper-imental therapies is regularly updated on the National Cancer Institute's Web site (www.cancer.gov).

Prevention

Can we learn to prevent cancer? We already know we can reduce the risk of cancer by controlling certain environmental factors, such as cigarette smoking. It is especially hard to tell our children not to take up the habit if we haven't kicked it yet ourselves. Teenagers are much more likely to begin smoking if their parents do.

Using effective sunscreens to prevent burning or deep tanning has been recommended to avoid skin cancers. This includes exposure in tanning booths. Minimizing the use of medical x-rays is another helpful step in avoiding cancer.

We also know that diet plays some role in the development of cancer. Beta-carotene, a substance found in deep-colored vegetables like broccoli, carrots, spinach, and pumpkin, seems to reverse the pro-cess by which normal cells turn malignant. Studies at Oxford University in England showed that people who eat a lot of food high in beta-carotene have a lower cancer rate than might be expected.

The National Academy of Science/National Cancer Institute has issued some guidelines for those who hope to limit the chances that they will develop cancer:

- Cut down on salt-cured, salt-pickled, and smoked foods high in nitrates (bologna, ham, hot dogs, dill pickles).
- Lower the consumption of saturated fats to 30% of the diet. Decrease, therefore, the intake of fatty meat, whole milk, dairy products, and saturated fat cooking oils while increasing the use of olive and other vegetable oils.
- Increase daily consumption of fruits, vegetables, and whole grains. Vitamin C (found in citrus fruits; dark leafy vegetables like Swiss chard and spinach; carrots; winter squash; tomatoes; and members of the cabbage family, including broccoli and cauliflower) is especially good.

The body converts beta-carotene to vitamin A, which is also beneficial in protecting against cancer. Taking vitamins A and C in pill form is not a good substitute; the effect may not be the same and elevated doses may be harmful. Total intake shouldn't be higher than 100% of the recommended daily allowance (RDA) of vitamins. Cereal boxes are a good source of that information.

A high-fat diet leads to increased rates of cancers of the colon, breast, and prostate in some people. Following this reasonable diet will help protect your family against future malignancies as well as other preventable illnesses like heart disease.

Further Resources

READING

Groopman, Jerome E., "Luck of the Draw", chapter in *Second Opinions*.
New York: Viking, 2000.
This chapter looks at interferon, so called because it "interferes" with the growth of viruses and cancers. Lucid and interesting discussion of testing the three types (alpha, beta, and gamma).

Hall, Stephen S. *A Commotion in the Blood: Life, Death and the Immune System*. New York: Holt, 1997.
Highly recommended report on various attempts to harness the immune system against cancer. Monoclonal antibodies, interleukin-12, and more, from a science journalist.

ORGANIZATIONS/WEB SITES

Cure magazine (www.curetoday.com)

This Web site provides the full text of the excellent quarterly periodical *Cure*. Issues have current information on all aspects of therapy and various cancer types. Not specific to pediatrics. Back issues are online and a mailed subscription is free. See the Summer 2008 issue for an update on pediatric cancer drug research.

21

Alternative and Complementary Treatments

When your child is diagnosed with cancer, friends and relatives (and sometimes even complete strangers) might approach you to suggest or promote nontraditional forms of therapy. Some of these treatments might well be beneficial, when combined with conventional therapies. For the purpose of this book, the unconventional therapies are broken down into *alternative* (unproven) and *complementary* treatments.

Alternative treatments are those whose proponents recommend using them in place of some standard therapies. These unproven methods can border on—or cross into—quackery. *Complementary* therapy is a course of treatment used alone or in conjunction with conventional treatments. The goal for this approach may be to increase the patient's chance of a cure or to alleviate side effects of the radiation or chemotherapy, for example.

While a full discussion of all (or even most) of the current alternative or complementary therapies is beyond the scope of this book, a brief look into several of the better-known modes is in order.

Alternative (Unproven) Treatments

Alternative therapy is a course of treatments undertaken by a patient instead of conventional modes in general use like surgery, radiation, and chemotherapy. Some patients switch from conventional to alternative treatments during therapy for a variety of reasons—perhaps with a hope of better results, a wish to avoid unpleasant or debilitating side effects, or a belief that a completely altered approach by a different sort of practitioner is desirable, particularly as the often-long haul of standard treatment looms through the foreseeable future.

These methods often involve theories that are either far out of the mainstream or, in some cases, based on reasonable-sounding theories that have not been, or cannot be, proven effective in clinical studies.

Beware of unproven methods. When things go wrong with conventional therapy, there is a temptation to try anything. This temptation might even arise when reading the lists of potential side effects from other treatments. Be skeptical of anyone promising a "sure cure," particularly if it is claimed to have no side effects; dishonest people will promise anything. This is especially cruel because doctors providing conventional therapy cannot guarantee results. At their worst, "quacks" draw patients who may have a real chance at a cure with conventional therapy away from their doctors and substitute questionable or worthless treatments. Parents owe it to their children to get the best help available to give them the best chance at a long and healthy life, even if there must be temporary disability.

Although the emphasis of this book is on standard therapies, several unproven cancer treatments are discussed here because most readers will undoubtedly have heard of some of them. Sources with more detailed discussion of unconventional treatments are given at the end of this chapter for those who are interested.

Laetrile

Laetrile is a well-known unconventional therapy, perhaps less common today. Made from apricot pits, the drug contains cyanide, a poison. Laetrile is claimed to work by releasing cyanide into the cancer cell and killing it, yet sparing normal cells. It is also said to relieve pain and the general sickness of late-stage cancer, to shrink tumors, and to prolong lives. Larger doses of laetrile taken orally can be fatal. It is possible that laetrile may indeed control some pain, but so do many other, safer, substances.

Laetrile, also called amygdalin, vitamin B-17, and Aprikern, is not approved for use in the United States, and people wishing to try it go to clinics outside the United States, particularly in Mexico. One proponent insists that hospitals in Mexico and Germany achieve nearly 100% recovery rates with those who "have not yet been burned up with chemotherapy and radiation."

At the urging of proponents, the National Cancer Institute completed patient trials with laetrile. No effect was found, even when it was given in conjunction with the special diets often prescribed as an adjunct. Supporters of the drug, however, have rejected the results of these tests and insist that they are entitled to freedom of choice. The courts have generally agreed that adults may choose unproven methods for themselves but not for their children.

Antineoplastons

Antineoplaston is a "safe, nontoxic" therapy developed by Dr. Stanislaw Burzynski to attack cancer at the genetic level. The approach is quite in line with some current hot theories in cancer research, but so far the actuality is unproven. Burzynski has been cleared of medical fraud charges but to date controlled clinical trials have not shown antineoplaston to be effective in treating cancer, except, perhaps, in very limited circumstances. Interestingly, antineoplastons have been awarded "orphan drug" status by the U.S. Food and Drug Administration. Trials indicate that some patients with high-risk or recurrent primitive neuroectodermal tumor or brain stem glioma benefit from the Burzynski preparation. The doctor continues to attract the attention of patients and parents, drawn by his insistence that "antineoplastons can help patients with… a wide array of different cancers such as prostate, brain, breast and lung…"

Shark Cartilage

The theory behind the use of shark cartilage in cancer therapy is the notion that sharks don't develop malignancies, and therefore a derivative of their cartilage should fight the disease in humans. Three possible means of effectiveness have been studied: as a direct killer of cancer cells, as a stimulant to the body's immune system, or as a blocker of a tumor's blood supply (angiogenesis) needed for growth. (This should not be confused with the late Dr. Judah Folkman's anti-angiogenesis studies.) Human studies are under way to investigate these claims for shark cartilage (also called Carticin, Cartilade, and BeneFin), with results to date inconclusive at best. The Cleveland Clinic suggests that the Neovastat form has some benefit with multiple myeloma patients.

Nutritional Therapy

Advocates of nutritional therapy claim that it cures cancer; processed foods are eliminated from the diet and careful preparation is required of the items that are permitted. Juices made from vegetables and cooked calves' liver certainly will not hurt you if they are taken as part of a well-balanced diet, but they will not cure cancer, either. A moderate diet is essential for all cancer patients, who need nutrients drawn from all food groups to rebuild damaged tissues and to gain strength to withstand the side effects of therapy. A low-calorie or low-protein diet can lead to malnutrition and subsequent deterioration in the patient. Some nutritional therapy regimens permit only raw foods; another stresses wheatgrass. There has been much research on links between diet and cancer, and the results are inconclusive. Contrary to some slanted news reports, no reputable doctor will deny patients the right to wholesome food.

Nutritional therapy, often undertaken with laetrile, includes the use of frequent coffee enemas to "clean out bad cells in the bowel."

Interest in nutritional therapy has had a beneficial effect because it stimulated the medical community to take a closer look at the role diet plays in our health generally. Doctors today may be more willing to accept a special diet, assuming it is not bizarre, as a compromise with nutritional therapy.

Harms of Unproven Therapies

Unproven treatments can harm the patient in more ways than physical. Quackwatch, an anti-unproven-therapies Web site, reports that billions of dollars are spent each year on what they term "cancer quackery." Insurance companies do not pay for these treatments, which can be very expensive; a single month's treatment of one alternative cancer therapy is estimated at $7000 to $14,000. Stories abound of families spending their life savings, even losing their homes, while trying to save a loved one's life.

Other treatments can cause dreadful side effects or delay conventional therapy to patients who have a very real chance of surviving their disease. Psychological harm can also result for the patient and the family who place their trust in methods that are untrustworthy and likely to cause more harm than good, including premature death.

It is important to remember that many of the people who testify that these therapies cured them have not had tests to determine whether they had cancer in the first place. Others had conventional treatments before turning to unproven methods, but insist on attributing the success to the latter.

Why do people choose unconventional therapy over standard treatments, particularly since such strides are being made now? Part of the blame must rest with the medical community. Some doctors are arrogant; others hold back or withdraw emotionally from the patient when the therapy doesn't work well. And no honest doctor can guarantee that conventional therapy will cure any individual patient. This contrasts sharply with many centers offering unproven treatments. They are often staffed with caring, warm, supportive people who will absolutely guarantee that they can help. Amazingly, families of patients who died despite unconventional therapy continue to sing the praises of these centers, their friendly staff, and the treatments themselves. Whatever else they may do, quacks make people feel good. Doctors could learn something from them.

Complementary Treatments

Some of the better-known complementary treatments are relaxation therapy, meditation, guided imagery, hypnosis, humor, acupuncture, biofeedback, massage therapy, prayer, and spirituality. Used in conjunction with traditional therapy, these efforts may indeed be a big help to the patient. They might lessen some side effects such as nausea and vomiting. They might stimulate the immune system to better fight the disease. They might help a patient feel more "in control" of his disease and the therapy. They might reduce stress, improve the patient's sense of well-being, and strengthen the will to live. They might be a bridge to a larger support community, such as a religious group. They may well greatly improve the patient's quality of life.

Indeed, alternative, complementary, and even unproven therapies may someday be proven effective in some way against disease. In the meantime, though, the wise consumer balances the orthodox with the unorthodox for the greatest chance for survival.

Whatever course of action is chosen, however, it is vital that the primary physician be aware of all treatments and drugs, even over-the-counter medications, that the child is taking. Adverse reactions can occur even with the most innocuous-seeming preparations.

Faith and Prayer

"There are no atheists in foxholes," it is said, and there may not be many in childhood cancer clinics, either. At any rate, whatever the religious background of the family, many turn to faith communities for support. Having faced crises both alone and with the practical and spiritual help of a congregation, I have found the latter to be infinitely more bearable. Some groups pray for patients, and clergy from all faiths are available, both in the community and likely on the hospital staff, to work with the patient and the family.

When Lisa was undergoing therapy and even afterwards, a favorite stop at the Massachusetts General Hospital was the lovely little chapel with its blue stained-glass windows. Medical centers have chapels for personal prayer and meditation, for regular worship services of many faiths, and for memorial gatherings. Recent research has suggested, interestingly, that patients who were the unknowing subjects of intercessory prayer actually had fewer postoperative complications and less pain than those in control groups.

Some groups rely on faith healing, in which case the therapy would be alternative rather than complementary.

Humor

There seem to be two major coping mechanisms for crisis: tears and laughter. While many can attest to the stress-relieving value of a good cry, a good laugh can provide the same benefits.

Research has verified the role of humor in medical therapy. The movie *Patch Adams* told the story of a physician with unorthodox methods of healing—low-tech, no insurance, no bills, just a fun-filled family practice.

Patty Wooten's *Compassionate Laughter* has many concrete ideas for using therapeutic laughter to heal body and spirit. She includes many suggestions for discovering and developing the humor in tragic or difficult circumstances—humor for hope, for stress relief, to combat staff burnout, even gallows humor to transform the intolerable into the bearable (which admittedly might not be appreciated by everyone). Wooten talks about a comedy cart to carry humor to the bedside, suggests humor baskets with toys and gadgets, and offers an extensive list of resources.

Researchers hypothesize that laughter stimulates the immune system, attacks the biological stress response, and increases tolerance to pain.

For Nausea and Vomiting

Psi bands are cool-looking bracelets that use wrist acupressure, an ancient healing art, to relieve nausea. Little research has been conducted on Psi bands for nausea relief in cancer patients, but the bands use no drugs and therefore cause no drowsiness. Specifically for children, SeaBands come in bright colors most kids would love to wear. More information is available on Web sites cited at the end of this chapter.

Hypnosis, Guided Imagery, and Mind/Body Therapies

Writing in the *Journal of the National Cancer Institute,* William Redd notes that research has shown hypnotic-type behavioral intervention—hypnosis, guided imagery and relaxation—to be effective in controlling anticipatory nausea and vomiting, anxiety, and distress. It shows great promise in pain management. Its use in post-chemotherapy nausea and vomiting, however, is less clear. Still, this behavioral modification has "an important place in the care of patients undergoing invasive cancer treatments."

Hypnosis and guided imagery have different but related approaches to helping the child cancer patient. Karen Olness and Gail Gardner, writing in *Hypnosis and Hypnotherapy with Children,* explain that "[h]ypnotherapy is a treatment modality in which the patient is in the altered state of hypnosis at least part of the time [and then] treated with any number of methods ranging from simple suggestion to psychoanalysis." Possible benefits include pain relief or reduction, dealing with needle phobia, helping to alleviate nausea and vomiting, facilitating ER procedures like anesthesia induction, and postoperative cooperation.

Hypnotherapy has benefits for the dying child as well as for the family and other supporters. As the patient's anxiety and depression decrease, so do the family's. Additional benefits that should please the HMO bottom-liners are studies that indicate hypnotherapy can reduce the number of ER visits for chronic illness, decrease the need for medications, and significantly reduce the overall health care costs for trained children.

Guided imagery, according to Dr. Roxanne Daleo, is "a powerful form of mind/body medicine...now helping people of any age...cope with difficult medical treatments and the everyday stresses of life... using relaxation exercises, positive mental images, and special breathing techniques."

Guided imagery, also called visualization, involves varied techniques, some going back to ancient times. One is the Simonton method, developed by a doctor and his psychotherapist daughter, in which patients imagine, for example, chemo drugs like missiles attacking cancer cells and winning the battle.

Potential benefits parallel those for hypnosis—alleviate chemo-related nausea and vomiting, relieve stress, enhance the immune system, help with weight gain, fight depression, and lower pain levels.

While hypnosis and guided imagery do not cure cancer, these therapies can make patients more comfortable and give them a greater feeling of control over the disease.

An excellent package of guided imagery materials for use with children has been published by Nancy Klein of Inner Coaching in Watertown, Wisconsin. Her practical manual is accompanied by a workbook for children from the ages of 4 to 12 as well as a CD with soothing stories, relaxation techniques, and music and a related activity kit with toys, stickers, and the like in a convenient carrying bag. Materials such as these are a real boon to parents and others who want to calm their children and ease their distress.

Storytelling/Journaling

Dr. Noelle Holly, writing on the "Mind/Body-Oncology Connection" on the Internet, cited storytelling as an ancient coping tool with modern applications. Researchers in Great Britain showed that cancer patients who share their stories understand their illnesses better and lighten their emotional burdens.

Massage Therapy

Many articles have been published demonstrating the value of light- and medium-touch massage therapy for childhood cancer patients. Massage can help relieve anxiety, pain, depression, and other side effects of treatment. Some researchers think massage may improve immune function. The noninvasive therapy is useful for physical as well as emotional relief. Parents and other caregivers can also benefit from massage.

Further Resources

READING

American Cancer Society's Guide to Complementary and Alternative Cancer Methods. Atlanta, GA: ACS, 2000.

A comprehensive and encyclopedic gathering of information presented in an easy-to-use and understandable format. Hundreds of therapies, from acupuncture to zinc, are evaluated—what they are, history, risk factors. See also the ACS Web site www.cancer.org for up-to-date information; use their internal search function.

Bogner, David. *Cancer: Increasing Your Odds for Survival.* Alameda, CA: Hunter House Publishers, 1998.

In-depth information and advice on combining mainstream, alternative, and complementary therapies in the battle against cancer. Not specifically pediatric in focus.

Bombeck, Erma. *I Want to Grow Hair, I Want to Grow Up, I Want to Go to Boise.* New York: Harper and Row, 1981.

The beloved humorist's discussions with childhood cancer patients. Delightful and encouraging.

Cassileth, Barrie R., PhD. *The Alternative Medicine Handbook: the Complete Reference Guide to Alternative and Complementary Therapies.* New York: W. W. Norton & Co., 1999.

A source with broad coverage but including an especially good section on humor therapy.

Daleo, Roxanne. "How your mind can help you feel better". *CCCF Youth Newsletter*, vol. 19, 1 (Winter 1997), pp. 1.

Gordon, James, MD, and Sharon Curtin, MD. *Comprehensive Cancer Care: Integrating Alternative, Complementary and Conventional Therapies.* Cambridge, MA: Perseus Publishing, 2000.
A thoughtful, careful, and authoritative discussion of the more experimental types of therapy for patients in every stage of the disease. Dr. Gordon is director of the Center for Mind-Body Medicine in Washington, D.C., and believes that combining standard and complementary therapies is the future of effective health care.

Holly, Noell (Dr.). "Mind/Body-Oncology Connection". Available at www.mdlinx.com, accessed July 25, 2007.
Holly cites A. Carlick, et al. Thoughts on the therapeutic use of narrative in the promotion of coping in an internet breast cancer support group. *Psycho-oncology* vol. 14 (2005), pp. 211–220.

Hughes, Deborah, et al. Massage therapy as a supportive care intervention for children with cancer. *Oncology Nursing Forum*, vol. 35 3 (May 2008), pp. 431–442.

Klein, Nancy. *Healing Images for Children, Healing Images for Children Activity Book and Healing Images for Children*, Relax and Imagine CD.
Available from Inner Coaching, 1108 Western Avenue, Watertown, WI 53094 (920) 262-0439; email kids@readysetrelax.com; www.innercoaching. com. A highly recommended integrated program written by a cancer survivor; the CD has relaxation exercises and stories that tie to the book, and the activity book is more than a coloring book, meant to be written and drawn in to serve as a memory book. The target age group is 4 to 12. There are games, writing suggestions, puzzles. The few illustrated human forms have neither gender nor racial identity. Some activities are also therapeutic in improving eye–hand coordination, for example.

Komp, Diane, MD. *A Child Shall Lead Them; Lessons in Hope from Children with Cancer*. Grand Rapids, MI: Zondervan, 1993. Also, *Hope Springs from Mended Places*. Grand Rapids, MI: Zondervan, 1994.
Dr. Komp is a pediatric oncologist. Her books explore the faith of sick, often dying, children. Highly recommended.

Olness, Karen, MD, and G. Gail Gardner, PhD. *Hypnosis and Hypnotherapy with Children*. Gruen & Stratton, 2d edition, 1988 (newer edition not seen).
In-depth discussion of the benefits of hypnosis in treating children or alleviating side effects.

Redd, William H., et al, "Behavioral intervention for cancer side effects." *Journal of the National Cancer Institute*, vol. 93 (11) (June 1, 2001), P. 810–823.

Wooten, Patty, RN. *Compassionate Laughter: Jest for Your Health*. Salt Lake City, UT: Commune-A-Key Pub., 1996.
Many suggestions for implementing humor in tragic or difficult circumstances. Has an excellent, comprehensive list of humor resources.

ORGANIZATIONS / WEB SITES

About.com
The Internet search engine has an interesting article about "How to Spot Fake Cancer Cures." Go to www.cancer.about.com and use their internal search engine.

Academy for Guided Imagery (10780 Santa Monica Blvd., Suite 290, Los Angeles, CA 90025; 800-726-2070; www.acadgi.com)
Check here for conferences and workshops, research reports on distraction and guided imagery for pediatric chemotherapy and surgery patients.

M.D. Anderson Hospital (www.mdanderson.org/departments/cimer)
The Texas hospital's Web site for complementary and integrative medicine.

Anti-nausea bands: Check these manufacturers' websites for further information:
http://www.psibands.com/
http://www.sea-band.com/

The Cancer Club (P.O. Box 24747, Edina, MN 55424; 800-586-9062; 612-944-0639; www.cancerclub.com)
Has a list of books, tapes, and other gift ideas for cancer patients as well as a quarterly newsletter with humor and patient stories.

National Cancer Institute (www.cancer.gov)
Check here for current clinical trials of new and yet unproven therapies.

National Institutes of Health, Office of Cancer Complementary and Alternative Medicine (www.nccam.nih.gov)
Extensive information on various unproven therapies.

Quack Watch (www.quackwatch.org)
"Your Guide to Health Fraud, Quackery and Intelligent Decisions." Unabashedly pro-conventional therapy, this Web site carries extensive essays by mainstream doctors who pull no punches in denigrating various cancer (and other) treatments that have not passed stringent clinical trials. Talkback "cheers and jeers" from the site's visitors add another dimension to the material.

22

Supporting the Child Through Therapy

B esides major treatments like chemotherapy, some other procedures and precautions are carried out on children with cancer.
The procedures described in this chapter are not specific to any one
kind of malignancy but apply to cancer treatment generally.

Central Lines and Other Catheters

Since the first edition of *Children with Cancer* was published in 1986,
one of the biggest changes in treating children has been the wide use
of central lines and other indwelling catheters. In cancer's "dark ages"
when Lisa was treated, children were constantly prodded and poked
with needles. Finger sticks or venipunctures for blood tests, intravenous lines for chemotherapy drugs, fluids, and blood transfusions—
these were a daily occurrence. In many of the patients, with their tiny
or uncooperative veins, multiple "sticks" were a given. Except for
bone marrow aspirations and similar "deep" procedures, no painkillers were used to numb the skin or injection site.

These daily sessions were agony for the staff and families as well
as for the patients. It is astounding how the kids usually developed a
stoic attitude, with plenty of tears and howls to be sure, but they were
very forgiving. After each IV was started, the doctor or nurse often

jury-rigged a protective device using torn Styrofoam cups and lots of tape.

Fortunately, those days are in the past. Today it is common for the child to have a catheter or other indwelling device implanted and left in place for months or even years. These appliances, of several types, save the patients from the endless sticks and pokes. Blood is drawn, drugs are administered, fluids are infused, all through these catheters.

The following information is by no means complete; it's intended as a quick introduction to these catheters. Your clinic or hospital will provide booklets and other instructions to explain insertion and care of the devices.

The uses and benefits of catheters and ports include the following:

- Give medicines: chemotherapy drugs, antibiotics, pain medications
- Draw blood for testing
- Transfuse blood
- Hydration, IV fluids
- Total parenteral nutrition (TPN)
- Useful in an emergency to give fluids or medications quickly
- Allow thicker medicines to be delivered to larger veins
- Allow larger doses of chemotherapy drugs because the risk of damage to small vein walls is eliminated
- Avoids skin and tissue damage from strong drugs that could burn
- Avoids the constant need for IV sticks, which can polarize the parent and child against the caregivers who must find useful veins

However, problems can occur with catheters and ports:

- The sites can become infected or the tubes clogged.
- Daily or regular care is required to keep them clean and functioning.
- The patient or the family/caregivers may be daunted by this sophisticated device. Despite training at the clinic or hospital, they may feel unable to care for it. Print brochures and online resources will reinforce the training, but some may still be wary.

Types of Catheters and Ports

Most familiar is the "peripheral venous access" IV, which is practical for short-term use, but after about 3 days, a new IV will be needed (perhaps sooner, of course). This is used primarily but not exclusively for inpatients, and their arm movement must be limited to prevent dislodging the IV tubes.

CENTRAL VENOUS ACCESS DEVICES (CVAD), CENTRAL VENOUS CATHETERS, CENTRAL VENOUS LINES

These are tunneled about 6 inches through the patient's chest skin, through large vessels to the superior vena cava, the large vein that empties directly into the heart. Placed during day surgery in the operating room, these devices are known as Hickman, Broviac, Leonard, or other names, and they can remain in place and useful for months to years for blood draws, stem cell transplants, and drug administration. One or more "tails" come out of the chest area for access; after the surgical wounds have healed, there is little effect on daily activities. Even baths or showers are acceptable as long as the dressing is covered with plastic and tape; if the dressing gets wet, it should be changed. Blockage of the catheter or infection is possible, and the tubing might be misplaced because of coughing or other movements. Several inches of tubing protrude from the skin and are looped, then taped to the dressing. Some clever parents make special tee shirts with pockets for the loops.

PERIPHERALLY INSERTED CENTRAL CATHETERS (PICC)

These devices are implanted under sterile but not operating room conditions, with skin-numbing but not general anesthesia; older children may be awake during the procedure. Placed in an upper arm vein, they are threaded through to the superior vena cava, where stronger drugs may be safely infused. They are more likely to be visible when the patient wears short-sleeved clothing. PICCs can remain in place for weeks or months and perhaps longer.

Short-term subclavian catheters are placed via the jugular vein, are not tunneled, and have a useful life of days or weeks. Deseret and Arrow are two brands.

Vascular access ports are internal catheters implanted during day surgery for intermittent use. Because they are completely under the skin, topical anesthetics like EMLA may be used when accessing them. Port-a-Cath is an example of this device. A reservoir about the size of a quarter is implanted under the skin to hold a small amount of liquid, to be carried via catheter into a vein for circulation in the body. This type of catheter has a life of months or even years for occasional use, like chemotherapy drugs given once a month. Two big advantages to this type of catheter: there is no external device for kids to grab, and it requires no home care.

When using the various types of catheters and ports, vary the tape location a little bit each time you apply it to reduce skin irritation. Products that may ease some of the catheter care procedures include Microdon (a soft paper bandage available in different sizes), Tegaderm (which covers a skin patch to help hold it in place), Detachol (adhesive remover), and Cavilon No Sting Barrier Film from 3M (put on before Tegaderm to make removal easier). Nurses in your clinic or hospital will likely have other favorites to recommend.

A survivor's discussion list online recently had a thread about children's varied reactions when the tubes are pulled for the last time (which will probably not be immediately after active treatment is completed, but within weeks). Some give the tubing an honored place in their homes or scrapbooks; one family hung it on the Christmas tree! Others just throw it away. Your family will no doubt know what to do when that happy time comes.

Hydration

With intravenous chemotherapy medication, flushing the drugs through the body is essential. Until recently that meant the patient had to stay in the hospital, often for days on end. Children's Hospital of Boston has a new program allowing families to give the fluids at home or in other non-hospital residences like Ronald McDonald houses.

Managing Infection

Infection is not as much of a problem today, given the number of antibiotics available, but for children with cancer, particularly those not in remission, it is the leading cause of serious complications and death. Infection may be caused by medical procedures such as finger sticks or starting IVs (much less frequent today than in the past), inserting catheters or drainage tubes, radiation, or surgical wounds.

Infections are generally caused by bacteria, viruses, and fungi. It is not usually helpful to isolate the patient in hopes that he will avoid bacterial infections, because we get sick from our own germs on the skin or in the gastrointestinal tract as well as from stray ones in the environment. Children with cancer, like other kids, often get colds and also are susceptible to skin infections in the rectal area.

Your doctor may suggest or take a few precautions to lessen the possibility of infection:

- Always wash your hands thoroughly before entering the child's room.
- Keep bottles of waterless liquid/gel antibacterial cleaner in your pocket or purse and use it regularly. Hospitals and clinics have dispensers available for a quick "de-bugging." (However, neither this product nor the packaged wet-and-dry napkins, while very useful in a pinch, is a complete substitute for soap, water, and a little gentle scrubbing.)
- Avoid inoculations of live viruses like polio, measles, and smallpox.
- Avoid taking temperatures rectally.
- Avoid enemas. (At last! Some good news for the kids!)
- Alternate the sites where IVs are started.
- Practice good dental habits (including flossing, after checking with your medical team if your child's blood counts are low).
- No roughhousing. Take special care when the platelet count is low to avoid hemorrhage.

New antibiotics have been developed that prevent or control infections in these children most of the time. Your doctor will watch your child's white blood count carefully and will alert you when the count is low so you can avoid crowds. Watch for any fever, cold or flu symptoms, rashes, or other signs that an infection may be taking hold.

Children are often affected by a "fever of unknown origin" (FUO). In a child with cancer, the doctor will assume that the cause is an infection until it is proven otherwise. The doctor will take cultures as appropriate for the symptoms (blood, urine, bone marrow, spinal fluid, throat, rectum) and look for telltale bacteria and fungi. If the neutrophil count is low, the doctor immediately starts the child on a broad-spectrum antibiotic—that is, one proven effective against a wide variety of infections—even before the laboratory results are available. The child may also need a transfusion of granulocytes if the antibiotics are not working, the neutrophil count is still low, and he has a life-threatening infection.

Infections can be frightening and frustrating, and they may be very serious indeed, but new drugs, plus supportive care like refrigeration blankets to bring down high fevers, have made it easier to treat children with malignancies. With a variety of drugs to choose from, switching medications can wipe out infections that in earlier years would have been fatal.

Managing Pain

Your child's pain may be from the tumor itself (affecting body function and tissues), from a procedure like a lumbar puncture or other needles, or from side effects of therapy like mouth ulcers or healing surgical sites. Another advance has been in the development of pain-killing drugs and procedures. If your child is as active as normal, or nearly so, you may be lulled into believing he is therefore not in pain. A study reported in a Candlelighters publication discounted this and other myths about pain in children. In fact, children may be active as a way to relieve their anxieties and also to keep one step ahead of the doctors and nurses. They may not admit they are hurting because they have gotten shots at some point to relieve the pain, although pain relief is effectively given via IV, central line, or other avenues. Rather than injections, some drugs may also be given through skin patches, an experimental mouth swab, or inhaled doses.

In fact, the false notion that children don't feel pain in the same way adults do has led too often to skimping on relief measures for them. (Pain control may also be skimpy for the elderly and for minorities treated in low-income-area clinics.) The medical team should also know how the child, especially a younger one, refers to pain. "Owie" and "boo-boo" are only two of the many expressions families use to talk about discomfort.

In children, the worst pain is usually caused by extensive, widespread cancer, but steps can be taken to ease discomfort in any stage. There may also be more than one simultaneous cause of pain.

Watch for the child who is being stoic, because there is no need to be brave, nor are there any badges for "toughing it out" where pain is concerned. It isn't "bad" or "demanding" to insist on effective pain relief around the clock.

Nor should the medical staff wait until pain is overwhelming to provide relieving medications. Pain is more easily managed on a steady basis, allowing the body to focus on healing rather than discomfort or even agony. Cultural differences, too, may affect how children and families react to pain. Some cultures react to discomfort in dramatic, expressive ways, while others may try not to react at all. A patient in pain is often not able to sleep or eat, and sleeping and eating are needed for healing.

Older children are quite able to show where it hurts and even to characterize the sensation: does it burn, tingle, ache? Different types of medications are used for different levels and types of pain. Younger patients can learn to use the Wong-Baker pain-rating scale based on faces.

You know your child best. Watch and listen to him. Good indicators of pain are clenching the jaw, hands, or fists; being restless; and twisting or arching the body. Try lowering the lights and noise level in the room. Perhaps he can be distracted with television, taped books, art supplies, a hand-held video game, or a DVD. Possibly a trip to the playroom and a visit with the play therapist or child life worker will change the child's focus. Hot or cold packs are sometimes effective. And loving is always a balm: hold, rock, and cuddle your child as much as feasible given tubes, drains, or whatever apparatus may be present. Play soft music tapes or sing quietly; your child doesn't care

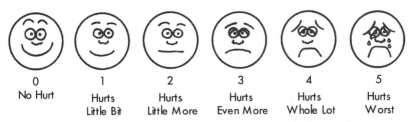

| 0 | 1 | 2 | 3 | 4 | 5 |
| No Hurt | Hurts Little Bit | Hurts Little More | Hurts Even More | Hurts Whole Lot | Hurts Worst |

FIGURE 22.1 Wong-Baker FACES Pain Rating Scale. From Hockenberry, M. J., Wilson, D., Winkelstein, M. L., *Wong's Essentials as Pediatric of Nursing*, ed. 7, St. Louis, 2005, p. 1259. Used with permission. Copyright, Mosby

if you're not a candidate for the Mormon Tabernacle Choir, he just wants to hear your soothing voice.

Different types of pain medications work in different ways, so some combination of them is usually appropriate. The types of medications you may encounter are:

- **Sedatives** relax the child and relieve anxiety and may allow him to sleep or tolerate some medical procedures. Doctors may try to complete more than one procedure at a time to take advantage of anesthesia. A side effect may be amnesia so the child doesn't remember the procedure.

- **Tranquilizers** relieve anxiety. (In times of crisis a tranquilizer may be helpful for the parents as well, but it is vital to recognize that these drugs are potentially habit-forming and must be used with care; an addicted parent is of little help to a needy child.)

- Mild **analgesics**, or **painkillers**, can help with the discomfort of mouth ulcers and other side effects, but remember that aspirin can depress platelet function, so it should not be used in cancer patients. Your doctor may want you to skip aspirin altogether and switch to acetaminophen, the generic name for Tylenol and similar preparations.

- **Codeine** is useful if the pain is not severe and is of short duration. Higher doses will increase the sedative effect without more pain relief. As with all narcotics, watch for constipation and try to head it off with fluids, fiber, laxatives, and stool softeners.

- **Strong analgesics** like Dilaudid and **morphine** are used in late stages when cancer is widely disseminated. At that point the sedative effect may not be a problem. When the body develops a tolerance for these drugs, higher doses may always be employed. Demerol is used for short-term pain relief, perhaps for 2 to 3 days after surgery, but there may be time-limiting side effects such as seizures.

- An **anesthetic nerve block** can be performed by an anesthesiologist or a neurosurgeon. These procedures block the nerves to specific body regions, providing long-term relief of pain.

- **Acupuncture** or variations are proving helpful in some instances.

- **Self-hypnosis, biofeedback, relaxation-imagery,** or **behavior modification** techniques often make the pain more bearable. If a deep breath is needed, have the child blow bubbles or a party favor. See Chapter 21 for an extensive discussion of these activities, which are not a substitute for medications but can be useful as an adjunct.
- Consulting a **palliative care team** may be helpful in treating your child's pain. These specialists no longer serve only hospice or dying patients.

Other advances have been made in the methods used to administer the medications. Far from the days of just giving "shots," clinics now use many avenues to relieve pain without inflicting more in the process. For example:

- Skin cream (EMLA is one type) is placed on the site of a planned injection an hour or more before the procedure and covered with an airtight bandage. The site will be numb by the time the needle approaches. (EMLA does not require a prescription in Canada.) Accessing a Port-a-Cath is rendered painless.
- Intravenous through an IV or central line
- Rectal suppositories
- Medicated lollipops
- Medicated skin patches
- Under the tongue
- Battery-operated devices to push the anesthetic through the skin without needles, done 15 minutes before a procedure to numb the skin
- Nose squirts
- Conscious sedation is used for procedures like a bone marrow biopsy, combining pain killers with sedation; the patient is drowsy but awake.
- Patient-controlled analgesia (PCA). Children as young as kindergarten can self-medicate as needed, using a pump that delivers drugs through their IV line. The doses are premeasured and metered, giving a small amount at a time, but the child decides when he needs it.

It is foolish to worry about a terminally ill child becoming addicted to painkillers. His comfort is the important thing at that point.

Besides, studies have shown that using narcotic drugs even in escalating doses is not addictive behavior. The patient's body may become dependent on them and experience withdrawal if the drugs are not given, but this is not "addiction." Addictive behavior includes the psychological urge to do anything to get a "fix," without there being a therapeutic need or benefit. Cancer patients rarely if ever become addicted in the classic sense. Tapering off the doses if necessary or appropriate will lessen the withdrawal symptoms and discomfort.

Blood Transfusions

A big step in the battle to control cancer in children has been the advance in blood transfusions, particularly of blood components. Whole blood is not usually given to children unless there has been a large blood loss. By separating the red blood cells, white blood cells, and platelets, several patients can be helped by a single donor.

Blood type is important when red blood cells, needed to carry oxygen throughout the body, are transfused into a patient with anemia. An exact match is not usually needed for transfusions of white blood cells, however, or platelets, unless they are given frequently, in which case the family may be screened for a close match. Potential marrow donors should not be used as blood donors.

Blood transfusions are not without some dangers and complications, some of which can be very serious. Destruction of the donated blood products by the patient's immune system can become a big problem with repeated transfusions. With each transfusion, the child develops antibodies that destroy donated blood cells, reducing the effect of the transfusion. If both donor and recipient have the same blood type, the body doesn't recognize the new blood cells as foreign and ignores them; if they're different, it will try to destroy them.

A rare transfusion reaction can be life-threatening, so report these symptoms at once:

- Nausea and vomiting
- Skin rash or itching
- Fever and chills
- Heaviness in the chest
- Jaundice
- Low back pain
- Red urine

Parents often fear that their children will get hepatitis or AIDS from transfused blood. While this theoretically possible, donated blood is screened for these diseases and today the risk is small or nonexistent.

Besides whole blood, patients sometimes receive transfusions of specific blood components: fresh frozen plasma (FFP), granulocytes, and platelets. Granulocytes are white blood cells found primarily in the bone marrow and tissues that use the bloodstream as a highway to rush to a site of inflammation. Most granulocyte transfusions are given to patients with ANLL to help them fight bacterial infections when they are critically ill.

Usually doctors transfuse granulocytes into a child with a fever and an infection that has not responded to antibiotics. Until the marrow recovers and begins manufacturing granulocytes on its own, the patient is still at risk of a fatal infection.

Side effects of granulocyte transfusion may be chills and fever, difficulty breathing, and potentially fatal graft-versus-host disease. Bone marrow transplant patients who receive granulocytes may also develop cytomegalovirus pneumonia, another life-threatening complication.

Platelet transfusions are given to children to prevent or stop bleeding associated with a low platelet count caused by the disease (such as leukemia) or the treatments (like chemotherapy). Patients can become immunized against later transfusions of platelets, sometimes after only one transfusion is given, or sometimes after a number of units. In that case a sibling or an otherwise compatible donor may be used to reap the maximum benefits from the transfusion. Platelets can also be collected from a patient in remission and preserved for later use if needed. A potential side effect of platelet transfusion is fever.

Doctors use special drugs to boost the patient's blood. Epoetin alfa (Procrit or Epogen) is given to chemotherapy patients to build red blood cell volume while reducing fatigue and the need for transfusions. Other drugs like filgrastim (Neupogen) and pegfilgrastim (Neulasta) are injected to build white blood cells. They are expensive but may be cost-effective in reducing hospital time.

Blood transfusions, as wonderful as they are, simply buy time until the child's own bone marrow and other blood-forming tissues can reproduce their own new cells. Advances in blood replacement techniques have been important features in improving the outlook for children with cancer.

Isolation

Sometimes patients are placed in isolation to minimize exposure to other people's germs. This may prevent infection, which is a common and potentially lethal complication of leukemia and cancer chemotherapy. It is not, however, without risks. Placing a person in extreme isolation is stressful and is therefore not done routinely with children. When children must be isolated for their own safety, doctors choose an appropriate degree of protection. One possibility is a clean hospital room with special air filters that carry germs away from the child in a steady flow. This also requires that the patient's own body be sterilized with antibiotics and antiseptics, since the major threat is from his own skin and bowel. Visitors may be required to don full surgical garb like gowns, shoe and hair covers, gloves, and masks before entering the room, or they may only have to wash their hands well and put on a mask (which has to be changed twice an hour or it loses its effectiveness). If actual physical contact is kept to a minimum, there should not be any unwarranted risk of infection.

Even given all those precautions, isolation will not protect the patient from the biggest infection source of all: his own natural germs.

Hyperalimentation

Hyperalimentation (also called total parenteral nutrition) does not treat the cancer itself but provides nutrition for the patient while the digestive system is temporarily unable to do the whole job. This special feeding method is helpful when chemotherapy, radiation, or invasion by the tumor itself has affected the gastrointestinal tract to the point that the body is not getting the fuel it needs to fight the invading malignancy, or when the child cannot or will not eat.

In the operating room, a central line is inserted into a large neck vein if the patient doesn't already have a central line in place. The hyperalimentation fluid is carried directly to the blood above the heart, where it is soon diluted and disseminated throughout the body by the bloodstream.

The fluid contains a special mixture of vitamins, minerals, carbohydrates, amino acids, and other nutrients to feed the child who cannot eat for himself, perhaps because of ulcers in the gastrointestinal tract caused by cancer treatments.

The hyperalimentation liquid is pumped into the child at a measured and controlled rate. Depending on how much the child can take by mouth and digest, the rate can be altered. The pump may be hooked up for 24 hours a day, or, sometimes, especially when the patient is at home, just during the night.

Particularly when the patient has a limited natural immune system because of chemotherapy or radiation, it is vital that the site where the tube is inserted be kept clean and sterile to avoid infection. Dressings are changed under sterile conditions.

Hyperalimentation does not cure but sustains the patient while other treatments go to work.

Rehabilitation

The young person who has faced cancer may need special help to gain the best possible level of physical and intellectual activity during and after treatment. Those involved with the oncology team in the patient's rehabilitation may include therapists, social workers, and perhaps a psychologist or a psychiatrist to motivate the patient or the family. Psychological rehabilitation and coping are discussed in detail in Chapter 23.

Side effects of chemotherapy may rarely include nerve damage so that a brace is required to boost weakened muscles. Other patients lose weight and strength through poor nutrition and loss of sleep, leading to temporary disability.

Long bones that are the target of radiation treatments may stop growing, may grow more slowly than their counterparts in an unradiated limb, or may bow. Shoe lifts may, for example, be necessary to correct the resulting gait disturbance. Muscles may need rebuilding, and a radiated spine may need stretching to maintain posture. Swimming is excellent for these purposes.

In preventing or correcting these and other physical disabilities, the physical therapist can help the youngster avoid psychological and social problems that may result. Rehabilitation is especially important today with the long-term survival and cures so many of the children achieve.

TABLE 22.1 Drugs used to control or treat side effects

Drug name	Alternate/trade names	Purpose	Route
Anti-emetics			
Chlorpromazine	Thorazine	Anti-emetic	Oral, IV
Dexamethasone	Methylprednisolone, Decadron	Anti-emetic	Oral, rectal suppository, IV, IM
Diphenhydramine	Benadryl	Anti-emetic	Oral, IV
Droperidol	Inapsine	Anti-emetic	IM, IV
Granisetron	Kytril	Anti-emetic	IV, oral
Haloperidol	Haldol	Anti-emetic	IM, IV, oral
Metoclopramide	Reglan	Anti-emetic	IV, oral
Ondansetron	Zofran	Anti-emetic	IV, oral lozenge
Prochlorperazine	Compazine	Anti-emetic	Oral, IV, IM, rectal suppository
Promethazine	Phenergan	Anti-emetic	Oral, rectal suppository, IM, IV
Trimethobenzamide	Tigan	Anti-emetic	IV, oral, rectal suppository
For pain			
Codeine	Opium alkaloid	For pain	Oral, IM
EMLA cream	Lidocaine and prilocaine	Numbs injection sites before procedures	Skin cream (needs an hour or so take effect)

Fentanyl	Actiq, Durogesic, Fentora	Prevent chronic breakthrough pain	IV, patch, lollipop, oral tablet
Hydromorphone	Dilaudid (narcotic)	For pain	IV, oral, rectal suppository
Meperidine	Demerol (narcotic)	For pain	IV, oral
Methadone	Narcotic	For pain	IV, oral
Morphine	Narcotic	For pain	IV, oral
Numby Stuff	Needle-free application of lidocaine and epinephrine	Numb site before procedures	Uses electrical currents to numb skin and tissue
Oxycodone	Percocet (narcotic)	For pain	
Other purposes			
Epoetin-alfa	Epogen, Procrit, EPO, erythropoietin	Stimulates red blood cell production	IV or subcutaneous
Mesna	Mesnex	Reduce urinary side effects of chemo drugs like Cytoxan	IV
Sargramostim	Leukine, GM-CSF	Cell-stimulating factor to help blood cell recovery	IV, subcutaneous

Some of this information was drawn from Shiminski-Maher, Tania, et al. *Childhood Brain and Spinal Cord Tumors: A Guide for Families, Friends and Caregivers.* Sebastapol, CA: O'Reilly, 2002, and from Ablin, Arthur R. *Supportive Care of Children with Cancer* (2d ed.), Baltimore: Johns Hopkins University Press, 1997.

Rehabilitation is a family matter. The parents and siblings, where appropriate, should understand the goals of the program and should be taught how to take part in it. They can help with the therapy in the hospital as well as at home—an excellent way to show their love and support for their child, and a fine way for them to make a genuine contribution to his care.

In the case of an amputation, rehabilitation may begin even before surgery by training in the use of crutches or by building one-handed dexterity. Parents are also trained in positioning the child and in the care of the stump. Consult the chapter on bone cancer (Chapter 8) for a more detailed discussion of amputation and aftercare.

Families needing help with rehabilitation may be put in contact with:

- The state division of crippled children's services or vocational rehabilitation
- American Cancer Society
- The local visiting nurse
- Public health service nurses
- Leukemia and Lymphoma Society
- Mental health service
- Occupational therapists (less likely with a young child)
- Physical therapist

The school should also be notified, preferably in conference with the medical team and the parents, of any disabilities or limitations on activities. Keeping teachers and school authorities informed will pay off. (This is not a one-time conference; in our experience, vigilance is essential. While Lisa's school knew of her background and late effects, someone decided that rather than having her run around playing field hockey and risking collisions, they would make her goalie!)

The child's progress will be evaluated regularly, probably a couple of times a year, and exercises may be changed, added, or dropped as appropriate.

Palliative Management

Even when cure is no longer a realistic possibility, the treatment team may still undertake some forms of treatment that either prolong the patient's life or relieve symptoms to increase comfort for whatever time the child has left. At this stage the child may be in the hospital or at home, working with a hospice team. Palliative management includes terminal care when prolonged survival or another good remission is unlikely, but it is also used today to "comfort" patients in therapy who have a very good prognosis.

In the case of end-of-life patients, many people are involved in the care of the child, but clergy members, a visiting nurse, or a hospice worker may play a larger role here. Everyone on the team must be careful to tell the child and family the same thing and to deal with the truth frankly and compassionately. The patient and the family have a right to know what is happening and what to expect in the future.

Chemotherapy may still be used when cure is not possible because of widespread disease or infiltration of vital organ systems, but only after all the potential risks and benefits have been carefully weighed. A good-quality life may be extended by relieving pain and symptoms of organ obstruction. This has been helpful in all types of cancers.

Surgery may help, too, although major palliative surgery is not often worth it unless there is a good chance for a long-term remission, perhaps aided by drugs and radiation. The doctor may operate to relieve obstructions in the gastrointestinal tract, the urinary tract, or the airways to make the child more comfortable. Another role of the surgeon may be to place a shunt in children with increased pressure in the skull caused by an inoperable brain tumor. In these cases vision may be saved, an early death due to the high pressure avoided, and headache or vomiting controlled. See the chapter on surgery (Chapter 16) for more discussion of palliative operations.

Other supportive measures may include giving the patient vitamins, antibiotics to fight infection, medicine to control vomiting, and other medications to ease itching. If the child is confined to bed, taking narcotic drugs, and eating poorly, he may be susceptible to severe constipation. Giving stool softeners and enemas (with the medical team's knowledge) before the problem becomes serious is helpful. The child may also lose bladder control if he is weak or on sedatives, which in turn can worsen any bedsores. The doctor may want to catheterize the child to avoid unnecessary complications.

Any palliative measures, of course, depend on the patient and the wishes of the family. The level of supportive treatments may change over time as the disease progresses.

Further Resources

READING

"Blood Transfusion," a booklet written in clear language explaining blood and its components, transfusion, blood donation, and complications of the therapy, is available from the Leukemia and Lymphoma Society (www.LLS.org).

"Cancer Pain Management in Children." Handbook from the Texas Children's Cancer Center in Houston, to read online or download from www.childcancerpain.org.

Gorfinkle, Kenneth, PhD. *Soothing Your Child's Pain*. Lincolnwood, IL: Contemporary Books, 1998.
The author, who works with hospitalized children, including cancer patients, discusses the process of pain and the root causes. Has suggestions on ways (distraction, play therapy, etc.) to handle, relieve, and bear pain. Also discusses alternative methods like acupuncture and herbal medicine. Not cancer-specific but broadly helpful.

Hilden, Joanne, MD, and Sarah Friebert, MD. Palliative or hospice care: Does my child need this service? *CCCF National Journal* (Fall 2001), n.p. Available online at www.childhoodcancer.org.

Keene, Nancy. *Childhood Leukemia: A Guide for Families, Friends and Caregivers*. Sebastopol, CA: O'Reilly, 2002.
Has an excellent chapter, "Choosing a Catheter," exploring the physical and psychological aspects of these devices.

McGrath, Patrick, et al. *Pain, Pain Go Away: Helping Children with Pain*. Online booklet from Izaak Walton Killiam Children's Hospital, Dalhousie Unit, Halifax, Nova Scotia, 1994.
A booklet available online from www.pediatric-pain.ca. Helps parents advocate for their children. Specific suggestions, tips, procedures (relaxation techniques, for example). A nice discussion on the complementary roles of parent, child/patient, and health care professional. This site also has a version of the Wong-Baker Faces scale for gauging pain in 33 languages.

"Pain Control, a Guide for People with Cancer and their Families." U. S. Department of Health and Human Services, Public Health Service, Institutes of Health, National Cancer Institute and American Cancer Society, 2007. Available online from the ACS (www.cancer.org) under "Treatment Topics and Resources."

Comprehensive and understandable booklet for nonprofessionals. Thoughtful discussion of pain's causes and relief methods, including types of drugs and side effects, biofeedback and other complementary methods. Referrals to other resources. A second booklet, "Making Cancer Less Painful: A Handbook for Parents" is also available.

Patt, Richard B., MD, and Susan S. Lang. *The Complete Guide to Relieving Cancer Pain and Suffering*. New York: Oxford University Press, 2004.

An authoritative and comprehensive guide to various forms of pain relief, with many references to children as patients. Lots of drug-specific data, with brand and generic names, comments, and precautions. Highly recommended.

How to Cope

23

Emotional Aspects of Childhood Cancer

Within recent memory, a diagnosis of childhood cancer meant swift and certain death. Today, fortunately, because of advances in treatment techniques, most children with cancer live for extended periods, long enough to be considered cured. Ironically, this has increased the stress on families, because months or years of uncertainty may be heaped on top of the shock of diagnosis and the disruption of family life patterns.

No family, no matter how stable, escapes this stress, and those already experiencing difficulties will especially need help. All members of the family are affected, too, whether or not they show it or are aware of it. Reading this section should reassure parents that their thoughts and feelings are shared by others in the same situation. The emphasis here is on *living* with cancer. The doctor has probably told the family to continue with normal life as much as possible. Partly drawing on my family's and our friends' experiences with childhood cancer, this section provides practical tips towards that end.

Initial Response to Diagnosis

The time of diagnosis is a very low point; parents feel fear, panic, shock, and guilt. A particularly common response among families is denial: the diagnosis must be wrong, they think; it cannot be our child. Up to a point, this is healthy; it can spare the parents thinking about cancer 24 hours a day and can give everyone some time to accept the diagnosis. Carried too far, however, denial can cause problems, such as when a parent takes a child to doctor after doctor seeking a softer diagnosis, thus losing precious time in beginning treatments. By all means, doubting parents should get a second opinion if they wish. But once two doctors or clinics have confirmed the diagnosis, the chance that both are wrong is extremely slim.

Hostility is another common reaction. Like the old days when the bearer of bad tidings was punished, it is not unusual for parents to lash out at the doctor or the hospital staff, or even at the child. I remember a brief flash of anger at my daughter Lisa for "rejecting" my mothering by getting cancer.

Another early sign of trouble is frantic activity that precludes a calm assessment of how to deal with the disease. Using euphemisms like "a blood disease" instead of naming the illness also indicates that the parent has not fully accepted the situation. A parent who cannot cry or at least talk about the sadness he or she feels may be in trouble. If, as is often the case, the two parents react in widely different ways, perhaps one disbelieving and the other prostrated by grief, they may need counseling. Fathers in particular, conditioned to suppress emotion, may need help to realize it is all right to show their feelings. Social workers and mental health professionals on the hospital staff can help. Your local clergy member may be another source of counseling. Parent groups may be helpful and some provide educational seminars or meetings and discussion groups.

Coping over Time

Response to the diagnosis and treatment of cancer in a child is not unlike the "grief stages" presented by Elizabeth Kübler-Ross in her research on death and dying. Most families pass through several stages before accepting the diagnosis of childhood cancer. Shock and denial, then guilt and anger (perhaps manifested by clashes with the medical staff), and eventually acceptance, meeting the problem head on and moving through it—these are common phases in the family's emotional reaction to diagnosis.

The time of diagnosis is accompanied by a sense of fear and isolation; in our case it lasted for a couple of months. This is perhaps the worst stage of all, as the world seemingly falls apart, and it may be repeated, unfortunately, if there is a relapse. As the family begins to accept the diagnosis, it becomes easier to turn outward to face the world again. Eventually, family members may develop a desire to take action to help others in the same situation. If the child dies, the blow will be felt after the death rather than during the terminal phase. Living with relapses and the death of a child will be discussed in a later chapter (Chapter 32).

Successful adaptation may require a shift in focus. Rather than worrying about getting the child into the best preschool or college, parents are concerned about shorter-term goals.

Beware of the emotional surges or shifts that may take place at the time of an "ordinary" life transition for other children: starting kindergarten, going to summer camp, having sleepovers. Parents as well as their child might be irritable, depressed, or moody at such times.

New concerns may arise when the child's period of therapy ends. If he has been on chemotherapy, parents may experience what one expert calls "drug dependence"—the fear that taking the child off the medication will lead to a relapse. This frightening thought can sneak up at a time when parents are beginning to breathe more freely—chemotherapy put the child into remission and has kept him there for some time; what will happen now? There is always a chance that the disease will return, but the doctor can help the family understand what the risk really is.

Another source of stress may appear as the family tries to resume normal life. Those members who experienced the least disruption during the therapy may assume they can continue with their regular activities. At the same time, the parent who carried most of the burden of taking the child to therapy may expect that the other will now make sacrifices while he or she rebuilds a career or re-establishes his or her own life. The discrepancy between the parents' assumptions and expectations can lead to conflict. Compromise is the key here, perhaps with the help of a counselor.

When the child successfully completes treatment and becomes a long-term survivor, an interesting problem may arise. If the child or a sibling develops any behavioral, emotional, or learning problems, therapists or school authorities may blame them on the cancer, perhaps even years later. Once the fact of cancer in the family is in the medical history, it stands out. Perhaps subsequent problems are indeed a result of the cancer, but perhaps they are not. Parents should make sure other causes are explored, too.

If the cancer survivor does develop learning problems, some educators are reluctant to blame either the cancer itself or the therapy, noting that a child who misses a great deal of school, whatever the cause, is likely to experience some educational consequences. It is reassuring that the majority of long-term survivors do graduate with their classes on schedule.

An article in *Parade Magazine* advised that patients and family form a support group (whether online or through your town or house of worship), keep laughing, and find a purpose to survive and thrive (family responsibilities, for example). A related article by a cancer survivor (speaking for patients and families) asks that others:

- Acknowledge our situation; don't ignore us or run away.
- Offer only help you can deliver.
- Guard our privacy.
- Listen to us.
- Allow us to hope.
- Ensure our dignity.

Let go a Little

Many people appreciate the emotional release of a good cry—or a good laugh. Having a child with cancer will tap these resources all the time. While tears are a regular lubricant for parents of sick children, humor is just as important and useful. The alternative and complementary treatments chapter (Chapter 21) discusses the therapeutic value of humor in more depth.

Discussing Cancer with the Child and Others

It is best to be honest when discussing the disease and the problems it is causing the family. The child with cancer should be told the truth, according to his age and level of understanding. A child who is told half-truths or nothing at all will probably discern the truth within a few months anyway, but by then may not be as trusting. The child may be reluctant to talk about the illness or his feelings to spare the parents pain or because he thinks it's a taboo subject for discussion.

It is important to create plenty of opportunities for the child to ask questions about the disease and to talk out his fears. This will also allow parents to dispel any false ideas the child may have. The youngest children are generally afraid they will be separated from their parents. Those approaching kindergarten age fear mutilation, and school-aged children fear pain and death. The child's anxiety will be eased by discussing the disease, and these are excellent opportunities for parents to express their love and commitment to the child's health and comfort.

Communication among all members of the family is important, whether siblings, grandparents, or other relatives. While it is not essential to inform everyone about the diagnosis, close family members should know, because they will inevitably be affected by the illness and will be in a better position to help if they understand the problem. All those who do know should have accurate information about the diagnosis, the prognosis, and the treatment.

Parents certainly are under no obligation to tell neighbors or acquaintances about the child's illness, but the family should recognize that it will be hard to keep such a thing secret. If the child or any siblings are in school, the teachers should be informed of the illness.

At the time of diagnosis every family feels alone. They may not know anyone else who has had this problem because it is, after all, very rare. As a matter of course, I think parents should be given the name and phone number (or e-mail address, if appropriate) of a family who has had experience with the same disease or a family whose child was the same age when cancer was diagnosed or who had the same treatments. This informal pairing can help ease the sense of isolation the family is likely to feel, although it should not replace the important relationships among the family, the doctor, and other clinic staff. If the family wishes such support and the hospital does not arrange it, parents can attend support-group meetings, contact the nearest Candlelighters chapter, or sign onto an Internet discussion group. Addresses and resources can be found in the Appendices.

Families must be aware that there are unfortunately still people who think cancer is contagious. Others do not know what to say and so avoid situations where they will have to say anything at all. This hurts, but it takes too much energy to worry about it. Parents should try instead to find strength and help through the caring people they already know or whom they will meet through this experience.

After the family has had some time to adjust to the idea that the child has cancer, they may well find themselves comforting friends and relatives as others come to terms with the diagnosis. At first this provides some emotional outlet, particularly for those who are helped by reaching out to others, but it can also become tiring once parents have accepted the news themselves. Still, it is worth the effort, because for the most part people who ask are genuinely concerned and interested. Those who are merely being nosy do not have to be told a thing.

Although every family will find its own way of adapting to the situation, I think it helped us to talk openly about our daughter's illness once she had started treatments. Her baldness did not look odd to us, because she had never had much hair anyway, but strangers who commented on it were likely to get a good-natured explanation about childhood cancer and the advances in its treatment. This happened in part because at that time there was a great deal of national publicity about a child with leukemia, and we could see from media coverage that people still thought a diagnosis of cancer was a death sentence.

As time went on we felt some frustration because there were people who simply would not believe that Lisa was surviving. She was admitted to the hospital numerous times for infections or corrective surgery, and at each admission we had to reassure people that she was not dying. For many years my mother had to deal with a neighbor who thought "it's just a matter of time."

Other people will say incredibly stupid or thoughtless things. When her son became ill with neuroblastoma, one mother was told (in church!), "Thank God he's only adopted." I read of a junior high school student who, after having a leg amputated, was told by a stranger, "Oh, you don't have cancer. Doctors just like to cut people up."

One woman who asked me about Lisa's illness responded, "Oh, my landlord's two daughters had that. They both died." It was not true, of course, but that did not make it any easier to hear. Some parents become reclusive, pulling into themselves to avoid such people, but this makes it harder to cope by magnifying the problem.

Cancer in the Media

After a child is diagnosed, it will seem as if every newspaper or magazine has an article about cancer. This is often true; cancer is "news," especially when scientific meetings are being held where researchers report on new studies. If parents read about new drugs, or new side effects from current treatments, they should discuss them with the members of the child's treatment team. Tabloids, magazines, even daily newspapers can sensationalize research reports and distort the findings. Parents should take copies of articles to the clinic so the doctors can respond appropriately to the issues they raise. Well-meaning friends and relatives (sometimes even strangers) may seize on these reports and urge families to take some action, whether it's to seek a new drug, to stop giving the child one reported to be dangerous in some way, or to try an unorthodox treatment like shark cartilage.

Articles that play up the unpleasant or serious side effects of certain therapies are understandably painful to read and occasionally result in a patient or parent halting the treatments. Although stopping therapy may be especially tempting when the child has been in remission for a while, the duration of treatments the doctors have prescribed is based on experience and research. And even though the child is healthy, relapses, like remissions, can happen very quickly.

Disruption of Normal Life

Early in the child's illness the family will make a fundamental decision, whether consciously or not, on how he is to be treated—like a sick child or, insofar as possible, like a normal child.

Nor surprisingly, an atmosphere of emotional stability will help. If the child is hostile, for example, it is hard not to respond in kind, but parents will be glad later that they restrained themselves. It is best to treat the child the same way as always.

Parents must guard against letting fears of infection or illnesses during periods of lowered immunity become an obsession. If the child is otherwise well, and the doctor approves, it is fine to take the child to stores, restaurants, or friends' houses.

The frequent clinic visits for chemotherapy and/or radiation cut deeply into the family's normal life schedules. It is important, if the parent's work will be affected, to sit down with the employer at the outset to enlist cooperation. Sometimes one parent has to take a leave of absence or quit a job to take care of the sick child. Not all employers are cooperative, but the doctor or a social worker from the hospital may be able to help. In dual-career families, parents might take turns going to the clinic with the child. In some fortunate cases employers permit parents to use their own accumulated sick leave to take care of a sick child. Maybe one parent can temporarily work either different or flexible hours or part time. However, quitting work, especially at such a crucial time, often leads to increased isolation and financial worry, especially if your health insurance is tied to that employment. See Chapter 26 for a brief discussion of the U.S. Family Medical Leave Act, which mandates unpaid leave to care for sick family members in some, but unfortunately not all, circumstances.

The disease itself and side effects from the treatments also disrupt schedules. Weakness, fever, diarrhea, vomiting, and hair loss make it hard to carry on normally. These are usually short-term or intermittent symptoms. Lisa was nauseated about 1 to 2 days a month and, except when she had urinary tract infections, was reasonably normal the rest of the time.

It may also be hard to live normally when relatives, neighbors, and friends want to indulge the sick youngster. Siblings will resent this, especially when the child is in remission and seems well. Parents may even be criticized by some for trying to live life as usual. But such criticism can be safely ignored.

A child nearing school age is old enough to take some part in his own care. The child can help keep daily charts of how he feels, pour juice to take pills with, collect urine specimens, or choose which finger will be "stuck" for blood samples, if necessary. The child can make simple decisions: will I take my medicine with orange or grape juice? But parents should beware: the child may also "give treatments" to the dog, a teddy bear, or a little brother, any one of whom may need a degree of protection.

Don't expect that at some point you will just "put the whole thing behind you." In a *New York Times* piece about post-traumatic stress disorder, Harriet Brown wrote, "A child's close call reverberates through the rest of a parent's life." After one very scary dialysis-related near-miss, for months I woke up every night at the slightest sound and had to check it out—even knowing it was probably made by one of our cats.

Take a Break

Despite health concerns and financial pressures—or perhaps because of them—it is important that the family get away when they can for vacations. With a little planning and maybe some help, it is possible to do so safely.

We took two out-of-state vacations while Lisa was on chemotherapy. The first, shortly after she began treatments, was to Denver to visit grandparents. Our doctor notified a Colorado doctor of our visit ahead of time, but we never had to contact her. The second vacation was a spring camping trip to the Blue Ridge Mountains. We went without a doctor's name but knew we could phone our doctor, and that he knew someone in Virginia if there was an emergency.

If the family cannot afford a vacation, there are quite a few organizations that pay for family trips if a child has a catastrophic or terminal illness. Summer camps have been founded for children with cancer and sometimes for their families. Organizations like Make-a-Wish provide fantastic escapes for children and families. See Appendix B for addresses.

Respite Care

People who have never spent hours "just sitting" in a hospital have no idea how exhausting the experience is. Hours of boredom punctuated by brief spurts of high drama can render the most stable caregiver a basket case. It's probably impossible to avoid this syndrome completely, but there are steps that can alleviate it somewhat.

The most obvious solution is to switch roles whenever possible. One parent stays with the hospitalized child while the other copes with daily life, siblings, work, whatever. Then they change places. Of course this will not work for everyone for many reasons. In those cases it is helpful to share bedside and clinic duties with trusted relatives and friends. They will be pleased to be able to pitch in and the break will work wonders for everybody.

Your state may provide financial assistance to get respite care for the child while the regular caregivers take a break. Ask the hospital or clinic social worker what's available. Other clinic parents who have become close friends may be another source of help when you need it. We became especially close to one family from the clinic who lived in a nearby town; when the mother broke her leg skiing, we took her daughter along with Lisa for chemotherapy visits. Be sure to have (or give) written permission if your child is going with a different adult for any health care. Planning and phoning ahead also smooth the way. To be sure, this strategy should only be used with trusted close friends who will contact you in the case of emergency.

We also "swapped" children on occasion with the same clinic family. One set of parents would get away for a day or two while the other babysat. Some time later the situation would be reversed. Again, it is essential that the temporary caregivers have written permission to take the child for medical help as scheduled or needed.

Discipline

It is hard enough to maintain family discipline when life is running smoothly, but when one of the children is seriously ill, it is almost impossible. It is a natural reaction to be either overly protective of the sick child or overly permissive. Not so many years ago, when the child was sure to die in a short time, this was not a problem; he was coddled and cared for, the remaining days made as comfortable as possible.

Today, with long survivals and cures, it is important to hold to normal standards of discipline, treating each child equally. If parents are more lenient with the sick child than with siblings, the sick child may think that they have written him off, or, alternatively, that he can get away with almost everything. Because sick children (like healthy ones) can be mean, parents will want to be just as sure that the child is not using the illness as a weapon as that others are not allowed to pick on him because of it. Discipline is a form of security, a setting of limits that helps our children become people we like to have around. A sick child deserves this as much as a healthy one.

Because it is a natural tendency to spoil a sick child, parents may have to persuade well-meaning friends, neighbors, and relatives that the youngster is to be treated as much as possible like other children. When Lisa was in the hospital she received many gifts (plenty of them from us), which we considered acceptable and loving on the part of our friends. When she began to exhibit signs of greed, however, we were careful to explain to her the need for sharing, and as an adult today she is sensitive and generous to a fault.

A sick child who is old enough should also be assigned household chores. The child may complain that he is tired or feeling ill to avoid them, but it is reasonable to expect him to participate in the family's life as much as possible. On most days the child should be able to keep his room picked up, set the table, sort socks, fold underwear, and generally perform "light duty." If the child is strong enough to play outside, perhaps he can also weed a row of the garden (watch for too much sun) or shovel a couple of inches of snow off the walk. Being loving, firm, and flexible throughout the illness should provide the family with a solid basis for the child's eventual return to normal life.

Adapted from an article in a Candlelighters publication, here are some wise suggestions for raising and disciplining a child with cancer:

1. Teach and expect age-appropriate behavior; don't treat a fourth grader like a preschooler.
2. Praise the child whenever you can to reward good behavior. Give the child attention for good behavior rather than exclusively when correcting "bad" behavior.
3. Recognize the child's current condition.
4. Spanking or similar physical punishment is especially unwise, given low platelet counts and similar risks.
5. Use time out or withdrawal of privileges to punish inappropriate behavior.
6. Don't make threats you can't carry through on. Don't make the hospital or the clinical staff into the "bad guys" ("Get back in bed or Nurse P will...*fill in the blank...*"). You will need their good will as time goes by.

Guilt

Virtually every parent or sibling of a child with cancer feels guilt, even knowing consciously that the illness is not his fault. This may be an effort to regain some control over the situation: if the parent feels responsible, through guilt, then he is not so helpless. The child may also feel guilty for disrupting the family's life patterns and for increased financial burdens. The child should not be allowed to dwell on these negative thoughts, just as other family members must not blame him for the disruptions and crisis. The family should reassure the child that the cancer did not result from anything he did or did not do. Gradually all the family members will come to accept this and put that stage behind them. That is a happy day.

Fear of Relapse

With the onset of every illness in the child with cancer, even a minor cold, parents will probably ask themselves whether it is a relapse. This is a perfectly normal reaction and one I felt frequently for longer than I expected. I was lucky to have a good friend, someone I met at the clinic, whom I could call to share my fears; this person could help me decide what was important enough to ask the doctor about and what I could handle myself. The parents of a sick child may lose confidence in their ability to care for him, but as time passes they will become more relaxed and self-assured. When in doubt, though, they should call the doctor; that is what he or she is there for.

Hope

Sustained hope is a necessity in beating cancer. The family should emphasize optimism, no matter how hard it seems. It is up to the parents to maintain a positive approach. They should not say that the child is cured if he is not, but they should make sure the child knows they are doing everything they can to ensure a healthy future. At every point in therapy it is important to plan for tomorrow.

And other family members must take care of themselves; that is one of the best things they can do for the child's health, although it may be one of the last things they think about. Good nutrition, enough sleep, and counseling, if necessary, are all important ingredients for their well-being, too. If others feel ill, they should see a doctor.

Some concise and excellent advice from Mark Chesler and Oscar Barbarin (see the bibliography at the end of this chapter for source):

1. Try to live as normal a life as possible.
2. Keep the lines of communication open among family members and medical staff.
3. Emotional swings, anxiety, depression, and anger are normal reactions to dreadful situations. A parent who gets stuck in one of those modes, however, may need counseling to move on.
4. Keep on keeping on, one day at a time. Do the best you can do with the information and resources you have at the time.

To this, Greg Anderson of *The Cancer Conqueror* would add:

5. Keep a positive attitude.
6. Exercise as much as you can, maybe just taking a walk.
7. Have a strong social support network.
8. Have a goal in life and fun in living.
9. Eat a healthy diet of fruits, vegetables, and whole grains.
10. Think creatively.
11. Have a strong spiritual (not necessarily religious) outlook.

Where to get Help

There are many potential sources of help, whether physical, emotional, or spiritual. Social workers, the clinic staff, and cancer organizations are of course a first line of defense, but parents should not shut themselves off from others. Many friends, neighbors, and relatives will offer sincere help; the family should accept it! Whether they babysit for the other children, provide a supper casserole on a clinic day, or take in the laundry when it rains (or to the Laundromat if necessary), helping is as important to them as it is for the family. They are offering a way out of isolation.

Twice, when the realities of life ran up smack against minor medical crises, we asked for unusual help. A group of friends helped me empty the kitchen drawers and cabinets before a badly timed renovation, and the same folks turned out in a cold November rain to plant hundreds of spring bulbs I had optimistically ordered but didn't have time to deal with.

Designate a good friend or close relative to screen help offers and provide an ongoing source of information for family and friends. Sign up for a free Web site to organize regular support. CaringBridge, Lotsa Helping Hands, and Share the Care are often useful. Contact information is given at the end of this chapter.

A family seeking spiritual support may want to talk with a local member of the clergy. The hospital or clinic will also have ministers, priests, and rabbis on staff who may be extremely comforting. It is not unusual for these people to develop strong supportive relationships with families, and they can be especially helpful to a family that finds itself in a clinic far from home.

While family and friends are sympathetic, they cannot understand the parents' feelings fully unless they have had the same experience, which is unlikely. This is where support groups come in. The Candlelighters, the Leukemia and Lymphoma Society, and other organizations have many local groups where families of young cancer patients and the children themselves can get together with others who truly understand. They can share their feelings, arrange for programs either to extend their own knowledge or to enlighten the community in general, and help each other in substantial ways, whether in venting emotions or in concrete sharing like carpooling or babysitting.

If there are no local chapters, parents can start one or can share their feelings with other parents they will meet at the clinic or the hospital. We spent a lot of time sitting around waiting rooms and parent lounges, and the one good aspect of this seemingly endless sitting was the chance it afforded to talk with others in the same situation. It is not easy to open up to people who are virtual strangers, but I found it well worth the effort.

Today, there is an even stronger ally in this search: the Internet. Families who are online or who have computer access at the local library, for example, can reach out to each other across the country and indeed around the world. See the chapter on the Internet (Chapter 33) for suggestions and warnings about this wonderful but challenging tool.

Further Resources

READING

American Cancer Society. "Listen with your heart, talking with the cancer patient." Available at www.cancer.org

This brief, pithy pamphlet has many concrete suggestions on how to really communicate with the cancer patient and the family. A copy or two of this pamphlet could be passed among friends and neighbors in advance of post-diagnosis meetings.

Anderson, Greg, *The Cancer Conqueror.* Kansas City, MO: Andrews McMeel Publishing, 2000.

Brown, Harriet, "My daughters are fine, but I'll never be the same." *New York Times*, April 8, 2008, p. F5

Chesler, Mark, and Oscar Barbarin. *Childhood Cancer and the Family.* New York: Bruner/Mazel, 1987.
A bit dated, but much of the advice still holds up today.

Fighting Chance: Journey through Childhood Cancer. Photos and story by Harry Connolly. Baltimore: Woodholme House, 1998.

Beautiful photos follow three childhood or adolescent cancer patients from diagnosis through therapy and beyond, providing a glimpse into a world foreign to so many people. Connolly's stunning pictures show better than any thousand words can what the world of pediatric cancer is like. Highly recommended for all.

Gordon, Melanie Apel. *Let's Talk About When Kids Have Cancer.* New York: Rosen Publishing Group's PowerKids Press, 1999.

For early and middle readers, although the patients in the photos seem a little older. A very basic information source for young kids.

Granet, Roger, MD. *Surviving Cancer Emotionally.* New York: John Wiley & Sons, 2001.

This book is helpful in handling the diagnosis of cancer, with its fears of treatments and death, the loss of control, and general uncertainty of such a life-altering event for a loved one. Written by a psycho-oncologist (a psychiatrist who treats cancer patients), the book is very reassuring and suggests both formal and informal coping strategies. There is an excellent chapter on cancer as it affects the patient's family.

Halpern, Susan P. *The Etiquette of Illness: What to Say When You Can't Find the Words*. New York: Bloomsbury, 2004.

The title suggests "Miss Manners/Emily Post does illness," but this small book goes beyond the superficial to brief but helpful suggestions on how to talk to sick friends, how to help, and how to figure out when to do or say little. Not specific at all to sick children, the advice nevertheless is transferable to families dealing with a child's cancer diagnosis. Many examples and anecdotes flesh out the advice, and one section discusses communication between patient and doctor. Preparing for death is handled with grace and compassion and not ignored. This is a book to keep around to read now and then as the child passes through different phases.

ORGANIZATIONS/WEB SITES

The Cancer Game (P.O. Box 13335, Reading, PA 19612; www.cancergame.org)
A free game for all ages to vent stress and anger in a fun way.

Cancer Kids (www.cancerkids.org)
A place for childhood cancer patients to tell their stories. Hundreds are here with varying diagnoses, in various stages of treatment, and honored in memorials.

CancerNet's Anxiety Disorder, PDQ (www.cancer.gov)
A "Cancer Topics" overview of various manifestations of anxiety, which is a perfectly normal reaction to a family's entry into the pediatric cancer world.

CaringBridge (www.caringbridge.org)
Provides a home page for families to share their cancer experience in words and pictures.

Chemo Duck (www.gabesmyheart.com)
A real-life lemons-make-lemonade story, Chemo Duck is a teaching toy provided free to hospitalized kids. This is a small organization with a big heart. The Web site has some good downloadable materials for kids and families.

Kids Cope (2045 Peachtree Road, Suite 150, Atlanta, GA 30309; 404-892-1437; www.kidscope.org)
This nonprofit organization develops and distributes materials to help kids understand cancer treatments and side effects. "Kemo shark" is a comic book hero designed to help children understand chemotherapy. Written for children whose parents have cancer, but the principle is the same. Free download. Also in Spanish.

Lotsa Helping Hands (www.lotsahelpinghands.com)

An Internet resource with a calendar-based system to organize help—friends, relatives, neighbors, etc.—with the feeling of a blog.

National Childhood Cancer Foundation/Children's Oncology Group (www.curesearch.org)

This joint Web site has a wealth of information on coping for friends, school, and community. Excellent explanation and advice on insurance issues.

Hershey Home Medical Guide: "Promoting Independence" and "Parent's Anxiety" (www.hmc.psu.edu/hematology/homeguide)

These are but two of the chapters in this excellent online publication. Advice is given in a reassuring but professional manner, with concrete steps to take in various situations. The Hershey Center is Pennsylvania State University's Hershey Medical Center.

Share the Care (www.sharethecare.org)

Post your needs—whether a ride to the clinic, laundry, meals, or whatever—so friends and family can see how they can help.

24

Siblings, Other Family, and Friends

How do people cope with the diagnosis of cancer in a beloved child? San Diego University clinical psychologist Dr. John Spinetta, who has researched and written extensively on living with childhood cancer, believes three factors influence how well the family survives the experience. First, those with a "well-established philosophy of life," religious or otherwise, will have that to draw on when illness strikes. Second, families who make an effort to educate their child and themselves about what is happening will experience less fear born of ignorance. And third, those with a strong support system, especially a good bond between the parents but including solid relationships with extended family and friends, will have an easier time.

The clinic or hospital will have social workers, psychologists, and psychiatrists on the staff or on call, and making these people part of the treatment team helps. Depression may come *after* crises are over, and these feelings may have to be worked out in therapy.

Parents

Mothers usually bear most of the burden in dealing with the disease itself—the clinic and hospital visits, the disruption of schedules, and helping the child with his disability. While the mother is thus occupied, perhaps to the exclusion of everything else, the father may well be retreating into his work. She begins to resent his absence; he feels left out.

This is a common pattern but not a universal one. Occasionally the mother carries on with normal life and the father takes the child for all medical care. Sometimes the parents alternate, and sometimes both are able to accompany the child to the clinic.

At the hospital, nurses will note in the medical record who accompanies the child on each visit and his or her state of mind. Then if one parent is consistently absent and perceived as "dropping out," the clinic staff will offer to arrange visits at alternate times, even after clinic hours if necessary, to allow both parents to talk with the doctor.

A father has too often been perceived as a peripheral family member, the stern disciplinarian who appears around dinnertime. The changes of the past few decades and the movement of so many women into the workforce are altering this perception, and many men today consider family relationships as important as rapid career advancement.

A small but revealing study at the University of Toronto looked at the father's role in his child's illness. The men were deeply concerned about their children and affected by the illness but received little support, whether professional or from family and friends, in contrast to the support their wives received. The fathers also had more trouble talking about the illness and had little opportunity to do so. They wanted to be included in discussions with the health care team but were not always able to attend. The men also worried that the child's illness was affecting family life, particularly the siblings' well-being, and about the effect the stress would have on their jobs.

It is important to keep the lines of communication between husband and wife open. One way to do this is by getting away by yourselves regularly for at least a few hours. There will be resentments and arguments, but they should be worked out rather than put off until the time seems more appropriate. Most studies have shown that the divorce rate among families of children with cancer is no greater than average and sometimes even lower. Every marriage goes through phases, and the added stress of childhood illness will complicate the relationship by intensifying its good or bad points, either weakening or strengthening the bond. On the plus side, many families come through the experience even stronger for having faced the crisis together.

Everyone needs time to himself or herself to rest, relax, recharge, and recuperate emotionally. This goes for both parents, together and alone.

Have goals, something you can think about and plan now and work toward "later." Plan a trip you will take, or a garden you will plant. The year I spent the most time sitting in hospital and clinic rooms, I knitted Christmas presents for everyone—afghans, sweaters, toddler dresses, mittens, hats. It gave me a real sense of personal accomplishment, which otherwise would have been sorely lacking those long months. That was also a period (before the Internet and e-mail) when far-flung relatives and friends got more frequent letters from me than ever before or since.

Siblings, or "What About Me?"

Siblings of the child with cancer experience problems, too. They may be afraid they will "catch" cancer, or that the child became sick because of ill will from a brother or sister. They are usually jealous of the added attention the sick child receives from their parents and others, and they may feel abandoned if one or both parents are spending a lot of time at the hospital or clinic, returning home in a state of exhaustion. The siblings may also feel guilty about the jealousy. The healthy children should not have to make too many concessions to the sick child over too long a period of time, or resentments will grow. Don't be fooled by a sibling who appears unconcerned about the family's situation. He or she may be hiding it, but it's certainly there anyway.

After diagnosis, siblings should have clear, age-appropriate explanations of the illness and what the family expects will happen. Parents should ensure that the brother or sister knows the disease is not a result of sibling rivalry. Some support groups also have chat sessions for siblings, and some camps have either integrated or dedicated programs for siblings of cancer patients.

Provide plenty of opportunity for the siblings to ask questions and discuss the situation. Don't be surprised if the same questions come up over and over again. Patience will pay off here. Be honest. If or when the question arises as to whether the child is going to die, admit that you don't know for sure, but that you are providing the best medical care you can to give the sick child the best chance there is.

They can, if they want, go along for clinic visits to see where the parents and their brother or sister are spending so much time. It is important to prepare them for the experience: the alien hospital environment will be frightening and the sick child's appearance may be changed a lot, too.

Expect changes in behavior. Perhaps a child who has been learning independence will become clingy. He may revert to younger behavior, like bedwetting in a potty-trained youngster. He may have nightmares or other sleep problems. Anger at being asked to do more chores than usual, or at being admonished to be quiet and considerate of the sick child, is very possible; tantrums are upsetting but rather normal in these circumstances. The sibling may tempt fate by adopting dangerous habits—riding a bike out of control or into unsafe circumstances, driving recklessly, doing drugs or alcohol.

It's obvious that the sick child's teachers need to be kept up on what's happening, but the siblings' teachers and coaches should be, too. Schoolwork could suffer, with poor grades and reluctance to go at all (which might be a fear that things will get worse while he is away). Social problems can arise at school, too; teasing or shunning behavior among classmates is not unusual and must be acknowledged and handled.

The sibling may lash out, withdraw, or suffer from "will it happen to me" anxiety. Let the child know that you realize his world is out of balance and that you're doing all you can to steady it. The sibling will see his parents in a new light; where he saw confidence before, he now recognizes fear, worry, and confusion.

Try to set aside time to do something special with the "left-out" siblings. Rent a movie and make some popcorn. Plan an outing like a picnic or a restaurant treat. Take a walk. Be very careful not to promise something you can't carry out. The "what" is not as important as the "who"—the focus on this child.

When Lisa was in high school, long after she'd completed chemotherapy, she had several difficult surgeries and her younger sister felt left out. At the end of the school year Mollie and I packed the car and went for a short camping trip at the Maine beach—just the two of us.

The nocturnal deflating air mattress, the flat tire when we had to empty the back of the car—these are things we still laugh about. It was our time.

Grandparents and Other Relatives

Grandparents, too, will need reassurance. If they live nearby, they can go to the clinic, to the hospital, or to support group meetings. If the situation permits it, grandparents can be important in keeping the household running smoothly and in caring for the siblings.

Grandparents are feeling double the pain—for the sick child, of course, but also for their child, the suffering parent. They can listen, hug, keep the rest of the family informed on a regular basis. They can visit the child and brighten his day. He's still their grandchild, not a diagnosis. Include grandparents as appropriate in hospital and clinic visits and meetings. Often they have the resources to be very helpful; if they are retired and in good health, they may also have time and energy that the parents simply lack.

Special Family Situations

Some families have special problems. Single parents are often stretched to the limit in normal life, juggling child care, visitation rights, home life, and jobs. Having a sick child must seem almost unbearable. They can ask family members, friends, and neighbors for help. Perhaps their town or neighborhood has an emergency social service agency that provides babysitting, transportation, or other help.

If the parents are divorced, it may require a special effort to keep both the father and the mother fully informed about the child's illness and therapy. If the divorced couple simply cannot communicate, perhaps a member of the health care team can be designated to keep an absent parent up to date.

Some families must seek help at clinics where they do not understand the language. Translators should be available on the hospital staff, on call, or in the community. Notifying the institution in advance of their arrival is the key here.

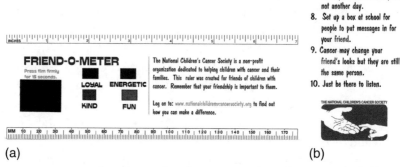

Friends Rule!

Good Friends Can Help
A Friend With Cancer:

1. Ask your friend if they want to talk.
2. Call to let your friend in on what's new at school.
3. Get classmates to send cards.
4. Connect through e-mail.
5. Start a phone chain.
6. Visit your friend often.
7. Just because your friend does not feel well enough to talk one day doesn't mean they will not another day.
8. Set up a box at school for people to put messages in for your friend.
9. Cancer may change your friend's looks but they are still the same person.
10. Just be there to listen.

FRIEND-O-METER

Press film firmly for 15 seconds.

LOYAL   ENERGETIC

KIND   FUN

The National Children's Cancer Society is a non-profit organization dedicated to helping children with cancer and their families. This ruler was created for friends of children with cancer. Remember that your friendship is important to them.

Log on to: www.nationalchildrenscancersociety.org to find out how you can make a difference.

THE NATIONAL CHILDREN'S CANCER SOCIETY

(a)   (b)

FIGURE 24.1 Friends Rule! Used with permission from the National Children's Cancer Society

Friends

It is difficult to know what to say to a family facing catastrophic illness, but it is even worse to say nothing. Do not avoid the family and the child patient for fear you will say something wrong. Be there. Listen. Keep your calls and visits brief until you fully understand the situation and what the family wants.

It is hard for many people to ask for help, but asking does not mean losing your independence, and it is not a sign of weakness; rather, it is a strengthening of ties, a sharing of burdens. Close friends can offer to go with the child and parents to important medical meetings. Another ear and a clearer mind is a benefit here; the friends can take notes, clarify information, and discuss it later, under less stress.

If the family is having financial difficulties, friends may wish to plan a fundraising event—anything from a yard sale to a golf tournament. If the family itself is all right with finances, friends can plan an event to raise awareness in the community and collect funds for cancer research. Many communities have carried out a bone marrow donor drive to identify potential matches not only for a specific child but also for information to bank for use with other patients down the road.

A national survey by Mark Clements in *Parade Magazine* gave some advice on how to help:

- Call to say hello.
- Focus on the person, not the disease.
- Stop in for a visit—and a laugh.
- Take a meal.
- Go with the family for medical visits.
- Run errands. Shop for food, carpool their kids, pick up their dry-cleaning.
- Entertain their kids, or help with homework.
- Provide financial assistance if you can and if it's needed.

A program called Baskets for Families in the Hospital (explained on the ACOR Web site—see the resource list at the end of the chapter) has wonderful ideas for a gift parcel that would be most welcomed by families whose trips to the hospital are often on an emergency basis and who find themselves without even the most basic needs such as toothbrushes, shampoo, and hand cream. While the hospital will probably be able to provide some of those things, a fancy little tube of fragrant moisturizer can be a real day-brightener. The Web site has many ideas on what to include. Do toss in something funny, too; a rubber pig nose or a wind-up bug are great for tension relief. The Archie McPhee Website (www.archiemcphee.com) sells amusing items like pirate-themed bandages and an armadillo handbag. Sometimes bright lights bother the patients, so a book light would be a great gift for the bedside parent who likes to read.

Here are some more ideas, from our experience and beyond. Give them a phone card to cover long-distance calls; a roll of quarters for tolls or other slots; a gas card to help pay for all those trips to the hospital; a gift certificate for groceries or perhaps for a restaurant near the hospital. Take their car for service. Throw in a load of their towels with your own. Take pets to the vet for checkups. Bathe Bowser if he tangles with a skunk. Help with transportation.

Lisa was once hospitalized during a big snowstorm. We dreaded going home, knowing we'd have to shovel to even get the car off the street. We were both touched and flabbergasted to turn the corner and find our driveway completely plowed. We still have no idea who did us this kindness, but we have tried to pass it on to others.

Gifts for the child need not be fancy or expensive. A fellow in an elevator on the way to deliver a lovely bouquet to the children's floor commented wisely, "The kid would probably rather have a coloring book and crayons." Hand-held electronic games need not be costly; for less than the price of a CD, we got pocket-size, battery-operated solitaire, Yahtzee, and similar games that have filled many boring hours.

Mostly: Listen. Be there. With hugs. Take chocolate or home-baked cookies. The family will never forget the kindness.

Further Resources

READING

Clements, Mark, "What we can learn from cancer." *Parade Magazine*, February 6, 2000, p. 12

Dodd, Michael. *Oliver's Story for "Sibs" of Kids with Cancer.*
Candlelighters Childhood Cancer Foundation, 2004.
Introductory material for parents by Rabbi Harold S. Kushner and for the siblings by the author/illustrator. Charming full-color drawings. The story is told in Oliver's words about his sister's treatment for cancer. Recognizes the sibling's own journey through the minefield of childhood cancer, validates feelings. Elementary school audience.

Halpern, Susan P. *The Etiquette of Illness: What to Say When You Can't Find the Words.* New York: Bloomsbury, 2004.
The title suggests "Miss Manners/Emily Post does illness," but this small book goes beyond the superficial to brief but helpful suggestions on how to talk to sick friends, how to help, and how to figure out when to do or say little. Not specific at all to sick children, the advice nevertheless is transferable to families dealing with a child's cancer diagnosis. Many examples and anecdotes flesh out the advice, and one section discusses communication between patient and doctor. Preparing for death is handled with grace and compassion and not ignored. This is a book to keep around to read now and then as the child passes through different phases.

Kalick, Rosanne. *Cancer Etiquette.* Scarsdale, NY: Lion Books, 2004.
This slim volume is packed with good advice for communicating with the patient and family.

Picoult, Jodi. *My Sister's Keeper.* New York: Atria, 2004.

This novel explores issues of medical ethics when one sister is conceived, as she feels, to provide healthy body parts (cord blood, stem cells, bone marrow, eventually a kidney) for a sister with cancer. The family dynamics especially rings true—the distracted mother, the acting-out brother. The legal aspect of bioethics is thought-provoking, although the final chapter is disappointing. Overall, a wise book by a good writer. The film version has a stronger conclusion, if even sadder.

Sonnenblick, Jordan. *Drums, Girls and Dangerous Pie*. Lehigh Valley, PA: Turning Tide Press, 2004.

A young adult novel. A 13-year-old boy's brother is diagnosed with ALL. This is a wise, readable account of a family nightmare from the point of view of the sibling, who feels invisible. Well-written and highly recommended. Sonnenblick has a new young adult novel, *After Ever After*, about survivor issues that promises to be as much fun and as honest as his earlier title.

Stewart, Gail B. *Alexandra Scott: Champion for Cancer Research*. Detroit: Kidhaven Press, 2006 (Young Heroes Series).

The heartening story of a young girl with neuroblastoma. For grades 4 and up.

Taking Time—Support for People with Cancer and the People Who Care About Them. National Institutes of Health, National Cancer Institute, 1997, 1999. Available at www.cancer.gov

Written for the cancer patient, this 60-page booklet is helpful for friends and others trying to understand what's happening emotionally (rather than focus on the physical).

"When Someone in Your Family Has Cancer." National Institutes of Health, National Cancer Institute, n.d. Available at www.cancer.gov

Excellent booklet to help children understand their feelings and the family's situation.

ORGANIZATIONS/WEB SITES

Gift baskets for families in the hospital: www.acor.org/ped-onc/cfissues/baskets.html

Hershey Medical Center: "Helping brothers and sisters cope" (www.pennstatehershey.org/web/childrens/patientcare/patientresources)

Chapter of a truly excellent online *Home Care Guide*, p. 69. Very thorough, thoughtful, and helpful.

SuperSibs (www.supersibs.org)

An Illinois-based nonprofit group with nationwide reach to "honor, support, and recognize brothers and sisters of children with cancer." Focus is on the "forgotten family members" who too often get lost in the shuffle—or feel that way. There are a lot of great links to other resources from this site.

Family Care Navigator (Family Caregiver Alliance; www.caregiver.org)

This state-by-state guide is a starting point to finding support programs both governmental and private.

OTHER

The Lion in the House. Five Families, Six Years. True Stories from the War on Cancer.

This powerful documentary film by Steven Bognar and Julia Reichert justifiably won awards from the Sundance Film Festival. Broadcast by PBS and available on DVD with an accompanying book, the film is extraordinary, real, true, sad, and a lot more. While I enthusiastically recommend this movie and book, be aware that there are extremely painful moments.

25

Handling Medical Problems at Home

The physical effects of cancer, both of the disease and its treatment, are especially difficult for a child to endure, and much of that unpleasantness is shared with the parents. But there are ways to help both patient and caregiver by easing the discomfort for the former and therefore also for the latter. Below are some practical tips.

Preventing Infection

To coin a phrase, it is far better to prevent an infection than treat one. While it is unlikely that all infections can be prevented while your child is on chemotherapy, there are steps you can take to minimize the likelihood.

- Have somebody besides your child clean bird cages, fish tanks, litter boxes, and the like. They are a source of bacteria.
- Wash your hands regularly but especially after using the bathroom and before touching your child or his toys, food, etc.
- Make sure everybody has his own toothbrush and oral thermometer.
- Keep your child out of crowds when his blood counts are low.
- Always use sunblock and protective clothing when the child is outdoors.

- Use creams and lotions to keep dry skin from cracking, which can allow bacteria to enter the bloodstream.
- Ask friends who are feeling "under the weather" to put off visiting until they are well again.
- Keep up regular dental care and brushing.
- Be careful of raw foods, especially meat and fish. (Skip the beefsteak tartare and sushi for now.)
- Make friends with someone at your child's school (probably the nurse) who will be aware of infectious diseases making the rounds and who will notify you to be on the alert.
- Invest in a supply of waterless antibacterial hand cleaners for use when handwashing is difficult. The cleaner is a good substitute for soap and water handwashing.

Getting "Shots"

Nobody likes getting needles, and especially for young children the very sight of a syringe can set off major fear and crying. Children facing repeated "sticks" can be given a local anesthetic in the form of a topical cream (EMLA) ahead of time to lessen the pain. Complementary therapies like guided imagery can relax the child and lessen the pain. Play therapy can address the dreaded needles, too. Try distracting the child with a party blower or similar small toy. Fortunately, with the central lines commonly used today, far fewer "sticks" are necessary for most patients.

Taking Temperatures

Although 98.6 degrees F (37 degrees C) is regarded as the normal body temperature, what is "normal" varies from person to person. It can even vary for the same person; for example, body temperatures are generally higher later in the day. Rectal temperatures, considered the most accurate, in younger children tend to run up to one degree higher than 98.6 degrees F and temperatures taken under the arm a bit lower. It helps to know what the child's normal temperature is. When a fever is suspected, the temperature is taken either by mouth (oral) or in the armpit (axillary). If the child has been physically active, he should rest half an hour before the temperature is taken to avoid a false high reading.

It takes 3 minutes for an oral temperature to register. These are accurate only if the child is old enough to cooperate and hold the thermometer under the tongue. Some newer models are shaped to help with that. To take the temperature in the armpit (axillary), the thermometer must be placed in the folds of the skin and not in clothing. The arm should be held firmly to the child's side for 5 minutes before the temperature is read. While less intrusive, axillary temperatures are not considered especially accurate.

Mercury is a poison, the main reason why the familiar mercury thermometers are no longer used. A new generation of non-mercury thermometers is now available, and your pharmacist can help you choose one, perhaps a digital type, with more precise and faster readings. For toddlers there are even "pacifier" thermometers.

A step up from the old "ther-MOM-eter," Mom's-hand-on-the-forehead method, is the temporal artery thermometer that uses a gentle stroke on the forehead to measure the temperature. They are sold by big box retailers and pharmacies. These measurements are more accurate than the ear thermometers. Studies have shown that temporal thermometers approach rectal temperatures for accuracy.

Hospitals are using paper thermometers to save on sterilizing glass instruments. The oral paper thermometers have liquid crystal dots that change color to indicate body temperature. Ear thermometers are pricey and not useful for infants.

Reducing Fever

These procedures should begin, of course, *after* the doctor or clinic is notified about the fever, which could signal a life-threatening infection. Besides infection, fever can be caused by an allergic reaction to a drug or a blood transfusion, certain tumors themselves, and other medical problems like hepatitis. The clinic may want to assess the child before therapy like Tylenol begins.

Avoid aspirin unless the doctor orders it, because it can interfere with the function of platelets. Instead, acetaminophen (Tylenol, Liquiprin, or less expensive generic brands) should be substituted. If the fever is quite high (over 103 degrees F) or if it seems resistant to medication, the doctor may suggest putting the child in a tepid bath. At the beginning, the water should be about body temperature, with cool water gradually added. This should continue for about 20 minutes, after which the youngster is rubbed dry. The blood vessels respond to this stimulation by dilating, bringing blood to the body surface for cooling. If the child's temperature is still elevated after half an hour, the bath can be repeated.

If the child is sweating with the fever, keep him dry by changing clothing and blankets, keeping him out of drafts (turn off that fan for now), and perhaps lowering the thermostat so he is more comfortable. Don't use ice water, ice packs, or alcohol sponges.

Tooth Care

The child should continue taking normal care of the teeth and gums when receiving chemotherapy or radiation. The child should brush after meals and at bedtime with a soft toothbrush, then rinse with a solution of salt and baking soda (1/4 teaspoon of each in a glass of water). If the child is too young to brush his own teeth, the parent should wrap a soft cloth around a finger, dip it in the rinse solution, and rub the teeth and gums. If the child's blood counts are low, ask your doctor about appropriate dental practices. With the doctor's approval, regular dental visits can and should continue.

Mouth Sores

Certain chemotherapy drugs and head and neck radiation can cause mouth sores; this is sometimes such a severe problem that the patient cannot eat or talk comfortably. The sores tend to appear a couple of weeks after therapy has begun. Besides the pain and nutritional difficulties, open oral sores can provide a pathway for germs to enter the bloodstream and cause infection. Drugs are in development for severe cases, but some steps can help prevent them in the first place:

- Good dental care (see above)
- Have the child floss unless the platelet level is so low that he could bleed.

- Do not use purchased mouthwashes, which contain alcohol.
- Give the child moderate foods—soft, chewable, not spicy, not too hot or too cold.
- If the child experiences dry mouth from a lack of saliva, have him sip water regularly and avoid sugary foods.
- Ask the doctor whether a fluoride gel would be helpful.

Constipation

The doctor may prescribe or recommend a stool softener such as docusate sodium (Colace) or a laxative like polyethylene glycol (MiraLAX) or senna (Senokot) to avoid constipation, but a careful diet may also prevent it. This diet should begin before the treatment (such as vincristine) is given and should be continued for a week after. Prune juice, whole-grain cereals and breads, and fresh fruits and vegetables help keep the digestive system working. Raisins, apricots, and apple juice are often favorites with children. Give the child plenty of liquids and do have him exercise, if that is feasible, perhaps with nonstrenuous video games. A constipated child on chemotherapy should not be given an enema unless it is specifically ordered by the primary doctor. Sometimes routine preparations for tests like an intravenous pyelogram (IVP) include an enema. If a different department at the hospital orders an enema, the primary doctor should verify the need for one first.

Morphine-type drugs like hydrocodone (Vicodin) and oxycodone also cause constipation. The child may be started on a bowel regimen at the time such drugs are ordered.

An older child or a teen may find the use of a bedpan so unpleasant or embarrassing that he or she can't "perform," so that constipation results or worsens. If possible, help him or her use a toilet or a bedside commode and provide privacy for the duration.

Diarrhea

Abdominal radiation and some chemotherapy drugs can lead to diarrhea. Again, diet can be an ally. The child should go easy on fruit in this circumstance, and eat lots of bananas (to replace lost potassium), rice, eggs, and potatoes. Cheese, cottage cheese, and yogurt may or may not be helpful, depending on the cause of the diarrhea. The clinic should know the child is having this problem because it might be alleviated by switching antibiotics, for example.

Ironically, one cause of diarrhea is constipation, so be sure to get expert advice before treating either of these conditions. Bowel impactions or obstructions are also common in cancer patients, caused by the cancer, by therapy, or by scar tissue after surgery. Prompt attention to any of these conditions is important.

Vomiting and Nausea

Many chemotherapy patients experience nausea and vomiting. This is one reason why doctors often give extra fluids intravenously at the time of treatments; another is to flush the medicines through the body. New anti-nausea drugs often appear on the market. Such medicines, like trimethobenzamide (Tigan), are given orally or rectally; they may cause drowsiness. Another drug called ondansetron (Zofran) does not cause drowsiness. The child may have to start taking these preparations the night before the therapy for maximum effectiveness. These anti-emetic medications may or may not work, and some have side effects as well. See the table in Chapter 22 for information on medications to alleviate these miseries.

What actually causes the nausea and vomiting? They are functions of the central nervous system. Vomiting is a reflex action controlled by the brain. Anxiety and fear of vomiting can indeed lead to vomiting itself. A child who has experienced nausea and vomiting after previous chemotherapy sessions may start to vomit even before receiving the next course of drugs—perhaps even before he enters the clinic. It can be triggered by smells (like alcohol swabs), taste, pain, motion, and more.

Anti-anxiety medications or nondrug intervention like relaxation or distraction may be effective in preventing this anticipatory nausea and vomiting. Radiation to the brain or abdomen and tumor growth in the gastrointestinal tract also stimulate vomiting.

The most effective way for the child to deal with the nausea is to sleep after treatments. Foods that may help include flat ginger ale, Popsicles, carbonated beverages or tea, fruit lollipops or hard candy, saltines, or bouillon. The child should avoid milk, which is not easy to digest; it is a shade easier to clean up vomited juice than milk anyway. Deep breathing and ice chips may also help control the queasiness.

Queasy-Pops are lollipops intended to ease nausea and vomiting. Made by Three Lollies, they are available on the Candlelighters Childhood Cancer Foundation Web site under "Comforts." The U.S. Food and Drug Administration has approved a medicated patch (Sancuso, a granisetron transdermal system) for adults with a high to moderate risk of chemotherapy-induced nausea and vomiting, although no pediatric research has been completed.

Some mind–body techniques may also help the child control nausea. Guided imagery, hypnosis, or acupuncture may help. See the chapter on alternative and complementary therapies (Chapter 21) for further information.

With vomiting and diarrhea, dehydration is a common problem. Some good old tap water will help alleviate it. The child might need sports drinks or similar fortified water sometimes, but for daily drinking, no fancy bottled water is necessary.

If the child seems to be getting too dehydrated from vomiting and diarrhea, offer ice chips, Jell-O, or a solution of Jell-O water and popsicles. Symptoms of serious dehydration include listlessness, lethargy, dry mouth, sunken eyes, a lack of tears or saliva, and infrequent urination. If these appear, call the doctor.

A recent technique that has helped many people is the slow administration of drugs with infusion pumps. The same dose of medication is given over the course of a week rather than in a few hours. Side effects like nausea and hair loss have decreased with this innovation, and there is a possibility that the constant administration is more effective in killing cancer cells than the quicker, larger doses.

Some hospitals are researching the use of marijuana to ease nausea and vomiting, with favorable results in certain circumstances. "Pot" also improved patients' appetites. An adolescent who wants to pursue this should discuss it with the doctor or another member of the clinic staff. Of course, no patient should experiment with this or any other illegal drug on his own: he doesn't need difficulties with the law in addition to the medical problems!

A drug called dronabinol (Marinol) has the active ingredient of cannabis and may be helpful, although it takes much longer to get into the bloodstream than the smoking route uses. Of course, smoked "pot" carries the toxins of inhaled smoke.

Preventing the onset of nausea and vomiting is certainly the best course of action. A snack prior to receiving chemo or an hour before radiation may be helpful, as well as packing food for long treatments. Small, frequent room-temperature meals may be better tolerated. Crackers, toast, or flat ginger ale may settle a queasy stomach. Avoid clothing that fits tightly around the abdomen.

Diet and Nutrition

Your child's nutritional status before and during therapy plays an important role in his overall response to treatments. A malnourished patient has more difficulty healing and recovering from illnesses and surgery. A child who was a picky eater before getting sick will pose special challenges.

If the child is nauseated, small high-protein, high-calorie meals and nutritious snacks several times a day served in a pleasant atmosphere may help. Protein is especially important for the regrowth of tissue. Although a good diet is important for any child, the period of remission will not be affected one way or the other by improper eating.

It is fine to cater to the child's likes; this is no time to insist on eating broccoli. Ethnic specialties may tempt his appetite. The child should drink plenty of water and other liquids to help flush the drugs through the body. Avoid greasy or overly sweet foods. Giving favorite foods to a nauseated child is not advisable, for he may come to associate them with sickness and refuse them in the future. The child may also develop unusual aversions to foods. Even today Lisa will not eat ice cream that is packaged in small cardboard cups, which she considers "hospital pack," and she has hated mint since taking an antibiotic with that flavor.

Some chemotherapy drugs change the sense of taste, making certain foods seem metallic, for example. The chapter on chemotherapy (Chapter 18) has a more thorough discussion of this problem.

There are several excellent books on diet for the child with cancer, some of them available free from the government or on the World Wide Web. These have recipes, special diet regimens, and lots of advice for the parent struggling to get nutritious food into a sick youngster. The bibliography has specific titles. The clinic or hospital may have copies for loan or distribution.

Enteral Nutrition

Sometimes children may not be able to eat normally for a period of time. Enteral nutrition, or tube feeding, may be an effective temporary measure to provide nutrients. A nasogastric (NG) tube passes from the nose into the stomach; a gastronomy tube (GT) is placed during surgery through the stomach wall. A child who can't digest food normally may be placed on total parenteral nutrition (TPN), which is administered intravenously.

Sleep

It is easy enough to say but hard to accomplish: the child needs adequate sleep. This may mean naps during the day even for older children and adolescents who may have long outgrown the need for them. Parents can do themselves a favor by taking a nap, too. This was another bit of advice I fought, even as Lisa awakened us nightly for months on end. I eventually learned to sleep for half an hour wherever I landed: on trains, in hallways, even slumped over a bedside table in the hospital.

Itching

Anyone who has had a close encounter with poison ivy knows how unpleasant it is to feel itchy. The medical term is pruritus, and it may occur in cancer patients as a result of certain types of malignancies (leukemia, lymphoma, and others). It may also be caused by some chemotherapy agents, by radiation, by bone marrow transplantation, and by some other forms of therapy, alone or in combination. It could also be a symptom of infection. While the impulse to scratch is almost overwhelming, the child should not be allowed to do so because skin broken by scratching can result in infection. Tell the doctor about the itching—when it occurs, how long it lasts, and so forth.

Relief may be gained by using lotions to moisturize the skin, by using mild soaps, by keeping the patient cool, and by soaking for half an hour in a lukewarm bath (to which perhaps some oatmeal has been added). Too-frequent and too-hot baths can result in dry skin that leads to itching, and the cycle continues. Dressing the child in natural fibers (but not wool) and using cotton bedding avoids the itching sometimes caused by synthetic fibers and wool.

Complementary therapies like relaxation techniques and guided imagery may distract the child and provide relief. Your doctor may prescribe medication to alleviate the itching. In the meantime, an ice pack or a cool wet washcloth over the affected area may also be soothing.

Giving Medicine at Home

Getting the child to take medicine at home can be a big problem. We have some not-so-fond memories of trying to get Lisa to take her long-term liquid antibiotic (the mint-flavored one). Until we redecorated the room where her changing table once stood, there were smudges of the stuff on the wall. The appearance of the drug in a new cherry flavor was our particular salvation. If the child dislikes the taste of his medicine, the doctor or pharmacist might know of an alternative brand with a more palatable flavor. One parent suggests that the child suck an ice cube (or perhaps a Popsicle) before taking oral medicine to deaden taste buds.

Most medicine will eventually go down if it is mixed with applesauce or a favorite treat. (Lisa tells me now that she was not fooled and knew that I had hidden pills in those spoons of chocolate syrup and grape jelly.) Tablets can be ground between two spoons and dissolved in a few drops of water for half an hour. Follow the dose with a drink. If the medicine is in liquid form, putting half of it at a time in the spoon will minimize spills. If the child spits it out or vomits within half an hour, repeat the dose. If the child fights taking medicines, perhaps his attention can be diverted with a storybook or a toy. A very young child can be wrapped in a blanket and held to soothe him.

Doctors advise mixing the drug with a spoonful of applesauce or chocolate syrup and following it with a drink rather than mixing it with the drink itself because the child may not drink the whole glass or bottle. Also, some drugs should not be given at the same time as milk; the pharmacist should explain this when the prescription is filled.

One mother, a nurse, melted chocolate, mixed in the oral medicine, and poured the candy into molds. (Ice cube trays would work, too, each cube having a single dose.) This is the sort of tip found in the Candlelighters' *CCCF Newsletter*. Parents should check with the doctor or druggist before doing this, though.

There are a couple of different devices available at drugstores that may be useful in giving liquid medicine. One is a "test tube" with a spoon-like mouthpiece on the end to measure and administer these drugs. The doctor can also provide syringes (without needle tips, of course) to accurately measure the dose. This is especially helpful if the prescription is written for cubic centimeters (cc's) since many homes have only measuring spoons. (In that case, remember that 5 ml = 5 cc = 1 tsp.) An added benefit of the syringe is that the parent can "shoot" the medicine into the back of the child's mouth with far less spillage. If the family has several syringes, your child might enjoy playing with one in the bath; they make nifty squirt guns and I have seen larger-sized syringes used in hospital playrooms with wall targets and lots of towels on the floor.

Giving anti-nausea medicine by mouth is an exercise in futility if the child vomits. The doctor may instead prescribe a rectal suppository. (If the dose is half a suppository, it should be cut in half lengthwise with a warmed knife. Storing it first in the refrigerator can make it easier to cut—but it should be at room temperature before use.) The tapered end is pushed as far as a finger will go, then the buttocks should be held closed for 5 to 10 minutes to allow it to dissolve.

Because Lisa had a series of urinary tract infections requiring antibiotics available only for injection, the nurses taught me to give shots at home. Neither of us liked this, but it did save Lisa many days of hospitalization, because the drug had to be given for 10 days. When injections have to be given several times a day around the clock, it will be hard to find a visiting nurse willing to come to your home to give the shots. We even ran into a lot of red tape looking for someone official to help me give Lisa shots, and when the town nurse agreed to come, she only held Lisa while I gave the injection. I eventually learned to hold her myself while giving the shot. We both became quite stoic about it, especially after we stocked up on fancy cartoon Band-Aids as rewards. With indwelling catheters, some parents can be taught to give IV medications, too.

The doctor should know what over-the-counter medications the child is taking. Some cough syrups, for example, have an ingredient called glyceryl guaiacolate (guaifenesin) that, like aspirin, can interfere with the function of platelets. The pharmacist knows the ingredients of different cold medicines if the labels seem unclear.

Immunizations

Parents can now be grateful that the child is up to date on his shots. If a booster is due, or if the child missed some immunizations, he cannot have any live vaccines while receiving chemotherapy because of the risk of serious illness. Live vaccines include those for measles, mumps, rubella (German measles) (sometimes given together as MMR), smallpox, chickenpox, and polio. Killed viruses like diphtheria, pertussis (whooping cough), and tetanus (sometimes combined in DPT) may be allowed by the primary doctor. If there is influenza in the community, the doctor may suggest immunization.

Chickenpox has been the most feared of these diseases because the usually mild illness can be dangerous for a child with a compromised immune system. Report any exposure to the clinic immediately. The child will be isolated during his clinic visits for several weeks to make sure other children are not exposed as well—or until the child contracts and gets over the chickenpox.

Doctors now recommend a single varicella shot (chickenpox immunization) between the ages of 12 and 18 months. Children with weak immune systems (such as those being treated for cancer) can become very ill if they do get chickenpox. If your child has a known exposure to chickenpox, a concentrated preparation of zoster immune globulin (ZIG) given within 3 days can prevent the disease or minimize its effects.

This is a good time to urge that the patient's friends and classmates get any immunizations they may have missed. The sick child may still be exposed to something at the supermarket or Disneyland, but every little bit helps.

Many schools require that a child have all shots before enrolling, but I have never heard of a youngster being refused admittance if he cannot have the vaccines due to cancer. The clinic doctor will deal with the school authorities if there are any questions.

Late-Stage Disease

If the child becomes increasingly disabled or bedridden, the parents' abilities will be taxed to the limit, and new skills will be required to provide for the child's comfort. The clinic or hospital staff will teach them what they need to know, and a visiting nurse may be provided for at-home professional care. If appropriate, hospice organizations help organize these services.

Here are just a few of the physical symptoms you may see in a terminally ill child.

Skin Problems

Meticulous skin care is required to avoid irritated skin and bedsores in bedridden children. The nurse will teach the family how to move a bedridden child to prevent bedsores from developing. The child's skin can be rubbed with creams or perhaps some lotion left over from hospital visits, or the pharmacist can recommend good products. Do not use skin-care products with alcohol, which is drying. An air mattress or a waterbed may help avoid the sores, too. If the child needs a hospital bed or other equipment, in many areas the American Cancer Society can loan it.

Bone Fragility

If the youngster has metastases to the bones, care should be taken even when turning him sover in bed, to avoid breaking bones. A firm mattress and small pillows to support the limbs can reduce discomfort.

Loss of Bowel or Bladder Control

Patients with late-stage cancer may lose control of their bowel and bladder functions. The bed can be protected with rubber sheets and disposable pads or diapers. Keeping the child dry will help prevent sores and rashes, as will frequent baths and powder. If there is a problem with odor in the room, this cleanliness will help, as will room sprays.

When to Call the Doctor

Parents will soon learn to recognize problems they cannot or should not try to handle alone at home. In general, call the clinic about any unusual symptoms or reactions, particularly in the early days of treatment. Even just a "gut feeling" that something is very different and wrong should be investigated. Parents should watch for:

- Fever over 100 or 101 degrees F oral that does not respond promptly to acetaminophen (Tylenol, etc.). Note: Your doctor may not want you to give your child any medications before being evaluated.
- Bleeding that cannot be stopped in 15 minutes by constant pressure
- Bruising easily
- Unusual pain, including headaches
- Shortness of breath
- Blood in the urine
- Excessive thirst or urination
- Excessive vomiting (a vomiting child may not be getting the full benefit of any drugs)
- Runny stools or diarrhea
- Sores or ulcers in the mouth, on the skin, or near the anus
- Jaundice (yellow tint to the skin)
- Rash, swollen hands or feet (signs of an allergic reaction)

It is important to call the doctor right away if the youngster is exposed to childhood diseases like measles, mumps, and chickenpox, or to adults with shingles. These illnesses are minor in most children but are life-threatening to those with impaired immune systems, such as those undergoing chemotherapy. Vaccination is the major preventive measure, of course. If there is an outbreak of contagious disease, the doctor might advise keeping the patient home from school.

Some unfortunate youngsters get these illnesses more than once after their immune system fails. Most commonly the varicella virus is reactivated as shingles (herpes zoster); it tends to localize on one side of the body but may also be widespread. The doctor should be notified of exposure to any contagious disease. (The very first day Lisa was home from the hospital and went across the street to her day care house to visit, she was exposed to roseola. She never got it, but we learned quickly about notifying other parents at day care about her situation.)

Further Resources

READING

Betty Crocker's Living With Cancer Cookbook New York: Hungry Minds, Inc. 2002.

Highly recommended source, partly arranged by specific side effects (e.g., metallic taste, nausea, mouth sores). Tips and tasty-sounding recipes that might appeal and help with side effects—or bypass them, like dry mouth. The book is also crammed with nutritional tips and notes, and the information will be useful for the entire family.

Clegg, Holly, and Gerald Miletello, MD. *Eating Well Through Cancer.*
Memphis, TN: Favorite Recipes Press, 2001.

Recipes arranged by symptoms and cross-referenced. One section for "day of chemotherapy" has simple, flavorful food even kids would like: strawberry soup, "pizza" with a potato crust, baked French toast; also recipes for days of low white blood cell counts, to handle side effects like diarrhea, constipation, etc. The authors are an experienced cookbook/food writer and an oncologist. Foods are both nutritious and generally easy to prepare with common ingredients. This book was a lifesaver to a friend whose husband was getting chemotherapy.

"Eating Hints for Cancer Patients Before, During and After Treatment." National Institutes of Health, National Cancer Institute, 1999. Order a print version or view online at www.cancer.gov/cancertopics/eatinghints

This booklet has many ideas for foods that will still appeal to a child (or an adult) whose nutrition is being affected by altered taste buds or appetite or just lack of interest. There are several simple recipes designed to help with specific problems; the Apple/Prune Sauce might appeal to youngsters.

Field, Joanne. *Toobie: Self-Cath Coloring Book for Boys and Girls.* Santa Barbara: Mentor Urology, 1992.

Booklet for kids who have to learn to catheterize themselves. Free copies are available through several websites, including www.sbhabc.org (under "Resources Available"). Also in Spanish.

Keane, Maura, J.S., & Daniella Chace, M.S. *What to Eat if You Have Cancer: A Guide to Adding Nutritional Therapy to Your Treatment Plan*. Chicago: Contemporary Books, 1996.

Detailed guide to food-related issues and side effects of various treatments. Has food plans (e.g., "diets") for various circumstances as well as suggestions to prepare for and handle problems. Food lists, etc.

Keim, Rachel, and Ginny Smith. *What to Eat Now: The Cancer Lifeline Cookbook*. Seattle: Sasquatch Books, 1996.

Descriptive subtitle: "easy to use nutritional guide to delicious and health eating for cancer patients, survivors and caregivers." Tips for shopping and preparing healthy foods (with recipes) as well as suggestions for handling side effects like changes in taste or fatigue.

ORGANIZATIONS / WEB SITES

American Cancer Society (800-ACS-2345)

"Home Away from Home" program provides free hotel rooms

Cure Our Children Foundation (www.cureourchildren.org)

Has a lot of information on specific nausea drugs and herbal antibiotics.

National Cancer Institute (www.cancer.gov)

This trusted U.S. government Web site has a wealth of information on supportive care for oral complications of chemotherapy and radiation. The PDQ section has excellent online resources for controlling and treating side effects (http://www.cancer.gov/cancertopics/pdq/supportivecare/nausea).

Oley Foundation (214 Hun Memorial, MC-28, Albany Medical Center, Albany, NY 12208; 800-776-6539; www.oley.org)

This Web site has a good range of unusual resources, especially for families of patients doing home IV and tube feeding.

Pennsylvania State University Hershey Medical Center (www.pennstate hershey.org)

Excellent "Home Care Guide; caring for young persons with cancer at home," readable online or available to download. Covers everyday problems of caring for a sick youngster (or anyone, for that matter) from fever to depression, school issues to sibling coping skills.

26

Money Matters

Most families realize quickly the impact that the cost of the child's illness is going to have on their budget and very likely their savings as well. For many, the blow is staggering. Even if they have good insurance (and some do not), the expenses will mount quickly for parking, transportation, meals eaten out, insurance co-pays, long-distance telephone calls to doctors and family, babysitters for their other children, temporary housing near the hospital, wigs, and new clothing if the child gains or loses weight because of the illness or the treatments.

Insurance coverage in the United States varies widely, as do the amounts families must pay as deductibles before the insurance takes over. If treatments are considered experimental (as some transplants may be), the insurance may not pay for them. Some plans do not cover medications given to outpatients, and chemotherapy drugs are notoriously expensive.

Health maintenance organizations (HMOs) can add a layer of bureaucracy between the patient and the doctors. While coverage with an HMO may be comprehensive, the specific doctors and hospitals that are used can well be limited. Childhood cancer is not an illness that can successfully be handled by community hospitals and general practitioners: the primary care must be given by trained and experienced specialists in related pediatric fields. It is advisable to ask as early as possible after diagnosis for an insurance company or HMO liaison who can be brought onto the team to advocate for needed care. It may also be advantageous to designate another relative or close family friend to deal with insurance matters. Having a seriously ill child is stressful enough without the added frustration of an uncooperative or stonewalling insurance company.

If they have good insurance, the parents may see actual bills only rarely, because the hospital and the clinic deal directly with the company. This may sound good on the surface, but in studying our bills, which I saw by the hundreds for outpatient visits, I found many mistakes and overcharges, and the insurance company would have had no way to spot them.

Parents who encounter difficulties in having insurance claims processed accurately and promptly should ask to speak with an insurance company representative, an advocate who will go to bat for them— and will persist until they receive the information and guidance they seek.

Although we were an active-duty military family at the time and therefore, we assumed, were entitled to "free medical care," we ended up paying many thousands of dollars in cost-share expenses because we were treated by civilian facilities near our home. If Lisa had been diagnosed by military doctors, we could have obtained free care, but it would have meant traveling great distances to service hospitals and maximum family disruption.

On the flip side, adolescents and young adults may risk the loss of their health insurance if they are covered by the family's policy only as long as they are full-time students (mostly college age). "Michelle's Law," which goes into effect in late 2009, allows students to take a 1-year medical leave from their studies without losing dependent insurance benefits.

If a family is having trouble paying the cost-share portion of the bills, a parent should speak to the social worker at the hospital. It is possible that there are special funds to help out in such circumstances. Hospitals are also required by federal law to provide a certain amount of care at no cost to those who cannot pay. Some hospitals may waive part of the payment. The Leukemia and Lymphoma Society has a co-pay assistance program. The National Children's Cancer Society provides some financial and other assistance. See the list at the end of this chapter for contact information.

If the family does not have insurance, the state may help. The clinical social worker should advise the parents on this. Different states have children's health services located in or near the state capital. These agencies, sometimes under the state maternal and child health division, may provide services directly or contract with a major clinic to treat patients. Eligibility is determined by finances, although not restricted to low-income families, and by type of illness. Since coverage varies from state to state, some cover cancer patients and some do not. Children with cancer may even be able to receive physician-ordered physical and occupational therapy under the program.

A family may qualify for welfare and Medicaid payments in some circumstances. If the youngster with cancer is approaching college age, some state rehabilitation offices may help with tuition and other expenses. Parents can look for a state Division of Rehabilitation or ask the hospital social worker. If all else fails, a local reference librarian can help determine whom to call.

Another program that helps pay medical bills is Supplemental Security Income (SSI), which is administered by the Social Security Administration. Within strict guidelines, the child may be declared disabled because of the illness, and monthly payments will then be made.

Be sure to ask your caseworker about treatment-related travel expenses if you must visit a clinic or hospital at some distance from your home. In some cases lodging, car rental, parking, and perhaps meals may be covered.

SSI payments may be supplemented by individual states. Low- and middle-income families may be eligible, depending on the parents' income and resources, their expenses, and whether there are other children. SSI payments may be reduced if income rises. SSI is intended to help meet current living expenses; an ineligible patient reaching the age of 18 may become eligible if he reapplies as an individual, even living in the family home. Those covered under SSI may be automatically eligible for Medicaid as well.

SSI covers disabilities expected to last 12 or more months or to result in death. Payments are not immediate, since a decision on eligibility may take some weeks or months, but coverage is retroactive to the day of filing. A call to the local or regional Social Security office will determine whether a child is eligible.

The National Cancer Institute provides free care for their patients, who must meet certain strict criteria, as does St. Jude's Hospital in

Memphis, Tennessee. Cancer centers often raise funds through well-publicized charities. This money may be used entirely for general clinic operation or research, or a portion may be earmarked to help defray individual bills. A hospital social worker aware of a family's financial problems will be aware of such sources of help.

Cancer drugs and other medications needed by patients can be frighteningly expensive. Sometimes they are not completely covered by insurance and government programs. Many pharmaceutical companies provide free or reduced-rate drugs to eligible families. Check out the Partnership for Prescription Assistance Web site for other options.

Friends and relatives may have fund drives, dances, or the like to raise money for a child's expenses or perhaps to take a special trip. Although it may be hard to accept "charity," a family should not refuse, for this is an offer of support. Some day they will be able to repay the kindness, if not financially, then by helping someone else in a special way. Appendix B lists several organizations that provide trips or fulfill other special wishes for sick or terminally ill children.

The suggestions in this section apply primarily to American children being treated at American institutions. Families from outside the United States seeking medical help here may have to pay a substantial cash advance before the child can be admitted for treatments. Anyone thinking about bringing a foreign child to the United States for cancer therapy must therefore plan ahead for that eventuality.

Official health care policies vary widely from country to country, and support in the United States often stacks up poorly when compared to other developed nations. The U.S. federal Family and Medical Leave Act of 1993 allows some employees to take unpaid leave to care for a sick child. Restrictions do limit the eligibility of workers in small businesses, and the loss of a paycheck will be an impossible burden for some parents. Still, this legislation provides job protection in difficult circumstances. Some states provide additional resources for sick children and their families. The hospital or clinic social worker should be able to help find these resources. A call to your state insurance agency may also be fruitful.

A family with a child who has cancer probably is short of funds for entertainment and such nonessentials, but it is also possible that they will develop, as we did, a new way of looking at money. As the bills rolled in, we examined the way were living, thought about our priorities, and came to feel that enjoying our daughter and doing things together outweighed most other considerations. While we kept up with the bills, we were not afraid to spend whatever was left over on adventures and pleasures.

Record Keeping

It is important for several reasons to keep accurate records of the child's symptoms, treatments, and expenses. Two little notebooks to tuck into a pocket or purse will help with this. A small calendar to keep track of appointments and home medication schedules also helps.

One notebook is used to keep track of medical information: questions to ask the doctor at the next visit; how long symptoms like vomiting or fever lasted, and how they were eased; appointment dates and whether the child will need x-rays at that time. This is a good place to put e-mail addresses and phone numbers of other families and professionals met at the clinic or in the hospital for later contact. Jot down, too, the e-mail addresses and URLs of Web sites recommended by knowledgeable people for additional research.

Another small notebook is essential to record all tax-deductible expenses—mileage, money spent on long-distance telephone calls to doctors, parking and tolls (get receipts), public transportation, prescription drugs, doctor and hospital bills, and the like. Federal tax legislation allows a deduction for daily costs like moderate hotel costs and plane fare incurred by one parent accompanying a child to treatments. For many of these expenses cancelled checks and other documentation provide proof, but the little notebook is a good way to double-check records and to record expenses as soon as they are incurred and before they are forgotten.

I found these two little notebooks plus the calendar important in dealing with the insurance company. I could see exactly when we went to the clinic or the hospital, what treatments Lisa got, what her symptoms had been (if there was any question why an outpatient drug was prescribed), and what tests she had. The information was also valuable in checking the hospital's lengthy bills (at one point they were about 55 pages of computer-generated itemization, sent monthly, although much of it was repetitious), which, as I noted earlier, contained errors.

Of course, keep copies of letters, evaluations, and similar important paperwork where you can find it quickly if you need it. Insurance records, bills, and so forth can be sorted into a large accordion file for filing ease. A few minutes organizing documents can save much frustration later.

Many parents also keep a diary or journal during this time. This is an excellent way to unburden feelings and get some of the fear out to look it in the eye. The diary need not be great literature, and nobody else ever has to see it. Some day parents may want to remember how they felt and what they were thinking at different stages of the child's illness. It is amazing what they will forget, which is perhaps part of the mind's defense against immense stress. Occasionally parents have also written for publication about the illness. Many books, magazine, and newspaper articles have appeared that help the general public understand what it is like to have cancer in the family and perhaps help raise funds for further research.

Transportation

A child who is getting radiation or chemotherapy will make many trips to the clinic or hospital outpatient department. Getting there will not be, to paraphrase an old ad, half the fun. If the family lives at some distance, it may be difficult to drive alone and still care for the child. If possible, the parents should try to share the driving with another family from the clinic. This will not work for many patients or even for most visits, given varying schedules for therapy, but the parent should ask who else living nearby is getting treatments at the same place at the same general time. Even if they can share only a few rides, it will help both financially and emotionally.

The family can also check with the local chapters of organizations like the American Cancer Society to see what help they offer. They may provide drivers to take the child and a parent to outpatient therapy, or they may reimburse travel expenses. This is also true if the family has to use public transportation.

We were lucky because Lisa was so small during her treatments that she could be transported easily with a stroller. Many families of older, heavier patients may find a temporary need for a wheelchair, whether just for getting around the notoriously long corridors in hospitals or for use at home as well. They may be able to borrow a wheelchair (again, check local organizations) or rent one. It is also a good idea to find out ahead of time where at the clinic a wheelchair can be found in an emergency.

Some families prefer to use public transportation if it is available. We know of many from our suburban area who took commuter trains to the city for treatments. This avoids the stress of driving in city traffic and is ideal when the family has only one car or if the available auto is on its last wheels. At the suggestion of a friend, we made "airsick bags." We needed them only a couple of times, but the peace of mind they offered was immeasurable. When traveling in our own car, we quickly learned to keep an "emesis basin" handy. Most families will probably need a bucket in case the child throws up. We recommend that an empty plastic pail, the kind that comes with 5 pounds of peanut butter, be kept in the car. These have tight-fitting lids, which is a distinct advantage. On non-chemotherapy days, they make great toys for the beach, too.

Incidentally, when faced with juggling a toddler, a fold-up stroller, and numerous changes of clothing and supplies on trains, I quit carrying a purse. Other mothers may want to follow suit and get some tough waterproof tote bags big enough to carry clothes, diapers, bottles, the daily newspaper, and so forth. Appendix B suggests several sources for help with housing and travel expenses.

Dressing the Disabled Child

Whether the child must learn to live with a long-term disability or is temporarily disabled because of the disease or its therapy, the parent may want to investigate ways to adapt his clothing to make it easier to dress the child. There are books with ideas on using Velcro and zippers, for example, to facilitate dressing the child.

Organizations for the handicapped often have catalogs of various aids like pulls to attach to zippers so a child with limited reach can still dress himself. These groups include the National Easter Seal Society. Addresses and further information are given in the Appendices.

Further Resources

READING

Jasper, Margaret C. *Healthcare and Your Rights Under the Law* (Legal
 Almanac Series: Law for the Layperson). Dobbs Ferry, NY: Oceana
 Publications, Inc., 2002.
 This book has chapters on insurance, HMOs, rights, and grievances and
appendices with addresses and sample letters or forms. Some state-by-state
information is included.

Lozowski-Sullivan, Sheryl. *Know Before You Go, the Childhood Cancer
 Journey*. Candlelighters Childhood Cancer Foundation, 1998.
 Short, informative chapters, lots of quotes from experienced people
(patients and parents), photos, facts, further resources. Encourages families
to take charge, laugh, and ask for help. Acknowledges feelings like anger and
how to deal with them. A really excellent section on insurance. Compact yet
crammed with information.

ORGANIZATIONS/WEB SITES

Free Medicine program (www.freemedicineprogram.org)
 This Web site is a gateway to pharmaceutical manufacturers' free prescription services to those who qualify.

Leukemia and Lymphoma Society (www.LLS.org/copay; 877-557-2672)
 Provides co-pay assistance for some cancer patients

Michelle's Law (www.michelleslaw.com)
 This federal legislation allows sick or injured college students to take a
year's medical leave without losing insurance benefits.

National Children's Cancer Society (www.beyondthecure.org)
 Awards some scholarships.

Patient Advocate Foundation (700 Thimble Shoals Blvd, Suite 200, Newport
 News, VA 23606; 800-532-5274; www.patientadvocate.org)
 Helps with appeals of insurance coverage denial. Serves as liaison between
the patient/family and creditors (not limited to health care costs). Some
scholarships are awarded. Information also in Spanish.

Partnership for Prescription Assistance (www.pparx.org)
 Search this Web site for programs for which you may be eligible.

The Sam Fund (www.thesamfund.org)
 Awards grants and scholarships for education and other needs.

U.S. Social Security Administration (www.ssa.gov)

27

The Patient at the Clinic and in the Hospital

The term "clinic" is used throughout this book for the sake of simplicity. In some sections of the United States, clinics care only for poor people, but here it means an institution's outpatient department, day hospital, or ambulatory care center.

According to the Candlelighters newsletter, the 5-year survival rate for young cancer patients treated at "centers of excellence" (health care facilities providing a full range of cancer care services and meeting national quality standards as set by the National Cancer Institute and others) is significantly higher than the overall childhood cancer survivor rate.

Choosing a Clinic

The first treatments given to a child with cancer are vital, because the initial therapy provides the best chance for a cure. After a child relapses, the likelihood of an eventual cure decreases. Pediatric oncologists generally agree that it is not useful to ship a child across the country to another clinic; they do not usually differ much. If a local pediatrician or general practitioner diagnoses the child's illness, he should discuss area resources and specialists with the parents and refer them to one for further care.

If there is a choice of nearby institutions and time to make the decision (which there may well not be), parents might check out both the outpatient clinic and the inpatient hospital. What are the visiting hours and practices? Do they allow sibling visits? If parents can stay over with inpatients, what arrangements are made for them? A family could try to talk to parents of children treated there and ask about the attitudes of the staff. They can look at the size of the rooms, the number of beds, elbow room, indoor and outdoor play areas for inpatients, play programs, and tutoring for school-age children. Are any publications available to explain procedures and the layout of the clinic? Are there comfortable chairs or couches for parents, both in clinic and inpatient areas? Can a mother heat a can of soup somewhere? Can a father hang up his coat? Are the physical surroundings cheerful? Where are the bathrooms?

Having listed ways to assess a clinic, I must note that we did not have time to think about it. We were referred to a city hospital by our suburban pediatrician, who sent us to a specialist she respected rather than the institution she knew best. The physical facility was appalling at that time. The clinic (now replaced) overlooked a prison (now an upscale hotel), and the inpatient building (now demolished) had been constructed early in the 20th century. Comfort was at a premium because the building had not been designed for parents, yet the hospital allowed them to stay and fit in where they could, despite the inconvenience. This reflects the hospital's commitment to 24-hour visiting, which most enlightened centers now allow. During Lisa's first hospitalization the July temperatures soared to meteorological records that still stand—especially memorable because the inpatient floors were not air-conditioned. Yet we have never regretted our doctor's referral, because we knew Lisa was at a hospital with a worldwide reputation. We traded our comfort for the excellence of care, and I think we got a good bargain.

The Doctor–Family Relationship

The relationships between the doctor and the patient and between the specialist and the family are very important. They will be spending a lot of time together, and in most instances a bond will develop.

The key here is trust—and it works both ways. The family must know the doctor will be honest with them, and the doctor must know the parents will carry out instructions to the letter. As advocate for the child, the parent will have a lot of contact with the doctor, but even the youngest patients should have their own one-to-one relationship with the physician.

In almost all U.S. clinics the daily patient care is carried out by house officers (interns and residents still in training in this specialty) under the supervision of staff doctors. The involvement of the staff doctors varies tremendously. Some are never seen, while others are highly visible. In a very few smaller clinics, the staff doctors may provide most of the daily care themselves. Most pediatric oncologists work in groups, although one may be identified as the key person. This ensures that if the primary physician is away, other team members can step in.

Before spending very much time at the clinic, everyone will no doubt hear the old joke: A pediatrician has two patients—the child and the parent. No one need apologize for this—the parent is the child's representative. The parent is part of the team, and he or she knows the child better than anyone else at the hospital, however caring the staff might be. The parent is entitled to information about the child's illness on a continuing basis. If it is difficult to talk with the doctor in depth in front of the child, but the parent does not want to be obvious by asking him or her to step out of the room, they can certainly communicate over the phone or by e-mail.

Doctors specializing in childhood cancer find it difficult if not impossible to hold themselves apart from their patients. They suffer the losses with the families and rejoice in the gains. The parent should allow the doctor time with the child. Lisa always adored her "Dr. Marty" despite all the pain she had with the chemotherapy itself (and she danced at his wedding).

Clinic staff understand the family's shock at the diagnosis and the changes it will bring to everyone's lives. They will repeat everything, whether facts about the disease or directions for care, until they are sure the parent understands. They will feed the family a little information at a time, allowing an opportunity to absorb the bad (and good) news. They may write down names of the disease or medications that are unfamiliar. That way the parent can learn to recognize them and look them up if he or she wishes.

Both parents should be present for important conferences, like the one at diagnosis or the briefing after surgery (in the latter case we were both on telephone extensions). It is unrealistic to expect one parent to remember everything the doctor says and to relay it accurately to the other parent. The family also has a right to privacy during conferences, no matter how crowded facilities are.

It is not uncommon for the parents to feel initial hostility toward the bearer of bad tidings, the doctor, but he or she understands that, and a good long-term relationship can still be salvaged.

But doctors are not perfect and sometimes they do make it harder to cope. Perhaps this happens because they lack skills they need to carry out their work. They are more likely to harm their patients or the families by a failure to explain everything carefully, in minute detail and repeatedly. Friends of ours were hurt terribly when their doctor refused to allow them any hope after their daughter responded well to therapy. He had no right to destroy their hope—and as it happened, he was wrong and the child is well today. Unfeeling, uncaring doctors who frighten the patient or the family are in a minority, but their effect on the emotional well-being of all concerned can be devastating.

The nurse–patient relationship is also important. Nurses' assistance in the clinic is vital, and they can become great allies. Nurses help give treatments, mix and measure medicines, check the patient's height and weight, take temperatures, talk to the child and the parents before the doctor begins the treatment, and are generally available to answer questions between clinic appointments.

There are a wide variety of nurses, from LPNs (licensed practical nurses) to RNs (registered nurses), nurse-clinicians, or nurse-practitioners. The nurse-clinician or nurse-practitioner has more education than a registered nurse so that, in addition to nursing care, he or she performs some duties that formerly were handled only by doctors. In some states nurse-clinicians may prescribe medications, but elsewhere they may not. In some clinics they start the chemotherapy IVs and perform bone marrow tests and even spinal taps, although in others only the doctors are allowed to do those procedures. Clinic nurses can also be a source of tips on nutrition, teething, and a myriad of other child care questions not directly related to cancer.

Parents should cultivate good relationships with these nurses and doctors and other important clinic staff such as the secretary or the x-ray technicians, because they will be seeing a lot of each other.

Although the frequency of outpatient clinic visits will vary over time, they will probably be there often, with adjustments according to how well the child is doing and how he reacts to the treatments. At first each of Lisa's monthly courses lasted for 7 days, with all chemotherapy treatments given in the outpatient department. She then had 3 weeks off. Eventually that dropped to 4 days per monthly course. Other diseases require a different protocol and altered scheduling. If there is a relapse or recurrence, the child may have to go more often for a while.

An Outpatient Visit

A preliminary or follow-up visit with a surgeon does not differ much from any doctor appointments, but chemotherapy sessions are a bit different.

First, if the child has been exposed to an infectious disease like chickenpox or measles that he has not had, the parent must phone the clinic ahead of time to warn them; the youngster will either be isolated from the other patients or told to delay the visit, if that is possible. If the clinic has not been contacted in advance about the exposure, the child should not even be taken into the waiting area because other children would be placed at risk as well. The family should stay in a neutral area like the lobby and contact the clinic before entering.

By all means healthy siblings can be taken along on clinic visits so they can meet everyone, see what goes on, and become part of the team. This will help demystify the sick child's experiences for the others and help alleviate jealousy.

An outpatient visit begins with tests of blood counts and other components. The doctor needs to know what the white blood cell count is before more drugs can be given. If the white count is too low, there may be a delay while the body recovers from the effects of earlier treatments; if it is high, the child may be coming down with an infection that would also mean a delay. In large institutions where pediatric and adult patients use the same laboratories, parents can check whether special dispensation allows youngsters to "go to the head of the line" when a lot of people are waiting. Any reduction in waiting time, and therefore stress on the child, is worth it.

Children with indwelling central lines or catheters will be spared many of the painful finger sticks and venipunctures needed to draw blood or inject medications, including chemotherapy drugs.

At the beginning of each course of chemotherapy, the nurse or a nursing assistant will take the child's height and weight to determine exact doses of medication and also to check how he is growing generally. His temperature will be taken every day before any medicine is given to make sure there is no infection. The doctor or nurse-practitioner will perform a physical examination, probing the abdomen, neck, and groin area to look for abnormal swelling or lumps and checking the ears for infection.

The child may enjoy helping with the instruments needed for an examination, using the stethoscope to listen for the nurse's heartbeat, for example.

Sometimes a visiting physician or one new to the staff will appear, perhaps to perform the checkup or other treatments. Changes in staff are inevitable, particularly in teaching hospitals as interns become residents and others complete their training and move on. It can be painful to see staff leave with whom a good rapport has been built, but others, who may become close as well, will probably arrive in due time. At the other end of the spectrum, it can be extremely irritating when new people, particularly medical students, bustle into the clinic and begin to examine the child without telling the family their names, why they are there, and how long they expect to be around the hospital. They may have a right to be there, but they should have the courtesy to introduce themselves. If they do not, ask. If a new staff person will be conducting a test, he or she should be introduced ahead of time.

The child may have regular x-rays, particularly of the chest, looking for any suspicious growth in the lungs that might signal metastasis. This can be a worry, because the dangers of x-rays have been well publicized, but the benefit of finding metastases early is greater than the risks. As time passes, the frequency of x-rays will drop.

In some diseases, notably leukemia, the child will need regular bone marrow aspirations, spinal taps, and sophisticated blood tests and cultures to check the status of the illness more accurately than is possible with a "finger stick" blood sample. These and other tests are described in detail in Appendix D.

The parent should expect to spend quite a lot of time in the clinic, particularly if the child needs intravenous chemotherapy drugs or extra fluid to avoid dehydration in a nauseated patient. They may have to wait an hour or more before the treatment can begin. Emergencies occur that throw off the schedule. It may take an hour or more for the therapy itself, and they should plan on more time for blood transfusions and other tests. This is an excellent opportunity to get to know the other parents. These friendships can help immeasurably to get through the child's illness.

Preventing Errors

Medical and drug errors happen every day and the cost, both in money and patient care, is enormous. No institution is immune. Everybody makes mistakes, and even the most experienced staff person at a hospital with the highest regard can do something wrong. Some hospital errors are relatively benign, but others can be lethal.

The parent should not be afraid to speak up to the clinic staff if something looks wrong. For example, if the medicine is a different color or the dose looks larger than usual, the parent should inquire. The medication may have been changed, but it is also possible that an error was made. Lisa once went through a period of puzzling lethargy. We discovered that the chain pharmacy had filled a prescription with an incorrect dosage that had kept her overdosed for days.

It is perfectly acceptable to make legitimate complaints. Nobody cares more about the child than the parent does, so it is all right to stand up for him. It may not be easy to speak up, but nobody will withhold care as a result of a complaint. A parent can be nice but need not be passive. Professional staff understand the parental role as an advocate for the child, listening to concerns and acting on them. If an error does occur, insist on a full accounting of why it happened and what effect it might have on the child.

Again: if something looks wrong or just different, it is okay to ask about it. If the pill is green instead of orange, ask. Take notes. Keep medicines at home in the original containers. Make sure the doctor knows what other medications your child is taking, including over-the-counter drugs, vitamins, and herbs.

The Joint Commission (formerly the Joint Commission on Accreditation of Healthcare Organizations) has a publication "Speak Up—Help Prevent Errors in Your Care." Briefly, the organization recommends the following:

- Speak up if you have any questions or concerns.
- Don't assume anything—question health care professionals, medications, or treatments.
- Educate yourself about your child's diagnosis, tests, and treatment plans.
- Ask a trusted friend or relative to be your advocate.
- Know what medications your child takes and why.
- Participate in all decisions regarding therapy.

Clinic Activities

It is wise to take things to the clinic to keep both parent and child busy during long waits, either before therapy begins or during treatments. There may be a staff play therapist or child life specialist, which is helpful, and there may be special toys for children whose activities are restricted by IVs.

Television may be available to distract the child. Many parents prefer other diversions, but kids expect TV. A video or DVD player to show good movies is another possibility. Books and magazines are excellent, but the sick child (or the weary parent) may just not feel like reading or even holding a book. Audiobooks can be another distraction.

Arts and crafts are a good way to pass the time if the child is well enough; it is pretty good for parents, too. Older children and teens will appreciate a radio (with headphones) or an MP3 player. Handheld videogames, whether the Game Boy type or simple inexpensive solitaire games, can kill a lot of time. Infants enjoy a fluttering or swaying mobile over the bed and books with bright colors and simple shapes.

Leukemia survivor Ben Duskin's "Make-a-Wish" desire was to create a video game for the other kids with cancer. Ben's Game is the result, a game that takes the patient's mind off the disease. The free game can be downloaded from the Internet; see the list at the end of the chapter for more information.

Most clinic activity will be passive because of the child's illness, the IV tether, and the confined area. Still, young children who have the energy may want to run and jump around. We did allow that to the extent possible, as long as there was no added risk of Lisa hurting herself or others. It does people good to see these kids so active, happy, and normal.

We missed plenty of meals while we were at the clinic, but I did try to take along a nutritious snack for both of us. The clinic also had coffee and tea for parents, juice and soft drinks for the patients, and often other goodies as well. If no parent provided a cake, brownies, or bread on a particular day, there was always a supply of crackers, jelly, and peanut butter. The clinic staff misses meals, too, when there is a backup, and we used to tease one of the doctors that chocolate chip cookies (which he considers the perfect food) are not a well-balanced meal.

Inpatient Stays

I know a young woman, now in her 30s, who was treated for leukemia for over 10 years, including a relapse and second remission. Amazingly, she never spent a single night in the hospital in all that time. Most cancer patients, however, are admitted to the hospital, sometimes repeatedly.

Much of the child's reaction to hospitalization and clinic visits will depend on how the family responds. A parent may feel that his or her role as the child's central authority figure is being usurped by the hospital staff and may fight against this loss of control. This struggle will color the child's acceptance of the hospital and its staff, increasing the child's apprehension and resistance to procedures. Occasionally hospitals restrict parental visits because children are easier to handle by sticking to a routine. This may work to cure the child's physical ailments, but he will surely suffer emotionally. Most institutions now recognize that parents are useful people to have around pediatric wards, whether to comfort the patients, to translate the toddler's language, to help the child dress, to fetch ginger ale, or to read to and entertain the patients. Parents and the nursing staff together are an unbeatable team.

How a child will respond to hospitalization depends also on his age. Children over 6 generally adapt well to the hospital, as do infants. Some young patients may have tantrums or nightmares, however, which sometimes continue even after they go home. Children from 2 to 6 tend to have more fears about pain and separation from their parents and may need a lot of reassurance that the hospitalization is neither punishment nor rejection. This group may be afraid that they will never go home, so they need help understanding how long they will have to stay. The parent should not lie—if unsure, he or she should say so. How devastated a child would be if he were promised he could go home on Wednesday, and the doctor decided to keep him until Friday! Children who cannot tell time may not be able to distinguish today from tomorrow, so marking days off on a calendar may help.

Preparing the Patient

Experts have many suggestions for choosing which hospital to use, assuming you have a choice and the time to look around. If your child must be hospitalized and you have a choice of hospitals, you might want to see which offer:

- Prehospitalization tours or other orientation programs
- A child life department
- Visiting privileges for siblings
- Permission for parents to be with a child during anesthesia
- Support groups or other psychological services for children
- Arrangements for parents who want to stay overnight
- A Ronald McDonald House or similar residence nearby

If the family knows in advance that the child will be admitted to the hospital, that time should be used to prepare him. If it is not the child's first inpatient stay, a day's notice should be enough for a preschooler. Adolescents and other school-age children, on the other hand, may need earlier notice so that they can consult with teachers and plan their school schedules around the admission.

If the child is being admitted for the first time, the hospital may arrange tours for pediatric patients. During these orientations, the youngster often has an opportunity to see where he will be treated; to try out some equipment like masks, gloves, and stethoscopes; to meet some of the hospital staff; and perhaps to explore a typical hospital room and the playroom.

If the child is age 4 to 6, the parent can tell him before admission what will happen and where the family will be during the hospital stay. It is important to be honest about possible discomfort and pain and to give the child a chance to express any fears, perhaps by drawing pictures or talking about the hospital. The doctor can give the family guidelines ahead of time to facilitate discussion and reassurance. Librarians either at the hospital or at your public library can recommend good books about children in hospitals for children of all ages.

A study at the Children's Hospital of Philadelphia reported that children prepared ahead of time for surgery show increased anxiety right after the explanation but a lowered level after the surgery, and little residual fear 6 weeks later. Children not prepared at all are calm until the preoperative procedures begin. Their anxiety then rises sharply and remains high even 6 weeks later.

Advising the family to prepare the child ahead of time is easy, but admissions for cancer are often emergencies, occurring at the time of diagnosis, or as a result of complications or a relapse. The lack of time to prepare mentally and financially, and to get the child physically and emotionally ready, adds stress and fear. In these circumstances, the parent's presence at the hospital is especially important to the child, so visits should be as frequent as possible.

Anger

A child in the hospital is likely to be angry and may refuse to eat, take medicine, or play. The child may ignore family members; in that case, a friendly nurse is a good ally. The child may also respond to another patient of a similar age, even when he is not civil to parents or other visitors. On the other hand, a child who is extremely compliant may be showing signs of depression. Even though he isn't saying anything, the child may not truly accept the hospitalization.

Whenever Lisa was hospitalized, I arrived at her bedside every morning before 7 a.m., usually just about the time the surgeons completed their rounds. But I also got a flexible part-time job for financial, social, and emotional relief. Just once I worked in the morning when Lisa, about 3 at the time, was hospitalized. Although I told her ahead of time I would be there in the early afternoon after her nap, she was angry and withdrawn, not only when I was not there but also after I arrived on schedule. She would not even respond to her favorite nurses and doctors, thawing only in the evening when her father appeared. I resented this but I could understand it.

The stress of hospitalization increases as admissions recur. Parents will feel angry at the disruption of their normal life, at the forced neglect of their other children, at the strain on their finances. The bond between the doctor and the patient will be important in easing this stress to whatever extent possible. Parents and child will have to trust the medical decision that hospitalization is required.

Fear

Hospitalized young children are likely to be afraid, whether of pain, separation, all the strangers, the unusual smells, or the array of intimidating equipment. Some children hide this fear because they think they are being hospitalized as punishment for being "bad." Parental recognition of their expressed or unspoken fear gives them a chance to share their feelings and get reassurance.

Youngsters are also understandably afraid of pain. Whether or not a parent can be present when the child has painful treatments, when IVs are started and when shots are given, will depend partly on hospital policy and partly on choice. Adolescents may or may not want the parent to stay for procedures and treatments, so a parent should ask the teenager ahead of time.

If a parent's presence is permitted, he or she will have to decide whether to remain in the room. Each parent has to decide this for himself or herself. Some think that the child, particularly an infant, will come to associate the parent with pain. Babies, the theory goes, are let down that Mom or Dad did not protect them. Other parents believe that their presence will comfort the child by showing they will not abandon him to pain. Still others cannot stand to see their children in pain and simply have to leave.

Perhaps a parent who finds watching the procedures too draining can sit or stand where he can touch, hold, and comfort the child but does not have to watch the test or treatment. If this is also upsetting, it is probably best to step outside the room, because the child will sense the parent's tension and assimilate it. Some parents become hostile to the medical staff when, for example, they think too many attempts are being made to start an IV without a respite for the child. A non-hostile parent who is present can suggest that another doctor try to start the IV if there have been several "dry sticks." Much of this particular pain and stress is avoided with the indwelling catheters used today.

The parent who is able to stand by during treatments can provide comfort and perhaps help calm a restless child or check that the IV is still dripping.

Discipline

Discipline of the hospitalized child is difficult. Some children regress to earlier behavior, like thumb-sucking, baby talk, and loss of toilet training, when faced with the stresses of the hospital environment. Others become angry and aggressive with their toys or dolls. This acting-out usually disappears when normal routines are again achieved when the child returns home. If it seems to continue for a long time, the family may want to seek professional help.

Our Lisa has always been a night owl, and in the hospital she raised this to a high art. The nurses were lenient with her, letting her take late walks around the floor, making phone calls for them to their friends, and emptying the wastebaskets at the nurses' station. Yet when she returned home, getting her to bed was no more of a problem than it had ever been.

Getting teenagers to cooperate with hospital routine will be easier if they don't perceive the rules as pointless. They should know the reasons for the various regulations. Lack of privacy is especially hard on adolescents. They (and their parents) should have a chance to talk to the doctor and to ask questions without eavesdropping roommates.

Parental Exhaustion

Parents who are sleeping over at the hospital are especially likely to be exhausted. Even if they are going home regularly, travel and stress added to the drain of sitting beside a sick child's bed for hours will be more tiring than anyone else could ever imagine. Sleep-over parents may have the added burdens of guilt over "neglect" of other children or for missing work. Should they stay? Some experts say yes, particularly if the child is an infant, toddler, or preschooler.

If work or other family responsibilities prevent the parents from being at the hospital as often as they would like, there are certain crucial times when they should make every effort to be present— just before surgery, through the first night, and for major tests and procedures.

Because there were limited sleeping facilities for families at our daughter's hospital and because we lived within commuting distance, we chose to head home every evening. During lengthy daily visits we tried to get some relief from the alternating boredom and drama by taking walks in the hospital and outside, weather permitting, and taking Lisa along when possible. We went shopping or to restaurants during Lisa's naps, always making sure she knew that we would be back shortly after she awoke.

Breaks from the hospital are essential. Sometimes we went out with friends, to a movie or to parties, when Lisa was well on the mend. We joked on those occasions that we had the most expensive babysitter in town.

Rarely, a child will refuse to let a parent out of his sight, carrying on whenever the parent even steps out for a bite to eat. This may be an act for the parent's sake. One child screamed hysterically from the instant her mother arose from her chair until she was out of earshot. One day the mother forgot something and had to return for it; she was amazed to see her child playing happily until, spotting Mom, she began screaming again.

We enlisted the help of our favorite nurses to distract Lisa at the time we were leaving each night. Sometimes they read a story, gave her a bath, or played with her. We were careful to let her know when we would be back, then kissed her, and she would cheerfully wave goodbye. I do not envy those parents whose children will not even let them go to the bathroom without raising a ruckus. An exhausted, malnourished mother or father cannot possibly cope with the fears or uncertainties of hospitals and serious illness. Perhaps grandparents, other relatives, and close friends can stand in on a regular basis so Mom and Dad can go home or just get away for a while.

If, on the other hand, hospital policy does not allow parents to sleep over and a mother or father really wants to stay with the child, maybe the doctor will "order" him or her to stay, in writing. Meanwhile, the family should complain in writing to the head administrator of the hospital. If the hospital is unswayed, the family may want to consider locating a center whose policies favor liberal parental visits.

The physical set-up will play a role in the parent's coping. Is there a real bed or convertible recliner for those who stay over, comfortable chairs for long hours at the bedside, a shower the family can use, a lounge to get away for a bit? A friendly staff person will know if parents are allowed to eat in the hospital cafeteria and what hours it is open. A social worker may be able to help parents sort out their feelings. Formal and informal parent group discussions are often beneficial. Is there someone parents can contact to get free or reduced-rate parking?

Parents who are at the hospital day and night may see patients whose families are not there all the time. Those who have the opportunity and the inclination may talk to these children and read to them, but should not give them food or try to care for them. I once watched a well-meaning woman give her grandchild's roommate some chocolate that the child's mother had to take out of the toddler's mouth because he was allergic to it. We appreciated reports from other parents who stayed all night, because they reinforced the nurses' reassurances, but we did not expect them to care for Lisa and would not have welcomed it if they did.

No modern American hospital will permit indoor smoking, so the problem of unbreathable indoor air is now moot. For those who do still indulge, it's unlikely that the designated smoking area will be either comfortable or convenient; at one of our hospitals, it was located next to the morgue exit used by funeral directors.

The Hospital Staff

Large medical institutions are likely to have a bewildering array of personnel, and the staff may not always be easy to identify. The house staff or house officers consist of interns, or doctors just out of medical school and beginning their training, and residents, who are receiving specialty training, in pediatrics or surgery, for instance. There will often be doctors who have completed specialty training who are learning a subspecialty like oncology. These are the physicians seen most often, although private and other staff doctors may well have the main responsibility for a child's care. In teaching hospitals—those affiliated with medical schools—parents are also likely to encounter medical students.

It can be annoying to see the child examined by many doctors, some of whom are not very experienced in patient care. When a hospital is connected with a medical school, however, patients receive the most current therapy, the trade-off being these numerous examinations. Parents might not appreciate the extra attention if the child has a broken arm, but when he has something as threatening as cancer, some additional prodding seems more acceptable. Perhaps the doctor can offer reassurance that no examinations will be made by any personnel not directly involved in the youngster's care; it would not hurt to ask. Lisa also asked that whenever possible examinations be conducted by female doctors, and the staff obliged.

The bond between the patient and the doctor is important, and so is that between the parents and the doctor. Physicians do need emotional distance. We were not always prepared to accept that, because we needed their support. Still, the dedication of the doctors, who seemed to always be there when we needed them, was striking and immensely reassuring.

Relationships with the nurses are important, too. Parents who stay with their children for the entire hospital admission, feeding them, caring for them, bathing them, and sleeping nearby, sometimes feel that nurses are neglecting their child because the parent is available for routine care. Others may feel that a dedicated nurse is doing too much, taking over the parent's role; this perception is less likely today in the age of managed care, with its nursing crisis. The best arrangement I have seen is when the hospital assigns a primary care nurse to each patient. Continued over subsequent admissions, this allows a good relationship to develop among the nurse, the patient, and the family. Some centers also assign inpatient nurses to the day clinic, which provides the patient and family with continuity after the child is discharged, keeps the inpatient staff updated during outpatient therapy, and means that there will be familiar faces both in the hospital and at the clinic.

The hospital staff must care for many patients at the same time. Except in emergencies, a family cannot expect a split-second response to requests, especially those of a non-medical nature. It is, however, appropriate to expect prompt help when a child is in pain, and parents should get reasonably prompt explanations of new procedures.

Nurses can teach parents some medical skills, which they can use to help out during the hospital stay or when the child goes home. These might include giving shots or collecting urine specimens. The parent can also help monitor a child who is "NPO" (not allowed any food or drink because he is scheduled for anesthesia or tests), watch to see that the correct diet is supplied, or make sure that the correct medication is given at the proper times. One specialist quipped that the parents of the child with cancer develop skills that would be admirable in most nurses.

Here, also, the child should be introduced to any new staff he may encounter. If personnel seem cold or brusque, they may be unsure of what they are doing. They may also be protecting themselves against personal involvements that could be painful if the child does not do well on the therapy. The child deserves and needs better than that. Although we never encountered that attitude, others unfortunately have. If a family is having a problem with anyone in particular, perhaps a substitution can be made. On the other hand, we knew of a doctor on the staff who was unapproachable, unkind, and uncommunicative; he was, however, one of the most skilled physicians in the country. Parents of his patients learned to find support and affection elsewhere, and the nurses tried to shield families from his unpleasantness.

Other regular visitors to the child's room are likely to include technicians who draw blood and perform other tests; dietitians who can help the parent plan well-balanced meals with foods the patient is more likely to enjoy; perhaps social workers or psychologists; and play therapists or child life specialists, who either take activities to the child or arrange for him to go to the playroom.

The hospital staff may also include a patient representative, an advocate who is not involved in medical care but who can help arrange matters of comfort for the child. This might be a good person to contact if the youngster is placed in a room with another patient with whom the family simply cannot cope.

Hospital Environment and Activities

Each patient's room should have a closet or locker to store personal things, a bulletin board for cards and posters, a bedside phone for older patients, and a television. At Lisa's most recent hospital stay, she also had an in-room safe, a little refrigerator, cable television, and a DVD player.

Hospitalized infants and toddlers may rarely be required to wear restraints whenever the parent is not at the bedside. This usually consists of a vest with straps that tie to the crib sides so the child cannot fall or climb out. While the child will be able to move some, he may also find it frustrating. These restraints can be avoided if the hospital has cage-top cribs, which look like they sound—like small zoo cages—with sides that can be raised and lowered for access. These cribs seem preferable to tying down an active youngster. We used to hang toys from the top with Velcro; mobiles also work if the baby is too small to reach them and possibly get tangled in the lines.

Taking the child a favorite blanket, stuffed toy, or other familiar item can make the hospital room less strange, but things do disappear. Cards, colorful posters, and notes from brothers, sisters, or classmates can help cheer the patient up. Flowers (if they are allowed) may be all right for older patients, but youngsters would probably appreciate a small gift more—such as a puzzle or box of crayons or, for a teenager, the newest CD from a favorite singing group, or extra batteries for the player. When Lisa was in the hospital recently for surgery, the hospital loaned her a laptop to use with their wireless Internet service. It's a new world.

In many cities a balloon-o-gram, a cheery get-well message accompanied by an enormous bouquet of helium balloons, can be delivered to the hospitalized child. (Ask ahead of time; some balloons are banned for safety reasons.) Once when Lisa was uncommunicative after surgery, a kind parent shared her child's balloons with several children on the floor. Lisa's pink balloon tied to her bed accomplished what all our prodding had not—she smiled and snapped out of her depression. On another occasion when we knew Lisa was going to be admitted for surgery and would be immobilized for nearly 2 weeks, my mother and I made a number of toys for her.

We always took along her pajamas, books, and snapshots of friends and the dog. If the family has an instant or a digital camera, a get-well "card" made with a photo of friends holding up a sign is nice to take to a later visit. Some public libraries loan such cameras.

The child will need shoes or slippers and a robe, a list of phone numbers where parents and other important relatives can be reached, and pencil and paper for messages and notes. A flashlight may be reassuring at night.

A huge assortment of audiobooks on cassette, by digital download or on CD is available, covering the whole gamut of interest and reading levels. The public library probably has these, and sometimes juvenile departments have book-and-cassette sets for early readers to follow along. The hospital may have a "boom box" to loan to the child or perhaps one can be borrowed from a friend. These can also be used to send messages to the sick child from those who cannot visit—maybe a tape from the whole class.

Other good in-bed activities are a chalk and slate; a "magic slate" that erases when the plastic is lifted; peg and board games; paper dolls; and a radio with headphones.

A word about television may be in order. Hospital rooms have them, either for rental or (in our more recent experience) free. I am sure that somewhere at the hospital is a color television we have paid for. I personally don't like television much and rather severely limited the amount my children could watch. But when Lisa was in the hospital and immobilized for long periods, I let her watch as much as she wanted. It was a treat for her, at a time when she really could not do much else. Pity, though, the poor families whose hospitalized children have to share a television; here is a major opportunity for conflict over program selection.

Parents should have some activity for themselves, too. My friends and relatives could always tell when Lisa had been in the hospital: one year I knitted sweaters, hats, mittens, a dress, and an afghan for Christmas presents. I wrote letters; read the daily newspaper, books, and magazines; and did some embroidery. If there is a kitchen parents can use, they can take tea bags, instant coffee and soups, and little snacks for themselves.

There should be a playroom or, for teenagers, a recreation room. Distractions include video games, perhaps a pool table, stereo system, fish tank, jigsaw puzzles, board games, books, arts and craft supplies, and possibly a computer with educational software to help with school work or Internet access for e-mail.

The playroom for youngsters will no doubt have harmless medical equipment for "treating" dolls, perhaps a water play table, stuffed toys and dolls, and a variety of playthings that can be taken to the patient's room. The playroom should be a refuge—*no* medical procedures should be carried out there, not even taking temperatures or giving medicine. On every surgical admission, Lisa would step off the elevator on the hospital floor and turn left toward the playroom, asking for her favorite play therapist, Susan. When she was admitted because of an illness, we knew she was feeling better when she asked if the playroom was open yet. Even children confined to their beds can be taken to a spacious playroom—bed and all. It makes a nice change for the child and the parent, too.

Trained play therapists help the hospitalized child deal with fears and anxieties. Listening to the child at play, they may pick up on fears that the child has not discussed with parents.

Hospital Food

Kids are notoriously picky eaters, and being in the hospital is not going to improve that in the least. While the institution probably offers a variety of meals to suit almost every taste, if the child eats only spaghetti, parents may be able to get that for him. Lisa was famous as a non-eater, and news that she was about to be admitted invariably sent our favorite nurse to the cupboards to check the supply of canned vegetable soup, about the only food we could be reasonably sure she would eat. A special menu was also available so kids could have hot dogs, hamburgers, French fries, fresh and canned fruits, peanut butter sandwiches, and other favorites even when those were not among the daily choices. Knowing what foods were available also made it a little easier to get some nutritious food into Lisa. We have had the opportunity to sample the food in four hospitals in recent years and discovered that for the most part it was actually pretty good.

Going Home

The hospital is a womb, a safe place where medical care is quickly available. Parents become accustomed to this safety and may be afraid at first to take the child home, as welcome as a return to normal would be. I found the transition a little tricky each time, but it got easier as time went on and we knew better what to expect.

Lisa always responded to a return home by waking at night, crying. At first it would happen several times every night, then less frequently. We would reassure her, give her a hug, and put her back down in her bed, changing her diaper if necessary. But we made it a policy not to pick her up and rock her once she had been put to bed. As time went on, we were able to call out to her from our room or the door of her room that we were nearby and she should go back to sleep. After her initial hospitalization, this lasted for months, and just about the time it disappeared, she was readmitted. With several hospitalizations the pattern repeated itself and we did not have any uninterrupted sleep for over a year. But toward the end of the second year, it eased off to just a few days.

Hostility or depression that begins at the hospital may continue after you go home, maybe even for months. The child needs parental support, but he has to understand that other people have rights, too. The family should work to reestablish normal life patterns when they can, once they are back together.

The family may need the services of a visiting nurse for a time after the child's return home; if so, the hospital can arrange it. If at all possible, families should take breaks and get away from their routine to relax and recuperate together. If it is not possible to take the child on every trip or excursion, and if there is no available friend or relative to take over his care, the clinic social worker should be able to provide information about respite care services by trained people in the community.

The doctor should be called if the child has any unusual reactions after going home. Once Lisa had rampant diarrhea for a couple of weeks, which I assumed was normal. I did not mention it until my nurse/aunt suggested I report it. The cause, it turned out, was antibiotics, and it was controllable through a changed dose and diet.

Today hospitals find it cheaper to purchase new equipment for each patient than to sterilize inexpensive plastic basins, pitchers, cups and the like. The nurse will know what will be discarded if it is not taken home. Wash basins, emesis basins, and bed pans have plenty of household uses. If there is no medical need for them, they make fine sand or bath toys.

Further Resources

READING

Buck, Jari Holland. *Hospital Stay Handbook: A Guide to Becoming a Patient Advocate for Your Loved One*. Woodbury, MN: Llewellyn Publications, 2007 (www.hospitalstayhandbook.com).
This serves as a workbook of sorts for family members advocating for a hospitalized loved one. While not directly pediatric, the sensible advice could save your child's life. An excellent source, with a diverse list of resources. Tellingly, the first section is about taking care of yourself and accepting help.

Center for Attitudinal Healing. *Advice to Doctors and Other Big People from Kids.*
With a foreword by Dr. Gerald Jampolsky. Berkeley, CA: Celestial Arts, 1991.
What kids want their caregivers to know. No big surprises here but reinforced good sense.

Keene, Nancy, and Rachel Prentice. *Your Child in the Hospital: a Practical Guide for Parents*. Sebastapol, CA: O'Reilly, 1999.
Good solid source with lots of anecdotal information on hospital experiences. Packed with facts and ideas, enhanced with anecdotes from other "been there, done that" folks.

Rey, H. A. *Curious George Goes to the Hospital* Boston: Houghton-Mifflin, 1966.
Little monkey, a favorite with the preschool to grade 2 group, swallows a puzzle piece and has to go to the hospital for an operation.

ORGANIZATIONS/WEB SITES

Ben's Game (www.makewish.org/ben)
Free download. Available in nine languages for international play.

Joint Commission (www.jointcommission.org)
Find the "Speak Up: Help Prevent Errors in Your Care" with the search function at their Web site (the URL is a long one).

The Wellness Community (www.thewellnesscommunity.org)
This organization offers "cancer support, education and hope." One of their excellent publications is "The Balancing Act: Tips for the Cancer Caregiver." Order a free copy at www.starcampaign.org or download it from the Internet.

28

Rights and Responsibilities

A ccording to Boston University professor and civil liberties expert
George Annas, parents have almost complete control over their
children except in cases of child abuse, neglect, and compulsory education. The rights of hospitalized children are usually the rights of
their parents.

For adolescents nearing legal adulthood, the assignment of rights
is governed by the state. Generally, parental consent is required for
treatment of children under the age of 18 living at home, although
the age of majority varies from state to state. An "emancipated minor"
(one who is under age but not in the care, custody, or support of his
parents or a guardian) may also be allowed to give or withhold consent. This is the case with married teenagers and those in the armed
services as well as any who are living on their own without support
from their families. Teenagers who accept responsibility for their own
care, however, must also accept financial responsibility, even though
minors are not legally held to financial contracts. In cases of neglect,
the parents may still be held responsible for payment. A lawyer may
be needed to sort out these complicated situations.

Rights

One area where there have been significant changes since the time of the first edition of *Children with Cancer* in 1986 is rights and privacy. As the computer and the Internet expand our ability to find and exchange information, fears about the loss of privacy are not unfounded. Recent legislation in the United States requires each provider to formulate a privacy policy and have each patient (or a representative such as a parent) sign it. Both parties keep copies of the statement. It remains to be seen whether this additional paperwork will actually protect patients.

The past few years have also seen a greater acknowledgement of the rights of individuals, children, caregivers, and others. While these creed-like statements carry little or no legal weight, they do shine a spotlight on issues that affect us all as families with sick children. Some of those are included later in this chapter.

Each patient and family have certain rights and responsibilities. Some are defined by law, while others are a matter of courtesy or effective care. This chapter is an introduction to the subject rather than an exhaustive discussion. Parents with questions or problems should check with the hospital's patient representative, the medical staff, or a lawyer familiar with the health care field. For example, a parent who wants to stay with a child during a time when visiting is not permitted by hospital regulations may have to seek legal advice. A parent's right to know that the child is dying, assuming he or she wants to know, and the child's right to die with dignity, however, are matters of good patient care rather than law.

Parents may need an attorney in some cases—sometimes even when they wish to see the child's medical records. The law on this varies from state to state, and institutional policies also vary. Some institutions never provide a copy of the medical record without a court order or some other authorization. This may be related to the privacy issue—the assurance that medical information will be kept confidential through limited access. Other institutions may make records readily available to parents or their legal representative upon request. This may depend heavily on the parents' reasons for wishing to see the records. If there is a hint that parents may want to sue for malpractice, access will probably be more difficult to obtain. In any event, a parent going over the records should do so with the help of a person with medical training, to avoid misinterpreting information.

If a parent refuses consent for conventional treatments and the child's life is in danger, the hospital may go to court to seek a guardian who will consent to the therapy on his behalf. There have been several well-publicized cases in which children with a reasonable expectation of improvement or cure had therapy withheld by their parents. The courts ordered the treatments, often citing the U.S. Supreme Court decision *Prince v. Massachusetts* (1943): "Parents may be free to become martyrs themselves. But it does not follow that they are free, in identical circumstances, to make martyrs of their children before they have reached the age of full and legal discretion when they can make that choice for themselves." In practice, this has resulted in court-ordered treatments for life-threatening disorders such as leukemia and bone tumors but not necessarily for a cleft palate.

Family and Medical Leave Act of 1993

Recognizing that many families face difficult choices when a child becomes ill, the U.S. Congress passed a law in 1993 requiring that employers allow workers leaves of absence (unpaid) to care for a sick youngster (among other family members). The Family Medical Leave Act (FMLA) requires covered employers to provide up to 12 weeks of unpaid, job-protected leave with certain eligibility standards. Length of service in the position, number of hours worked in the previous year, and the number of employees at the company are among the qualifiers. Advance notice may be required but health insurance must be maintained during the absence. Contact the U.S. Department of Labor for additional information.

HIPAA

The U.S. Health Insurance Portability and Accountability Act, passed in 1996, provides for continued insurance coverage when an insured person loses or changes jobs. The security and privacy of medical information, data, and records are also addressed—especially important in the electronic age. When a doctor tells a woman he can't reveal her husband's medical information without permission, HIPAA is cited.

Informed Consent

Parents have a legal right to know if the treatments offered are experimental, and they also have a right to refuse such therapy. The doctors must tell you both verbally and in writing why these treatments are being offered, what they are, their risks, side effects, what tests will be done before and after the treatments, what monitoring procedures will be done, and what expectation there is of improvement. If parents agree to the experimental therapy, they must sign a consent form.

The governmental policy also requires that consent be obtained without coercion or undue influence, nor may those who consent be required to waive their legal rights concerning any liability for negligence.

Americans with Disabilities Act

One major advance in the years since the first edition of this book appeared was the passage in the United States of the Americans with Disabilities Act (ADA). With this law it became illegal to discriminate against a person because of a disability. The law does not directly mention cancer, pediatric or otherwise, but the guidelines cover major physical or mental impairments, amputations, and learning disabilities, among other specifics, which surely expand to cover cancer in its many forms.

Children (and adults) who have had cancer cannot be denied jobs for which they are otherwise qualified because of their medical history. Their parents can't lose their jobs because their employer's insurance premiums are affected by the illness. These are but a few of the protections the ADA offers.

The law also covers reasonable accommodations that can be made to meet a cancer survivor's needs and also spells out exclusions and "separate but equal" arrangements that are no longer acceptable or legal. Parents, siblings, and spouses are also protected under some of the ADA's provisions.

A Child's Bill of Rights

This statement has been adopted by many hospitals and other institutions. This particular version is reprinted with permission from the Children's Hospital of Columbus, Ohio (now Nationwide Children's Hospital):

As a patient of Children's Hospital, I and my parents/family/guardian/ visitors have these rights…I have the right to
- Be identified correctly and called by name
- Receive a smile and loving care
- Be given careful evaluation, and courteous, prompt treatment
- Know the names of my doctors, my nurses and any others who help care for me
- Have my basic needs met—to be clean, dry, safe, comfortable and without restraints whenever possible
- Have a schedule for my tests and procedures that doesn't keep me hungry or thirsty any longer than necessary
- Have as normal a schedule as possible—uninterrupted sleep, quiet times, playroom, school, the comfort of my parents and members of my family, and the schedule should be designed for my convenience as much as possible. Sometimes schedules do not permit this and I understand that this can occur.
- Make choices whenever possible when they do not interfere with the quality of my care
- Cry and make noise, or object to anything that hurts me
- Have my parents with me at any time that they are able to stay as long as it doesn't interfere with my care
- Have an interpreter for my family and me whenever possible
- Be told what's happening to me, and have my questions answered honestly, in words I can understand
- Have confidentiality about my illness
- Have access to an ethical review
- Understand that doctors will be professionally discussing my situation so that I can get the best care. Sometimes these discussions take place over my bed, in my room or in the hallway. My parents or I have the right to know what's happening whenever possible.
- Be discharged from the hospital as soon as possible without harming my health

The Children's Hospital statement continues:

I have the responsibility to:
- Wear... hospital identification at all times
- Give information about my health
- Report changes in my condition
- Tell those who care for me when I do not understand the plan of care or what is expected of me
- Follow my plan of treatment
- Know, if I choose not to follow my plan of treatment, the consequences
- Know, if I refuse treatment, that the outcome is my responsibility
- Follow... hospital rules about patient care and conduct
- Be considerate of the rights of other patients and staff
- Help control noise and smoking and distractions
- Help provide an interpreter for my family and me whenever possible
- Respect the property of others and Children's Hospital

Caregiver's Bill of Rights

While the child/patient is certainly the central figure in treatment and beyond, he is not the only one whose feelings and well-being should be considered. The following document, used around the United States and across the Atlantic to the British Isles, and perhaps beyond, is reprinted with permission of the author, Jo Horne:

I (the caregiver) have the right:
- To take care of myself. This is not an act of selfishness. It will give me the capability of taking better care of my (child).
- To seek help from others even though my relatives may object. I recognize the limits of my own endurance and strength.
- To maintain facets of my own life that do not include (my child), just as I would if he were healthy. I know that I do everything that I reasonably can for (my child) and I have the right to do some things just for myself.
- To get angry, be depressed, and express other difficult feelings occasionally.
- To reject any attempts by (my child), either conscious or unconscious, to manipulate me through guilt and/or depression.

- To receive consideration, affection, forgiveness and acceptance for what I do for my (child) for as long as I offer these qualities in return.
- To take pride in what I am accomplishing and to applaud the courage it has sometimes taken to meet the needs of my (child).
- To protect my individuality and my right to make a life for myself that will sustain me in the time when my (child) no longer needs my full-time help.
- To expect and demand that as new strides are made in finding resources to aid physically and mentally impaired persons in our country, similar strides will be made towards aiding and supporting caregivers.

Responsibilities

Along with these rights come responsibilities. The parent (or the patient) has a responsibility to make an informed decision whether to sign a consent form for treatment. That means he or she must read the entire form and obtain answers to any questions it leaves unanswered. Only then can he or she responsibly decide whether to sign the form.

Parents have a responsibility to take their child to all scheduled treatments and tests. They must also see that their child takes medication as prescribed and follows any other home treatment programs, such as physical therapy. Parents have a responsibility to tell the doctor if their child misses any treatments at home or has an unusual reaction to them. They must also tell the doctor if the patient is exposed to a contagious disease, is taking other medications (including over-the-counter, herbal, and homeopathic preparations), is following a special diet, is taking vitamins, or is receiving any counseling that could affect his acceptance of therapy. In short, parents should report anything they think could have an impact on therapy, whether positive or negative.

Further Resources

READING

Annas, George. *The Rights of Hospital Patients* (an American Civil Liberties Union Handbook). New York: Avon Books, 1992.

Jasper, Margaret C. *Healthcare and Your Rights Under the Law* (Oceana's Legal Almanac Series: Law for the Layperson). Dobbs Ferry, NY: Oceana Publications, Inc., 2002.

Comprehensive coverage of various rights, including informed consent, refusing treatment, dealing with insurance (private and government), privacy, and considerations when the patient is a minor. Appendices have state-by-state information and referral addresses, sample forms and letters. A clear, intelligent source for information that is understandable by non-lawyers.

Keene, Nancy. *Working with Your Doctor: Getting the Healthcare You Deserve*. Sebastopol, CA: O'Reilly, 1998.

The author, whose child is a cancer survivor, covers a lot of territory here, including rights and responsibilities of patients and physicians. Anecdotes and examples clarify the information.

ORGANIZATIONS/WEB SITES

Cancer Legal Resource Center (Loyola Law School, 919 South Albany St., Los Angeles, CA 90015; 213-736-1455; http://www.lls.edu/academics/candp/clrc.html)

Provides information and educational outreach to consumers in all states on cancer-related legal issues.

HIPAA (www.hipaa.org)

U. S. Department of Labor, Family Leave Medical Act (www.dol.gov) Search "FMLA."

29

The Patient at School

Concerns about educating children with cancer are quite recent. Not so long ago, our focus was on saving lives or at least providing comfort during treatments and terminal illness. Many more children are surviving malignancies now, and with that success come new challenges. Education is one of them.

It is important that patients keep up with their studies as much as they can, whether in the hospital or at home. This is an investment in his future. A child who is an inpatient may have an individualized lesson plan and a tutor. If the child is being treated as an outpatient but cannot go to school, a tutor should be provided for as long as necessary. This is the child's legal right. Accommodations depend on the school district in which the hospital is located and what arrangements can be made with the home school district. When possible, participating in the regular classroom is best, however, because it provides the social contact and intellectual engagement necessary for the child's fullest recovery. Computer technology with webcams may provide a temporary link to the classroom as well. Even terminal patients should continue with lessons, although they may prefer to concentrate on a special subject rather than the whole gamut of courses. Choosing what they wish to learn is one of the few ways they can remain in control.

Teenage cancer survivors returning to school will have a different perspective on life than they had before they became ill; their health may seem more important than top grades (although many cancer patients receive top honors), and they may even drop out. On the other hand, a youngster who has lost athletic prowess may be able to compensate for a loss of self-esteem by concentrating on academic work or favorite extracurricular activities.

Children who have missed a lot of school or who have experienced significant physical changes (weight gain, hair loss, scars, perhaps an amputation) may find it very hard to go back to class. Many youngsters experience either temporary or long-term learning disabilities as a result of either the cancer or its treatments.

Children may, with good reason, fear teasing from classmates or feel frustration at falling behind the others. They may even refuse to go to school, although this is more likely in older children or teenagers. Younger children, on the other hand, may fear the threat of separation from their parents posed by a return to school. They may even develop genuine physical symptoms of fear, such as stomach aches or headaches. A child who tires very easily may do better with a shortened school day, at least temporarily.

Sometimes healthy siblings also experience school phobia. They are afraid to go, out of fear that their brother or sister with cancer will get worse or die while they are away.

The single most important step in a successful return to school is to enlist the teacher's support. The parents should have a conference with the teacher, school administrator, and nurse. The parent must tell them what the child knows about his illness. Most teachers and school nurses, who are often terrified at the prospect of having a "dying child" in class, need information and encouragement. A discussion ahead of time with the child will determine what he wants other children to know and whether the child wants to tell some of them himself; this information should be passed on at the meeting as well. Some re-entry programs include classmates' parents, too.

This first conference is just a beginning; the school should be kept informed about treatment schedules, what side effects to watch for and how to deal with them. The teacher should be urged to contact the family if there seem to be inordinate adjustment problems or if acting out takes place. The school nurse should be warned about giving any medication to the youngster, even aspirin. In our experience, these conferences must be repeated at the beginning of every school year whether or not the situation has changed. For privacy or whatever reasons, we found that teachers do not pass on this type of information to those who succeed them in higher grades. Don't assume that gym teachers and other support staff will be kept informed; contact them directly to be sure.

Some institutions and organizations like the Candlelighters and the National Children's Cancer Foundation sponsor programs, including clinic and classroom visits, for teachers so they can understand what the child is experiencing and how they can help. The treatment center personnel will work with the schools, too—by telephone or personal visits, as the parent requests. There are also several publications available written especially for educators.

The teacher should be urged to treat the child normally, just like the rest of the students. This includes discipline. The patient should not be given special privileges unless there is a sound medical reason. The child should not be isolated from the other students, nor should he be smothered with pity. As one parent noted, our kids need empathy, not sympathy. The school should notify the family if another student develops a contagious disease like chickenpox or measles, whether or not the patient has had the disease. Even sibling exposures should be reported to the parents. Time is of the essence if the child is to be treated to lessen the effects of these illnesses.

Teachers' reactions will vary. Some may fear contagion, classroom disruption, or the physical limitations imposed on the child by cancer. In the rare case that all efforts to enlist the teacher as a member of the team fail, it may be necessary to request—insist on—a change of classroom.

Other students should also be prepared for the child's return. If they understand what is happening, they are less likely to tease the youngster, but teachers must be on the lookout for such abuse and put a stop to it. "Just ignore it" is no response at all when a child is being tormented—and it happens.

Teachers can use the child's illness as a learning experience by devoting a class to the symptoms and treatment of cancer. Various organizations provide audiovisual materials and scripts as well as classroom visits to help with the re-entry process; some are sponsored by drug manufacturers. Check with your local Candlelighters or the clinic social workers. Older students can write papers on their experiences, do experiments or research for science courses, and give oral reports on related topics. Our other daughter Mollie did a science fair project on kidney failure based on Lisa's late effects. Younger students can also do projects to help their friends learn what is going on with them. Some children might feel uncomfortable being singled out in this way, but overcoming that reluctance can lead to a better understanding among other children and a resulting improvement in the way the patient is treated by classmates.

When Lisa returned to nursery school classes after an operation, I went along for a show-and-tell so the others would understand why she still wore diapers. We took along equipment like syringes (without needles!) to show her classmates, some of whom then told about going to the hospital for tonsillectomies or broken bones. When Lisa was in the first grade, the Massachusetts Division of the American Cancer Society made a videotape about her, so we prepared the classes for the presence of cameras and strangers. By then the story was old hat to them.

Even so, we had a long struggle with our small local school system. Teachers ignored teasing and were slow to recognize and accommodate Lisa's physical aftereffects. Despite the fact that her major therapy was finished long before she started school, she had many years of migraines and tears before, in desperation, we moved her to the next town under school choice. In the last 3 years of high school, she made huge advances socially and she did manage to graduate despite a lot of educational issues.

A Wish With Wings, Inc., of Arlington, Texas, conducted a survey asking, "How can teachers be most helpful when a sick child re-enters school?" and "What have teachers done that is least helpful?" Highlights of the responses were reprinted by the Candlelighters Childhood Cancer Foundation:

The Best Teachers (A Parent's View)...
1. Call or visit my child during times of absence.
2. Know that parents need a little TLC, too. Cards, phone calls, visits—all are appreciated.
3. Listen to my concerns and fears.
4. Take time to become familiar with treatments given my child and their effect on school performance.
5. Visit with my child before re-entry to talk about any fears he may have.

6. Adjust regular lesson plans to account for change in my child's ability to complete lengthy tasks or assignments.
7. Gently encourage my child to reach his *current* potential.
8. Follow my and the doctor's instructions regarding bathroom visits, snacks, wearing a hat, etc.
9. Accept the sometimes hard-to-accept side effects of cancer or its treatment (slurring words, falling asleep in class, diminished temper control, or ability to accept discipline, etc.).
10. Are supportive of us during setbacks in the illness.
11. Encourage classmates to call or write my child during periods of extended absence.
12. Prepare the class for physical and emotional changes in my child as a consequence of treatment; suggest ways to be helpful.
13. Treat my child as normally as possible, given the restrictions imposed by disease and its treatment; don't impose their own limits.
14. Are supportive and encouraging, but not phony in their praise.
15. Know when a situation is over their heads and call the parents, doctor or administrators for help.
16. Include my child in as many class functions as possible. He may not have the stamina for a full day of school, but may be able to come to the holiday party or class outing.

The Worse Teachers (A Parent's View)...not only don't do the above but:

1. Show fear about having my child in their class.
2. Allow pity for him within the classroom.
3. Fail to share information about my child's appearance, special needs, etc., with colleagues, substitutes, and aides.
4. Convey an attitude that assumes my child won't be able to do things.
5. Fail to educate themselves about the disease, its treatment, and possible changes in a child's appearance, mannerisms, etc.
6. Make an issue of my child's differences in front of the whole class.
7. Ignore problems classmates have in adjusting to their friends' disease, which may manifest as teasing, mimicking, etc.
8. Do not give my child an opportunity to at least try whatever the others are doing.
9. Do not give my child the benefit of the doubt whenever possible on assignments or homework.

Relaxing regulations like "no hats" for other students can go a long way toward helping a child with cancer fit back into the classroom without being "odd man out."

Further Resources

READING

Bessel, Ann G. Children Surviving Cancer: Psychosocial adjustment, quality of life and school experiences. *Exceptional Children*, vol. 67 (3) (Spring 2001), pp. 345.
Reports research using 51 survivors aged 8 to 17, studying their school re-entry issues, successes and challenges.

Keene, Nancy, ed. *Educating the Child with Cancer: A Guide for Parents and Teachers*. Candlelighters Childhood Cancer Foundation, 2003. Free from www.candlelighters.org
Real-world experience backs up this essential book from the CCCF and respected "cancer mom" and writer Keene. Anecdotes, lists, and lots of advice both for families and education professionals. Especially good at empowering parents to advocate for their children during and after diagnosis. How the various diseases and therapies affect learning over time.

Hamilton, Virginia. *Bluish*. New York: Blue Sky Press, 1999.
A novel for middle readers about an alternative New York City class, told through the eyes and journal of Deenie, one of the new kids. The other new kid is Natalie, who is clearly ill. The story introduces the basic concepts of leukemia in a multicultural setting. By an award-winning author who covers a lot of territory with a light but sure touch.

Keeney, Susan Nessim, and Ernest R. Katz. *A Parents' and Teachers' Guide for Kids with Cancer*. $40 from www.cancervive.org

ORGANIZATIONS/WEB SITES

American Cancer Society: "Children Diagnosed with Cancer: Returning to School" (www.cancer.org)
Good succinct information; search "school."

"Band-Aids and Backboards: When chronic illness...or some other medical problem... goes to school" (www.lehman.cuny.edu)
This is a program created by Joan Fleitas, associate professor of nursing at Fairfield University in Connecticut. "The goal is to help people understand what it's like, from the perspective of the children and teens who are" living with cancer and other illnesses. Choose from kids, teens, or adult level of

information and approach. Search "Band-Aids" or "Fleitas." The URL is a very long one.

Individuals with Disabilities in Education Act (IDEA): "Legal rights of cancer patients in the public education system" (http://www.acor.org/ped-onc/cfissues/backtoschool/backtoschool.html)

Explains this federal law and individualized educational plans (IEPs). IEPs vary; contact your state department of education for specifics.

Lance Armstrong Foundation/ LiveStrong and the Leukemia and Lymphoma Society: "Learning and Living with Cancer: Advocating for your child's educational needs" (www.livestrong.org)

Search "Living and Learning with Cancer." This is a terrific roadmap for navigating the regular and special educational needs of children with cancer—now and as late effects might appear.

Leukemia and Lymphoma Society (www.schoolandyouth.org)

Has a package of booklets and the Trish Greene Back to School Program for the Child with Cancer.

National Information Center for Children with Disabilities (NICHCY) (P.O. Box 1492, Washington, DC 20013; 800-695-0285; www.nichcy.org)

A federal government site to answer questions about health coverage and rights under HIPAA.

30

The Adolescent Cancer Patient

As noted in the chapters on specific diseases, adolescents (defined by the National Cancer Institute's SEER Pediatric Monograph as aged 15 to 19) are more susceptible to certain cancers. Most common are Hodgkin disease, germ cell tumors, central nervous system tumors, non-Hodgkin lymphoma, thyroid cancer, malignant melanoma, and ALL. These older patients rarely if ever are affected by neuroblastoma, Wilms tumor, retinoblastoma, hepatoblastoma, and ependymoma (a form of brain tumor). While the overall male-to-female ratio is equal, boys are more likely to get ALL, non-Hodgkin lymphoma, Ewing sarcoma, and osteosarcoma, while girls have higher rates of Hodgkin disease, thyroid carcinoma, and melanoma.

Some racial differences are seen as well. While blacks have a slightly higher rate of soft tissue sarcomas, whites have a significantly higher rate of acute myelogenous leukemia and non-Hodgkin lymphoma. Whites have an 18-fold risk of Ewing sarcoma and a 54-fold risk of melanoma.

It is especially hard for teenagers to cope with a diagnosis of cancer. Resistance to authority, rebellion, and rule-breaking are common in this age group anyway, and having cancer is likely to accentuate this behavior. Teenagers are seeking independence, and those with a serious illness are instead forced into dependence on doctors, clinics, and parents.

The first decision will be where to get treatment. Is the child an "old kid" or a "young adult"? While their age might suggest using an adult facility, teenagers have a lot more in common with younger cancer patients than with adults. Experts note the importance of using pediatric hospitals and clinics for students still in high school. There state-of-the-art treatment, including participation in clinical trials, improves the cure rate for adolescent patients.

Unfortunately, a significant number of older U.S. adolescents are uninsured, and they tend to fall in the "no man's land" between pediatric and adult cancer patients. The NCI's Dr. Malcolm Smith noted, "Recent publications have reported that adolescents and young adults treated on pediatric trials have better outcomes than similarly-aged [patients] using adult protocols for ALL."

Dr. Wendy Stock, in the same article, was quoted as saying there is a "tremendous disparity in outcome"; those patients treated by pediatric specialists had almost a 30% better chance for long-term survival.

Teenagers are very concerned about their sexuality and their body image; those with cancer may have puffy faces, bald heads, or amputated limbs. Their physical disability may limit their career choices, and they may fear losing their friends, their athletic and academic skills, and their social contacts. It may, in fact, be hard for them to keep up with their classes and to engage in athletic activities.

Parents should allow teenagers plenty of opportunity to express their anger and fears. They deserve a full explanation of their illness and therapy, as well as love, support, and reassurance. Teenagers are modest and need privacy; intimate examinations should be done in a private room rather than just behind a curtain if at all possible. Discussions with the doctor should also be out of the earshot of roommates. Sometimes a number of "extra" doctors and staff appear, especially in teaching hospitals; ask if it is necessary that all be present for examinations. There may be some room for negotiation here.

Sick teenagers may be more worried about their appearance than about the illness itself. They may want to get a wig before their hair falls out in order to get the best match in style and color. On the other hand, they may refuse to wear a wig, no matter how expensive it was.

Teenagers are old enough to recognize the financial strain that their illness is putting on the family. They need to be reassured that they are worth it. As with any serious budgetary problems, the family should decide openly how they will adapt to any changes and what steps can be taken to cope.

The teenager might also resent clinic visits and the doctor's control over his life. If the teen's health and strength permit, he may want to go to the clinic alone for treatments, perhaps on public transportation. Or the patient may want the parent to wait outside or go shopping while he is with the doctor or getting treatments. Parents should be careful not to stand between the adolescent and the doctor. The family is, of course, entitled to information about the illness and the treatments, but the doctor/patient relationship here is important. The adolescent can answer questions during the doctor's examination or when admitted to the hospital. He can call the laboratory to get results. He can also talk with newly diagnosed teenagers, telling them what to expect, and he can probably help medical students to understand better the impact of the disease. If the teenager is hospitalized, it may be better if he is placed with others of similar age rather than by specialty.

An adolescent about to undergo a procedure for the first time might want to read about it or look online for a video of it in advance, so he should know where information is available. He may want to look at slides under the microscope to learn about normal blood counts. The more a patient understands, the less threatening the treatments will be.

Noncompliance

Teenagers in the throes of rebellion are much more likely to be noncompliant with medical orders than other patients. Parents must be vigilant to ensure that they take their oral medications, and adults should also monitor other individual therapy like exercises. If problems arise, a referral to a trained counselor is appropriate—the sooner the better. Watch for moodiness, overly anxious feelings, stoicism, conflicts at home or elsewhere, and school problems. Relationships with peers are especially important, so if the patient seems to be isolated from friends and classmates, some counseling is in order.

As with anyone, be aware of suicidal symptoms or signs (withdrawal, giving away prized possessions, expressions of hopelessness, refusal to look at the future). Talking about suicide, perhaps making plans for suicide, or even attempting to take his own life—these frightening behaviors are more likely at the time of initial diagnosis or at relapse, if the youth is in unrelieved pain, or if he has arguments with friends or family members. Do not assume "he doesn't mean it." Seek professional help immediately.

Help Is Out There

Now more than ever before, there is help for adolescents with cancer. There are clinic "rap" groups, online discussions and chats among teen cancer patients, camps to connect with others in the same boat, and other opportunities. Check the lists of organizations in Appendix B and at the end of this chapter, and talk with social workers and other staff at the clinic or hospital. Don't give up. On the rare occasions that my daughter Lisa was able to talk with someone with similar medical problems, I could see a real improvement in her attitude and emotional health.

How teenagers ultimately cope with the illness will depend to a great extent on how their friends react. Many respond with a heart-warming show of love and caring. News stories repeatedly report on groups of friends who shave their heads to show solidarity with a sick friend on chemotherapy. The NCCF (www.curesearch.org) has a fund-raiser on St. Patrick's Day dubbed "St. Baldrick's Day" when many people go hairless for a cause. Finally, for all of our kids: Bald is In!

Hope Lab's "Re-Mission" video game aimed at adolescents and young adults combines accurate scientific information with fun technology. In tests, quality of life for the players increased along with a clearer understanding of cancer and the treatments. While it is a useful tool, it works in an entertaining way. "Re-Mission" is available on CD or by download from the Cigna Corp. Web site (see contact information at the end of this chapter).

Edith Pendleton, in *Too Old to Cry, Too Young to Die*, tells of one girl whose friends planted a flower garden in the backyard to lure her outside to care for it. Close friends can go to the clinic for visits, too, and can help the teenager who is missing school to keep up with the work by carrying assignments and schoolwork back and forth. Many tech-savvy teachers also put assignments and related materials on Web sites accessible from remote sites, like hospital inpatient rooms.

Teenagers may need special reassurance, either from the doctor or parents, that the illness was not caused by adolescent experimentation with drugs or sex. Many teenagers are sexually active but fail to use contraceptives. If a teenager insists on being sexually active, this should be discussed and appropriate contraception advised. Should a teenager with cancer become pregnant, the doctors must be informed immediately, because the drugs and radiation used to treat the tumor can be devastating for the fetus, especially in the early stages of development. Any course of action should be discussed fully with the adolescent's doctor as soon as possible.

It is important to maintain self-esteem, both for the patient and the family, as part of the coping process. A loss of positive self-image may lead to increased hostility and anger. It may be hard to handle daily stress. The teenager may respond to the illness by being overly compliant or angry, or by seeking a scapegoat (perhaps holding the family responsible for the illness or the doctor for being unable to cure it). He may feel entitled to special favors to make up for the ordeal. To a certain extent this behavior is understandable, but if it gets in the way of daily life or if it continues for an inordinately long period, seek help through the doctor or clinic staff.

The adolescent can try to compensate in other areas for losses. A patient who cannot play championship basketball anymore may still be able to work out with the team, coach, or be a manager or sportswriter. School and local newspapers usually welcome stories by students. During recovery, perhaps the teen can develop artistic talents or an interest in chemistry. The teen can also learn that there is pleasure in being a spectator, too. Teens can use this opportunity to develop their strong points: Is he creative? Does he have a wonderful sense of humor? Can he write? Does he do well at crafts?

Teens should have useful household chores to do, both as individuals (watering the garden, perhaps) and with the family (meal preparation and cleanup). The family's expectation that they will carry on as normally as possible will go a long way toward bolstering their self-esteem, so they should not be overprotected. People who are overly sympathetic or who lower their expectations may damage the youth's ego.

How does the teen want to be treated? Most likely, just like he always was. "I'm still me!" is a common comment from teens with cancer. They don't want pity. They don't want to be the subject of speculation; if a friend or classmate wants to know something, he should just ask. (Play this one by ear; a few don't want to talk about it at all.) Some less empathic classmates may resent the additional attention and special favors the patient receives (like being able to wear a hat where others aren't allowed to).

If there has been a strain in the parent–adolescent relationship, which is not unusual, the family may need counseling to learn how to use this adversity to strengthen ties. As long as the family is stuck with this disease, they might as well use it to their advantage in any way possible.

Cancer survivors often worry about being able to obtain health or life insurance, jobs, or promotions in later years. As more people survive and prosper, this concern should fade, but probably not very quickly. The U.S. government, too, has taken steps to help those in this situation. The Americans with Disabilities Act (ADA) makes it illegal to discriminate against persons with disabilities, and that includes cancer patients and survivors. Employers are required to make reasonable accommodations for otherwise qualified candidates and employees. The clinic staff and your local library can help you find information on the ADA and referrals to helpful legal sources. And as always, document everything in writing. A paper trail is important.

Teenagers old enough to seek jobs may be perceived as unemployable, or they may have trouble enlisting in the military or getting into some schools. If this happens, seek help from the American Cancer Society, Candlelighters Childhood Cancer Foundation, NCCF, or the Leukemia & Lymphoma Society. Publicity in the local newspaper may be helpful, and the American Civil Liberties Union (ACLU) sometimes takes on cases of injustice.

Changing health insurance may be risky while treatments are under way; anyone considering such a move should ask a lot of questions first. Even if the waiting period before a new policy's benefits begin is as short as a month, a cancer patient can pile up a lot of bills in a very brief period if there is an emergency. The U.S. federal insurance program COBRA may provide coverage in the interim; again, check with clinic staff and social workers. The Health Insurance Portability and Accountability Act (HIPAA) ensures that coverage is transferrable from one job to another.

Further Resources

READING

Abrams, Annah N., et al. Psychosocial issues in adolescents with cancer.
Cancer Treatment Reviews, vol. 33 (2007), pp. 622–630.

    This review article examines the adolescent cancer patient conundrum from the point of view of autonomy, compliance, and social issues. Well worth seeking out.

Albritton, Karen, MD. Age matters: The problems of teen cancer care.
Candlelighters Childhood Cancer Foundation Quarterly Journal
(Spring 2005).

    This is just one of several excellent adolescent-related articles in the issue, which is available online at www.candlelighters.org/journals/Spring2005.pdf

Azevedo, Marilyn, RN. *Defending Andy, One Mother's Fight to Save Her Son from Cancer and the Insurance Industry*. Deerfield Beach, FL: Health Communications, 2001.

    A lovely, moving, and beautifully written book about one mother's—one family's—and ultimately one community's fight against both the Big C and Big Business. While the former eventually won, the latter did not. An honest, self-revealing book that carries every mother's love and wishes for her sick child.

Carter, Alden R. *Sheila's Dying*. New York: G. P. Putnam's Sons, 1987.

    Don't be put off by the "downer" title. Although the (brief) medical therapy aspects of this well-written teen novel are outdated, the emotions felt by the sick girl's friends are as fresh as morning.

Dorfman, Elena. *The C-Word: Teenagers and Their Families Living with Cancer*. Portland, OR: NewSage Press, 1994.

"Improvements needed for adolescents and young adults," *NCI National Cancer Bulletin*, vol. 5 (6) (March 18, 2008), p. 9.

Grinyer, Anne. *Cancer in Young Adults Through a Parent's Eye*. Cambridge (UK) and Philadelphia: Open University Press, 2002.

    The young adults referred to in the title are ages 18 to 25, so they fall just at the far reaches of childhood cancer. Still, with discussions of sexuality, independence, and the like, this British publication has some interesting material. The financial section is quite European and not as helpful for Americans. Lots of anecdotes.

Stewart, Gail B. *Teens with Cancer*. San Diego, CA: Lucent, 2002.

Part of "The Other America" series. There is some background information, but the bulk of the book focuses on the stories of teens who have been treated for different kinds of cancer. A thoughtful presentation of their hopes, fears, and emotions. A good source for friends to read, too.

Pendleton, Edith, ed. *Too Old to Cry, Too Young to Die*. Nashville: Thomas Nelson Publishers, 1980.

Three dozen teenagers share their experiences battling several forms of cancer, including breast cancer and neuroblastoma, both rare in this age group. A highly recommended book, if a trifle dated. Includes practical tips.

Trillin, Alice. *Dear Bruno*. Illustrated by Edward Koren, foreword by Paul Newman. New York: New Press, 1996.

Probably most useful for teens, this short book is a letter to a new adolescent cancer patient named Bruno, from an adult lung cancer survivor (since deceased). Koren's illustrations are delightful and the book is both witty and wise.

ORGANIZATIONS/WEB SITES

Fertile Hope (888-994-4673; www.fertilehope.org)

Provides reproductive information and hope to cancer patients who may be facing infertility due to therapy.

I'm Too Young for This Cancer Foundation (www.imtooyoungforthis.org)

An organization to empower cancer patients age 15 and up. Interesting gift selections. Plus the Stupid Cancer Show on radio. Many great links and downloadable resources.

Lance Armstrong Foundation/LiveStrong: "Planning for Life After Cancer: A Guide to Survivorship for Teens and Young Adults" (www.livestrong.org)

Addresses teen concerns about the present and the future, using teen patients and survivors.

Planet Cancer (www.planetcancer.org)

Real-world information and contacts for cancer patients ages 18 and up. Amusing text, funny gifts (check out that thong!).

Re-Mission, the Game (www.re-mission.net)

Video game for adolescents and young adults. Order for free or download. Also in Spanish or French. Windows only; no MAC version.

The Sam Fund (www.thesamfund.org)

A nonprofit organization for young adult cancer survivors; scholarships and other financial support.

Starbright Foundation (www.starlight.org)

Steven Spielberg is co-chair and Jamie Lee Curtis is national spokesperson and chairperson emeritus of this organization. The Starbright World (SBW) is an online program for chronically ill adolescents. Lots of online fun and information to entertain and distract patients.

Teens Living with Cancer (www.teenslivingwithcancer.org)

A very cool Web site with basic information, discussion boards, peer online support, and a lot more. Partially sponsored by the Children's Oncology Group.

Ulman Cancer Fund for Young Adults (www.ulmanfund.org)

This Web site serves "young adults, their families and friends, who are affected by cancer, and to promote awareness and prevention of cancer." The site is a nice gateway to several teen-oriented sites to facilitate communication among patients, raise awareness, and just plain have fun.

Wellness Community (Group Loop) (www.grouploop.org)

This is a great site for ages 13 to 19, with support, resources, and information. Connect with other teens fighting cancer.

31

The Survivors

The need for this new chapter on childhood cancer survivors is one of the brightest spots of the past two decades. Today an estimated 75% of all childhood cancer patients, about 300,000 strong and growing, have survived for 5 or more years after diagnosis, a benchmark some call a cure. The improvements in treating ALL and Hodgkin disease are among the most positive developments in the cancer field.

In 1985 I wrote, "What will happen to the survivors? It's really too early to say..." and "Long-term survivors will have to be followed throughout their lives to...insure that no recurrence or late effect surfaces."

The latter is as true today as it was then. Long-term survivor clinics are following many thousands of former childhood cancer patients, assessing their current health, the consequences of their malignancies and treatments, and generally how their lives are playing out compared to their healthy siblings and friends. Extensive information on late effects and long-term follow-up has been printed in the *Candlelighters* newsletter, available at the CCCF Web site (www.candlelighters.org). Checking this Web site on a regular basis will give you much valuable, current information. The results have been heartening.

In 1981 Gerald P. Koocher, PhD, and John E. O'Malley, MD, of Harvard and the Children's Hospital Medical Center of Boston published the first major study of childhood cancer survivors, collecting the findings of a number of investigations. They found that more than half of the patients they surveyed had adjusted well after their ordeal. Of those who said they had had problems adjusting, most were living normal lives—affected only minimally—perhaps worrying about the return of the cancer or hiding their medical history from new friends. Many felt "special" for surviving the disease and were trying to enjoy each day fully. Just a few suffered serious emotional reactions—depression, anger, and bitterness that cancer had affected their lives. Koocher and O'Malley also reported that psychological problems tended to diminish with the passage of time. Children from families with higher incomes tended to adjust better, as did those who were younger at diagnosis, particularly neuroblastoma and Wilms tumor patients. Survivors of bone tumors, acute lymphoblastic leukemia, soft tissue tumors, and the lymphomas tended to have more trouble adjusting, as did those who had suffered recurrences, even though the relapses were successfully treated. The patients interviewed for that study received therapy for longer periods than more modern treatments require, so researchers have been interested to see whether those patterns would hold true for more recent patients.

To a great extent, the issues and problems today parallel those of 20 years ago, although the 21st-century experts recognize a more extensive range of potential challenges and disabilities in varying degrees. Unfortunately, the only major study reported covered patients treated from 1970 to 1986. Surely newer reviews are ongoing to quantify late effects in patients treated more recently with newer protocols.

Health

Risk factors for later health problems include the duration, timing, and intensity of the therapy and the age (and possibly gender) of the patient at the time. Some cancers may also carry genetic factors that predispose to new malignancies. Overall, about two out of three survivors report at least one chronic health problem, and many have several. The combination of different therapies like chemotherapy and radiation can increase the late effects on the survivors.

Among the health issues is the possibility of recurrence, in some cases even many years after the initial treatment is completed.

Many of the therapies, too, are themselves carcinogenic, with the risk that between 3% and 12% of former patients will develop a second type of cancer within about 20 years. These second malignancies are primarily radiation-related, striking greater numbers of Hodgkin disease, retinoblastoma, and ALL survivors. The second cancers are often breast (in female Hodgkin survivors), thyroid, brain, colon, lung (all diagnosed at a young age), and acute myelogenous leukemia (AML). Patients radiated in the chest could develop cardiac symptoms or a decrease in lung function. Brain tumor radiation can lead to obesity and high blood pressure. Spinal radiation can result in a shorter stature than might otherwise be attained, and certain fields of radiation can result in deformities (one limb shorter than the other, for example).

Some cancer drugs, too, cause cardiac, liver, kidney, and bladder problems. Infertility for both male and female survivors is a possibility with some forms of therapy and with some specific cancers. Growth problems treated with growth hormone have been suspected of increasing the risk for recurrences, but recent studies have dispelled that fear. Patients who had head and neck radiation are more susceptible to thyroid problems, and vision difficulties (such as cataracts) and hearing problems (ringing in the ears) are other potential late effects.

Adding the proverbial insult to injury, life-saving blood transfusions in earlier years often led to further illnesses. Some children contracted AIDS through blood products, and those who had transfusions prior to July 1992 (when screening began) often were infected with hepatitis C, an incurable liver disease.

At 30 years after diagnosis, over 70% of long-term survivors have a late-effect chronic health condition. As survivors reach middle age and beyond, they may well be at risk for increased chronic health conditions because of their earlier therapies. Time will tell.

Social

Social adjustment of survivors can be another concern. Not only have these children and adolescents missed a lot of school and other normal childhood activities, but they also may have obvious differences like amputations or learning difficulties. They may be overly dependent on their families and need to learn greater independence (and the families may need help learning to let go, too). Studies show cancer survivors are less apt to have close friends. Above all there is the fear of a recurrence, a second malignancy (lightening does strike twice!), and a fear of passing cancer on to their own children, if they are indeed able to have any.

Psychiatric

Psychiatric problems include post-traumatic stress disorder (PTSD), not unlike that suffered by battle veterans, with anxiety, nightmares, sleep problems, and flashbacks to the days of active treatments. These periods of PTSD are greatest during, but not limited to, the time of therapy and the time leading up to a major event like a bone marrow transplant. Many survivors have depression and anxiety disorders of varying severity.

Life Issues

As if all that weren't enough, survivors have life challenges that their healthier siblings and classmates never have to think about. Will they be able to finish school, get additional education, find satisfying and well-paying work, acquire life and health insurance? Some of these problems are addressed by legislation like the Americans with Disabilities Act, which provides a legal antidiscrimination basis in jobs. Check the resources listed at the end of this chapter for potential allies in any struggle regarding job, education, or health insurance discrimination.

Learning Problems

"Cognitive" means the ability to learn, to think, and to understand new material and information. When the child successfully completes treatments and becomes a long-term survivor, one interesting problem may arise. If the child or a sibling develops any behavioral, emotional, or learning problems, therapists or school authorities may blame them on the cancer, perhaps even years later. Once the fact of cancer in the family is in the medical history, it stands out. Perhaps subsequent problems are indeed a result of the cancer, but perhaps they are not. Parents should make sure other causes are explored, too.

On the other hand, if the cancer survivor does develop learning problems, some educators are reluctant to blame either the cancer itself or the therapy, noting that a child who misses a great deal of school, whatever the cause, is likely to experience some educational consequences. It is reassuring that the majority of long-term survivors do graduate with their classes on schedule, although cancer patients are more likely to repeat a grade than their healthy siblings and friends.

Learning difficulties may be the effects of chemotherapy and/or radiation on brain cells. These problems may appear later, even up to 5 years after therapy is completed. Unfortunately, those that arise do not tend to lessen over time. The younger the child is at the time of diagnosis for leukemia or brain tumor, for example, the greater the risks are for learning disabilities. Infants and toddlers carry the highest risk. Head radiation raises the risk, but modern therapy avoids this as much as possible in treating leukemia, for example, substituting drugs to diminish the possibility of central nervous system relapse.

Brain tumor survivors may also have learning and vision problems, may have trouble remembering, and may have seizures or a lack of coordination. Some studies show girls have a higher possibility of learning disabilities than boys. Planning and problem-solving skills may be weaker.

Whatever the disabilities that arise, it is vital to enlist the support of educational specialists to lessen the impact as much as possible. Long-term survivor clinics should be able to help identify professionals who can help.

Reproductive Issues

Chemotherapy, radiation, and surgery that save the lives of cancer patients can also affect their fertility in later years. Alkylating agents can lower sperm counts, for example. Radiation can kill eggs and sperm. Surgical removal of reproductive organs or scarring after regional surgery also reduces or eliminates fertility in boys and girls.

Survivors who reach adulthood are likely to want their own "natural" children but may be afraid of passing along their cancers to their offspring. Happily, studies show that in most cases this fear is unwarranted. In a few instances, genetics play a role; retinoblastoma, for example, sometimes has a familial origin. These survivors are more likely to see the cancer appear in their own children. A Scandinavian study of children born to survivors of childhood and adolescent cancer found that they are otherwise unlikely to "pass on" their illness. Many survivors have perfectly healthy children.

A new article reports on research that showed female survivors who had abdominal or brain radiation had considerably fewer offspring in later years. Those who had abdominal radiation are at a much higher risk for premature delivery of infants and low birth weights and show a small increase in miscarriage.

Adolescent boys may sometimes bank sperm before therapy starts in case of future infertility. Sometimes ovaries can be moved out of the radiation zone temporarily to avoid egg damage; although egg banking has not proven as viable, research is rapidly improving this potential. While the children born to survivors are generally healthy, women who have had pelvic radiation are more likely than the general population to miscarry before term, and birth weights tend to be lower.

The organization Fertile Hope (see the list at the end of this chapter for contact information) has excellent, up-to-date publications and suggestions both for the time of your child's cancer therapy and for survivors who are concerned with reproductive issues.

It is important to note that laws vary from country to country. As a result, not all reproductive technology is available to everyone. While the United States and the United Kingdom, among others, are quite liberal, some countries such as Italy and Switzerland ban many treatments available elsewhere.

The Good News

This is all pretty daunting, but it is well to remember that current therapies (including radiation and chemotherapy) are usually fine-tuned to target cancer cells while sparing healthy tissue. Drug doses are lower and the length of treatment is shorter. With each succeeding year and generation of childhood cancer patients, therapies improve and side and after effects are decreased.

Nor are all late effects negative. Survivors are often more compassionate, have different life values, are less shy, and have better job performance and stronger relationships than their healthy friends and relatives.

The Advice

Advice from the experts to childhood cancer survivors will sound pretty familiar to almost anyone:

- Don't use tobacco.
- Use sunscreen and avoid long sun exposure.
- Eat a healthy, low-fat, high-fiber diet with lots of vegetables rich in vitamins A and C.
- Watch your weight.
- Do regular self-examinations (breast and testicular).
- Get regular checkups with doctors who know your history.
- Keep your medical records complete and share them with any new medical people.
- Both moderate strength and endurance training are helpful, as well as exercise in general.

The really good news, of course, is still that there are so many survivors today and there will be even more tomorrow. Vigilance on the part of parents, doctors, and others will ensure that their health is optimal.

Further Resources

READING

Dorfman, Elena, and Heidi Schultz Adam. *Here and Now—Inspiring Stories of Cancer Survivors*. New York: Marlowe & Co., 2002.
Photos and first-person stories of people who have survived various types of cancer, including some childhood forms, from 11 months to 40 years. How they found the treatments, who supported them, who made a difference.

Inspiring reading. Some famous people are included, some "just regular folks," but all are touching.

Childhood Cancer Survivorship: Improving Care and Quality of Life,
Report from the Institute of Medicine. 2003. (Available for sale by the
National Academies Press, Washington, DC; www.nap.edu).
   Candlelighters recommends this publication. You can purchase the whole book or separate chapters online. There is an especially detailed and helpful section on employment and insurance issues that survivors face; discusses several U.S. government programs and laws that may help.

Hoffman, Barbara, JD. *A Cancer Survivor's Almanac: Charting Your*
Journey. New York: Wiley and Sons, 2004.
   A comprehensive discussion of employment and insurance rights issues, with commentary by experts in legal and oncology circles.

Keene, Nancy, et al. *Childhood Cancer Survivors: A Practical Guide to Your*
Future. Cambridge, MA: O'Reilly, 2000 (available from www.childhood
cancerguides.org).
   Comprehensive.

Landier, Wendy, and Smita Bhatia. Cancer survivorship: a pediatric perspective. *The Oncologist,* vol. 13 (11) (November 2008), pp. 1181–1192.
   Written for professionals, this article has extensive recommendations for screening survivors. If you are not working with a long-term survivor clinic, this article would be a good resource to share with your general practitioners.

"Long-Term Follow-up Study, Surviving Childhood Cancer" (CCSS). (Was
University of Minnesota, now at St. Jude's Web site: www.stjude.org)
   This is the *crème de la crème* of the survivorship studies. The authors have been gathering data on 20,346 survivors diagnosed between 1970 and 1986. Funded through 2004 by the National Cancer Institute, the study relies on cooperation from 31 cancer centers in the United States and Ontario. Results are disseminated to the many long-term survivor clinics around the country and internationally.

Oeffinger, Kevin C., MD, and Melissa M. Hudson, MD. Long-term
complications following childhood and adolescent cancer: foundations
for providing risk-based health care for survivors. *CA: A Cancer Journal*
for Clinicians, vol. 54 (4) (2004) pp. 208–236.
   This article has tables detailing late effects from various therapies, includ-ing radiation and drugs, for patients treated between 1970 and 1986.

Wallace, W. H. B., and D. M. Green, eds. *Late Effects of Childhood Cancer.*
London: Arnold, 2004.

Published in the United Kingdom but a collaboration of American and British institutions, this scholarly collection of specialist-written chapters is packed with helpful information. A comprehensive source for early and late effects from dental development to learning disabilities. Keep a medical dictionary handy—it's worth the effort.

ORGANIZATIONS / WEB SITES

Association for Cancer Online Resources (www.acor.org; www.acor.org/ped-onc/treatment/surclinics.html)
  Clinics for long-term survivors and a lot of other good information.

Beyond the Cure (www.beyondthecure.org)
  Information for survivors of pediatric malignancies from the National Children's Cancer Society. General information plus the opportunity to create a personal profile based on your own therapy and experience.

Cancervive (9006 Rosewood Avenue, Los Angeles CA 90048; 310-203-9232; www.cancervive.org)
  Broadly defines survivors as anyone who has been diagnosed with cancer and is still alive. Resources, support, and advocacy services.

Children's Oncology Group (www.survivorshipguidelines.org)
  "Long-term follow-up guidelines for survivors of childhood, adolescent, and young adult cancers." Has detailed information on health risks to various body systems, such as dental and hearing. Detailed and authoritative.

CureSearch (www.curesearch.org)
  Another Children's Oncology Group site with excellent information on health and other issues survivors may face. Includes *Establishing and Enhancing Services for Childhood Cancer Survivors, Long-Term Follow-Up Program Resource Guide*, edited by Wendy Lanier. Addresses all facets of late care, including employment, educational, and insurance issues.

Fertile Hope (888-994-HOPE; www.fertilehope.org)
  Cancer survivor fertility issues. Partnered with the Lance Armstrong Foundation/LiveStrong, among others, Fertile Hope is an excellent source for trusted information about childhood cancer and fertility issues. Downloadable brochures are available on the Web site.

National Coalition for Cancer Survivorship (NCCS) (1010 Wayne Ave., Suite 770, Silver Spring, MD 20910; 301-650-9127; 888-650-9127; www.cansearch.org)
  Cancer patient advocacy organization with information on insurance, community support groups, and employment discrimination as it affects

cancer survivors. Offers a "Cancer Survivor Toolbox" in English and Spanish. Free CD—order online.

Passport for Care (www.txccc.org)

Search for "passport." This innovative resource for survivors of chronic illnesses, developed by Baylor, has started with childhood cancer patients. A Web-based resource for survivors and caregivers from the Children's Oncology Group and Texas Children's Cancer Center/Baylor College of Medicine.

Survivor Alert (www.survivoralert.org)

A Web site with a lot of links for young adult survivors of cancer, this is an outreach program of the documentary film "A Lion in the House."

32

Death

Unfortunately, no book on childhood cancer can avoid a discussion of death. It is almost inevitable that those involved with this illness will be touched by death, whether of their own child or of a clinic friend. Some researchers think that by the year 2015 cancer will be a chronic rather than often-fatal illness. It will be a happy day when we can leave out this chapter completely. For now, though, this is intended only as an overview with some suggestions on sources of further help.

"My Wishes"

Doctors urge adults to sign "living wills" that detail what steps they wish to have taken on their behalf when they are not able to make the decisions themselves. Signing such a document can spare families and medical staff the kind of ugly, wrenching legal disputes that are played out in the courts and in the media on occasion as loved ones face off over heroic medical measures that might keep a comatose patient alive.

While living wills are probably not meant for pediatric patients, a new document called "My Wishes" may indeed be helpful for families facing the death of their child. An outgrowth of the "Five Wishes" program for terminally ill adults, these wishes indicate, in workbook format, how the patient wants to be treated, by whom, who he wants to see, and similar directives. Explanations of "My Wishes" are available online; a Google search for "my wishes" and "pediatric" will locate discussions. "My Wishes" is available from Aging with Dignity. (See the resources list at the end of this chapter for addresses.)

Death of a Child

Experts now generally agree that a child who is dying should be told if he asks or if the parent senses he wants to know. The child will perceive a change in attitude of those around him and may realize why, whether he says so or not. This can increase the child's fear. If the family provides an open, honest, and loving atmosphere, the child will understand that he can ask about death. He may not ask a parent but rather choose a friend or a trusted nurse or doctor. This does not mean the child is rejecting his parents. He must be able to talk about it openly, and this free discussion will increase the trust between parent and child. If no one talks to the child about it, his expectations may be worse than the reality.

Most children have some experience with death, whether of a pet or a relative. Frank discussions at such times will have given the family a basis for further talks as needed while the child is undergoing treatment for cancer and if he does not respond to therapy. The child may become more concerned with death than others of a similar age or may act overwhelmingly uninterested. The family should talk to the child about it and read from books that attempt to explain death in terms children can understand. It is most important that the child not feel he will be abandoned. Questions should be answered in the same spirit in which they are asked. A curious child deserves facts. A grieving child needs comfort.

Adolescents who are dying need plenty of opportunities to see their friends and anyone else they want to tell themselves, but they should not be pushed. As long as they are able to go places, the parents should not be overprotective. Putting the teenager in a glass cage, however loving the motive, may lead to conflict and resentment without any real benefit. Above all, patients need reassurance that any pain can and will be relieved.

That point deserves repeating: *any pain can and will be relieved.* Unfortunately, this is not always the case. A recent article reported that dying children suffer needlessly in the final month of life because the focus has always been on cure rather than quality of life. The study, carried out at two major Boston hospitals, showed that the children suffer from pain, fatigue, breathing difficulties, nausea, vomiting, and constipation. Treatment for these problems was rarely successful. There was little attempt to ease the problem of fatigue, which results from the disease as well as nutritional deficiencies, depression, and anemia.

Distressingly, the study showed that children are less likely than the elderly to die at home in comfort. "The discrepancy leads some experts to conclude that doctors are willing to concentrate on making older patients comfortable at the end of their lives, but they feel compelled to try to save the lives of children." Parents and other caregivers need to recognize that stopping ineffective treatments is not "giving up"; there should be no guilt attached. Pain relief is achievable and there should of course be no concern about developing an addiction to painkillers. The child needs reassurance that everything possible will be done to relieve any pain he may feel.

Another common problem is shortness of breath, which can be controlled by oxygen, a change in the patient's position, and dealing with fluid retention in the lungs, among other steps.

Explanations of death, as of the illness, should be age-related. People of all ages think about death, it appears, but children may not ask about it in order to spare their parents' feelings.

Preschoolers are afraid they will be separated from their parents. Honesty is important. They should be allowed to see the family's sadness. If they are concerned about the death of a friend, they may mull it over for a long time without actually talking about it. Lisa announced in odd places at odd times that her clinic friend Tommy died. Children need plenty of time and an opportunity to share their worries. These youngsters may view death as temporary. Several months after a beloved elderly neighbor's death, Lisa suddenly prayed for him to come back and sobbed brokenheartedly when she realized he was actually gone for good.

Children in elementary grades may see death as a person, a ghost, angel, or bogey man. They may decide they can avoid death through superstition. As their health fails, they may withdraw, feeling an increased separation from their parents and the hospital staff.

Older youngsters are especially aware of impending death, whether their own or that of a friend or loved one. They may "act up" to see if they will be disciplined as usual. Adolescents may fantasize that they will be saved at the last minute by some miracle. Again, the lines of communication must be kept open. The dying teenager still has many of the same concerns as his peers along with the problems caused by the illness.

The child may want to create something special to leave behind for others. This may be letters, pictures, works of art, a diary, pottery, or whatever interests him. The family can talk this over, if they wish, and make sure the child has any materials that he needs or wants. The child may write a message, maybe even tape it, for the funeral service or to comfort family and friends.

As time passes and the end nears, the child may or may not pass through the stages of dying theorized by Elisabeth Kübler-Ross: denial, anger, bargaining for life, acceptance, and detachment. He may pass through some of the stages in reverse order.

Dying children have three basic needs: relief of pain and other discomforts (discussed in detail in Section II of this book), contact with people, and control over their remaining days. They also need to know that their life, however short, has had meaning. The family can talk about special memories and what the child has meant to them, and his friends, the church, clubs, whatever has been important to the child. Parent and child can share sadness, too.

Family Reactions

There are many emotions when a child is dying, perhaps including anger: Does he not deserve to live after all he has gone through? This is understandable and helps vent feelings to some degree, but carried to extremes, parents could damage their relationships with some of the caregivers whom they will need to have on their side. Anger seems to depend on whether the family has had time to work through feelings, as well as on how much the child suffered and on the family's religious beliefs.

If the parent denies that the child is dying (again, a common temporary reaction), the resulting tension can lead to more stress. The child might start to act younger as a result, cutting himself off even more than would otherwise be the case.

Mourning begins before the child actually dies, and parents may draw back gradually from him and turn their attention back to their other children and to their work. In rare extreme cases, the parents may visit less often or stop going to see the child entirely. This of course is the realization of the child's worst fears of abandonment. More commonly, the dying child becomes the focus of the whole family. If this continues for weeks or months, it will be harder to pick up the pieces after the child's death.

The family may have an opportunity to choose where the child will die, whether at home or in a hospital. In an institution, the care will be good but may result in efforts to prolong the child's life after all hope is gone; clear discussions with the doctor ahead of time about the family's wishes regarding resuscitation and use of life-support equipment are essential. Just having the discussion is not enough; make sure your wishes are clearly written and kept with the child. A recent report in a daily newspaper noted that many DNR (do not resuscitate) orders are unavailable or unknown at the time of a medical crisis, resulting in unwanted heroics.

Home care could be a problem if the family cannot get the proper support. The hospice movement, imported to the United States from England, is a compromise between the two, but few inpatient hospices (particularly for children) now exist in North America. Where they have been set up, they provide a homelike setting with medical care but relaxed regulations regarding visiting.

Often the child wants to die at home, in familiar and non-threatening surroundings, with pets, toys, and friends nearby. This could be appropriate in many circumstances. Dr. Ida M. Martinson at the University of San Francisco School of Nursing has studied the topic and suggests that home care is appropriate when:

- No further efforts are being made to cure the child.
- The child and the parents want the child to be at home.
- The parents are confident they can provide care.
- Nurses and the doctor are willing to be on-call consultants.

The child's security and sense of being loved at the time of death are comforting for him, and the parents may feel less guilty, finding satisfaction in knowing they did all they possibly could.

Home care is much less costly than hospitalization. However, some insurance companies may not cover home care. If that is the case, advance negotiation, pointing out how much money they will save if the child goes home, may help. Any agreement should be written, of course.

Whether at home or in the hospital, as the child weakens, there will be a range of physical problems, depending in part on the type of cancer. The medical staff will discuss ahead of time what to expect and how to get help with these problems.

It is possible the family will detect a change in the doctor's attitude as the child is dying. Some parents report that the physician pulls away, also feeling guilt and distress, a sense of failure, and a loss of self-image. Other hospital staff may also distance themselves to protect their feelings. These people have been closely involved with the child and the whole family and will have their own period of mourning, which should be respected if they are grieving for another child. They should not completely withdraw, however, for their work is not yet done.

After the child dies, the parents may be asked to consent to an autopsy. The doctors may want to assess the child's response to different forms of treatments, particularly if any experimental steps were taken or if the disease is an especially rare one. The doctors know it may be hard for families to understand this. A doctor once told a Candlelighters group meeting how hard it is to ask.

The family can quietly begin making plans and arrangements for the funeral before the child dies. This will avoid hasty and possibly costly decisions made in a moment of extreme stress and confusion. Some children will want to help with these plans and some will not; parents will have a good idea by this stage how their youngster feels. Just as pregnancy and birth require long and careful preparation, the child's death is of at least equal importance in the family's history, and requires the same loving planning. The child can help decide who will participate in the service, where he will be buried or, if cremated, where his ashes might be scattered, and what favorite prayers and hymns should be part of the service, if the family is a church-going one. Working together on these plans may bring the parents closer together and show them ways to support each other. Parents may be dazed and crying for a long period after the child's death, feeling they have "lost our minds." They may still be angry, have strange thoughts, and even wish for death themselves. Many feel relief that the child's suffering is over, an honest and loving response that should carry no guilt. It is fine to mention the child—he is not forgotten and others need reassurance that it is all right to talk about him. Open channels of communication are important.

The two parents usually respond differently, which makes it hard. If one is silent, the other may feel he or she cannot discuss feelings openly. Because men in particular are expected to be stoic, people may urge them to "take care of" the child's mother, implying that the mother is more the wounded party. Men are therefore more likely to hide their grief. Other children need to share their grief too; they may regress to younger behavior temporarily. Parents may have a sense of emptiness and loneliness, and perhaps even physical symptoms like fatigue. Parents who are angry should take care not to drive a wedge between themselves and potential supporters. Instead, that energy can be turned into constructive activity like working for better facilities or equipment for other patients.

There are a number of support groups for grieving parents. The hospital or clinic staff will know if there is one meeting locally. Other sources of information are a chaplain or a member of the clergy, a social worker, or perhaps another parent. Meetings may be listed in local newspapers' calendars. Some support groups contact parents when they hear of a child's death. These groups may help and they may not. Some will find them a good outlet but some people will not be able to open up at all. This is a matter of finding one's own way.

When a Friend's Child Dies

If a friend from the clinic dies, other families will have to discuss it with their children. Even if they do not mention it, the children have probably realized that the friend is no longer there and are wondering why or have worked up some fantasy to avoid the reality. Children need to be part of the mourning, and their sadness may last a long time, too. If they do not take part in the funeral ritual and grieving, they may feel isolated. Taking them to the funeral home or to visit at the house will help satisfy their fears and curiosity, so by all means they should be allowed to go if they want to—but of course they should not be forced.

In talking with the grieving parents, friends should avoid saying things like "she is better off now." They should just say how sorry they are, how frustrated that the child died when so many are being saved, how angry they are. Some might write a condolence letter. It does not have to be a publishable literary masterpiece, but a letter is something the parent can keep and refer to over time. Sympathy, love, and sadness can be shared.

There are concrete ways others can help parents who have suffered the loss of a child. Depending on how close they are, they might:

- Offer to housesit during the wake, funeral home visiting hours, or funeral. (There are people who rob houses after reading obituaries.)
- Take some food for the family and things for their visitors. A casserole or pastry is good, but not a lot of perishable food, because they may have more things given to them than they can store safely. A friend might phone ahead and tell them that on the night of the wake, he will provide supper for the family. They are not thinking about food at all, of course, but they will have to keep their strength up, too.
- Visit. Sit, talk, weep, and hug. Keep it short—up to half an hour, unless there is something to be done.
- Help with the family's household chores—wash the dishes, run the vacuum, clean the bathroom, shovel the walk, mow the lawn.
- Read to siblings.
- Shop for groceries.
- Fill the family's car with gas.
- Listen, and let them mourn as long as they need to.

The youngster's toys can be put up out of the way, perhaps in a box in a closet, but *should not* be packed up and "gotten rid of" to spare the parents that chore. For most families that is an important step in the grieving process that they must carry out when they are ready. Friends can offer to help with that if they wish, but on the family's own schedule. The parents may, however, prefer to do it alone.

Down the road, the child's death anniversary and birthday should be commemorated. These days will be hard for the parents. Particularly if some months have passed, people may either forget the dates or not mention them for fear of reminding the grieving parents. But they remember quite well and will welcome a chance to talk about the youngster.

Friends of ours lost a toddler suddenly (not to cancer) and on her birthday they provided flowers for church—and balloons. After the service, the child's 3-year-old sister took the balloons outside and released them, "sending them to Katie." It was a lovely and moving gesture.

If friends have or know of a book that might help the parents, loan it or borrow it from the library for them. The family may not want to read a word, or they may find it very comforting.

Further Resources

READING

Andrae, Christine. *When Evening Comes—the Education of a Hospice Volunteer.* New York: St. Martin's Press, 2000.
   A readable memoir written for adults by a mystery novelist. Touching and informative.

Bennett, Amanda, and Terence B. Foley. *In Memoriam, A Practical Guide to Planning a Memorial Service.* Simon & Schuster, 1997.
   For adults. Religious and secular service, formal or informal. Selected readings, suggested music selections from classical to gospel to rock. An excellent resource, a good place to start.

Cure (Cancer Updates, Research and Education) magazine (back issues available online at www.curetoday.com)
   Often has articles on death and dying, hospice and palliative care. See especially the Winter 2006, Fall 2007, and Spring 2008 issues. Free subscription.

Hilden, Joanne, MD, & Daniel R. Tobin, MD, with Karen Lindsay. *Shelter from the Storm: Caring for a Child with a Life-Threatening Condition.* Perseus Publishing, 2003.
   No death of a child can be considered "good," as may be the case with an elderly person who has had a full life. There can, however, be a "peaceful" death, and this book prepares the family for such acceptance. There are many sad stories at pediatric oncology clinics, but the saddest was the 13-year-old

boy who died without his parents being able to face it. No one had a chance to say goodbye to this youth, who certainly understood his situation, unspoken or not. This book is a wise and useful source for patient, family, and friends—what to expect, who will help and how—and may you never need it.

Hood, Ann. *Comfort: a Journey Through Grief.* New York: W. W. Norton & Co, 2008.

This beautiful and sobering memoir details the sudden death of the author's young daughter from "ordinary" strep. Hood shows her slow acceptance of grief and return to joy.

Housden, Maria. *Hannah's Gift: Lessons from a Life Fully Lived.*
New York: Bantam Books, 2002.

This beautifully written, thoughtful, and moving book details a mother's (and a family's) struggle when almost-3-year-old Hannah is diagnosed with rhabdomyosarcoma. By turns funny, touching, and heart-wrenching, this is ultimately a hopeful book. Highly recommended for all parents—bereaved or not.

Johnson, Christopher M., MD. *Your Critically Ill Child: Life and Death Choices Parents Must Face.* Far Hills, NJ: New Horizon Press, 2007.

Written by an experienced pediatric intensive care unit physician, this readable and honest book walks parents through the PICU experience, noting the limits of medical technology and including anecdotes of his patients, always with hope.

Kübler-Ross, Elisabeth. *On Children and Death.* New York: Macmillan, 1983.

Valuable source in understanding how children think about death—their own or that of a loved one. Particularly encouraging in its discussion of afterlife, with many brief histories of death and hope. A lengthy bibliography includes unpublished material.

"A Lion in the House" (www.mylion.org)

This lovely, heartbreaking, and hopeful book-and-DVD combination includes a Web presence with many resources for families and communities. Years in the making, the video follows five patients on their cancer journeys. Some of the children die. Recommended for ages 12 and up. Many links to sources for all ages. Excellent section: "Facts and Resources: Pediatric Palliative, End-of-Life and Bereavement Care."

Orloff, Stacy, and Susan M. Huff, eds. *Home Care for Seriously Ill Children: a Manual for Parents.* Alexandria, VA: Children's Hospice International, 2003.

Just what it sounds like—a primer of skills, guidance, and support.

Rando, Therese. *How to Go On Living When Someone You Love Dies.*
New York: Bantam, 1991. Readable, encouraging, and supportive book
by a psychologist.

Schiff, Harriet Sarnoff. *The Bereaved Parent* New York: Crown Publishers,
1977.
Wise counsel from a mother whose young son died after heart surgery.
How to go on with your life. Highly recommended reading.

*When Children Die: Improving Palliative Care and End-of-Life Care for
Children and their Families.* Washington, DC: Institute of Medicine,
2002 (free 16-page summary is available from www.nap.edu).
A comprehensive report on palliative care for children who are dying.

Wogrin, Carol. *Matters of Life and Death: Finding the Words to Say
Goodbye.* New York: Broadway Books, 2001.
A librarian friend recommended this extremely helpful book. Many
suggestions on working with a dying friend or relative. Laced with anecdotes
that illustrate the principles and reassure the reader/caregiver. A good
chapter is "Helping Children Say Goodbye."

CHILDREN'S BOOKS

Brown, Laurie Krasny, and Marc Brown. *When Dinosaurs Die: A Guide to
Understanding Death.* Boston: Little, Brown, 1996.
For preschool and early elementary children.

Brown, Margaret Wise. *The Dead Bird.* Reading, MA: Addison-Wesley
Publishing Co., Inc., 1958.
Timeless picture book for preschoolers on death.

Buscaglia, Leo. *The Fall of Freddie the Leaf: A Story for All Ages.*
New York: Henry Holt, 1982.
An allegory of the cycle of life.

Coerr, Eleanor. *Sadako and the Thousand Paper Cranes.* New York:
G. P. Putnam's Sons, 1977.
Fiction, based on the story of a Japanese child who died of leukemia after
the World War II bombing of Hiroshima. Ages 11 and up.

DePaola, Thomas. *Nana Upstairs and Nana Downstairs.* New York:
G. P. Putnam's Sons, 1973.
Picture book for preschoolers through about grade 2. A simple, moving
story about a young child's special relationship with his grandmother and
with his great-grandmother who dies.

Joslin, Mary. *The Goodbye Boat*, illustrated by Claire St. Louis Little.
Grand Rapids, MI: Eerdman's Books for Young Readers, 1998.
Reminiscent of the well-known "Parable of Immortality," this very simple text with paintings in muted colors suggests the death of a loved one is a passing to another existence. The book can spark conversation even in preschoolers, who will be able to "reread" the book to themselves many times. This is a very simple poem with a profound message of comfort.

Lowry, Lois. *A Summer to Die*. Boston: Houghton Mifflin Co., 1977.
Fiction. A young teen's popular older sister dies of leukemia. Ages 10 to 14.

Viorst, Judith. *The Tenth Good Thing About Barney*. Boston: Athenaeum, 1971.
For children in mid-elementary grades. A boy learns about life cycles when his cat dies.

White, E. B. *Charlotte's Web*. New York: Harper and Row, 1952.
This wonderful children's classic is appropriate for even early elementary school-aged youngsters as an introduction to the idea of mortality.

Zolotow, Charlotte. *My Grandson Lew*. New York: Harper and Row, 1974.
Mother and son talk about Grandfather's death.

ORGANIZATIONS/WEB SITES

Association of Cancer Online Resources (www.acor.org/ped-onc/timetogo/timetogo.html)
End-of-life concerns. Many links to useful resources, some spiritual, some practical. ACOR also has many online discussions, including one on pediatric hospice. Go to www.acor.org, follow the links from "mailing lists" to PED-HOSPICE.

Compassionate Care Hospice (http://cchnet.net)
Provides in-hospital and home services in many states. Most services are covered by insurance. With limited exceptions, not pediatric-specific.

Children's Hospice International (www.chionline.org; 1101 King St., Suite 360, Alexandria, VA 22314; 703-684-0330; 800-2-4-CHILD)
Nonprofit organization providing education, training, and technical assistance for families of children with life-threatening illness.

Compassionate Friends (www.compassionatefriends.org; 900 Jorie Blvd., Suite 78, Oak Brook, IL 60523; 877-969-0010).
National organization to help grieving families who have lost a child (to any cause, not just cancer). Many local chapters with regular meetings. See Web site for "Supporting the Family After a Child Dies."

Good Grief Program (1 Boston Medical Center Place, Mat 5, Boston, MA
02118; 617-414-4005; http://www.bmc.org/pediatrics-goodgrief.htm)
Helping schools and community groups become a base of support for
children when a friend dies. A program of the Judge Baker Children's Center,
Boston Medical Center.

Kids Aid (www.kidsaid.com)
Part of www.griefnet.org, with age-appropriate help for the grieving—
not just death but divorce and other issues. Online community with memorial pages. For middle- and high-school students.

Love, Grief and Bereavement (PDQ) (www.cancer.gov)
A comprehensive source of information from the National Cancer
Institute on grief and loss, this government Web site has many suggestions
on helping children at varying ages. Also a list of appropriate publications
and a table showing what to watch for at different ages from infant on up.
Reassuring. Has resources for health professionals, too.

My Wishes (www.fivewishes.org/mywishes)
From Aging with Dignity; this organization helps people express how
they want to be treated during a fatal illness, when they can't speak for
themselves. The Five Wishes encompass spiritual, medical, emotional, and
personal aspects of a person's death. Serves those age 18 and over, although
the content could be altered to fit some children. They sell publications in
23 languages and Braille as well as a DVD that can generate discussion and
get a family talking about an impending death.

Poetry relating to death (www.photoaspects.com/chesil/death/)
A collection put together by a poetry lover. Lots of choices by well-known
writers and others.

33

Using the Internet

The difference between researching childhood cancer in the early 1980s and in the early 2000s is a huge one. For the first edition, finding and obtaining books and articles was very time-consuming and as a general rule involved several long-suffering interlibrary loan librarians. There were virtually no books written for laypeople interested in finding out about their child's (or their student's, or their neighbor's) illness. Most of the material gathered in the first edition of *Children with Cancer* was collected from professional articles and books, painstakingly digested and rendered into language accessible to the rest of us.

Now, hundreds, maybe thousands, of Web sites are devoted to childhood cancer. Some are presented by government agencies (U.S. and international) and others by organizations, by parents, by patients helping other patients, and by individuals.

Web pages tend to be relatively static, perhaps updated on a regular basis and perhaps not; they can be written by one or more people. E-mail discussion lists, blogs, and other two-way communication services provide a moving target—people talking to each other (often with potentially the whole world listening in). E-mail discussion list posts are often saved in searchable archives that members can find as needed. There is no guarantee of validity on the lists, nor can there be any expectation of privacy.

Sometimes e-mail lists morph into Web sites, which can be helpful, particularly if the material has been edited. But as a way for people to "talk to" each other, often at great distance, e-mail is unbeatable in its immediacy and range.

With this embarrassment of riches comes a warning. As one "net expert" writes, on the Internet there is "stuff" and "good stuff." Evaluating anything found on the Internet is essential. Just as thoughtful parents search for the best doctors and clinic for their children, they must also learn to choose the best information out there.

Information on the Internet can be characterized as "the good, the bad, and the ugly." Putting the good aside for the moment, let's look at the bad. Company Web sites can be bad, promoting their own products and services without providing any opportunity to compare them with others or to look at potential negative aspects. Organizations with an Internet presence can fall into the same narrow-minded group, perhaps pushing an agenda of questionable scientific or social validity. One organization comes to mind that insists all cancer is diet-related and if we all would just eat right, cancer would be history. Complete blather, as any parent knows whose child was fed only organic foods cooked in bottled water yet still developed a malignancy.

The ugly on the Internet has gotten plenty of media attention— the all-too-visible and growing "bandwidth" of X-rated pornography. Using the Google search engine (www.google.com) seems to have eliminated those "yikes!" moments that used to occur when using other search engines. Gross and upsetting pictures and words pop up because savvy pornographers use innocuous keywords that are picked up by mechanical "spiders" searching the Web for content. There isn't room here to explain all about the Internet and how to use it, but those who want to learn are urged to visit their public libraries, where books and articles, and probably training sessions, are available.

While the bad and the ugly are not completely avoidable (and filtering the content can screen out valid "hits"), the good on the Internet redeems the whole Web. Good sites are homepages for respected organizations and government agencies, and their information and sources of assistance are indeed invaluable. Some personal Web sites also have excellent links to professional information while providing a first-person perspective on some aspect of cancer or a related topic. Many families have developed their own Web sites where they share news, pictures, and other information on their activities; these don't often turn up in Google searches, so you will find these by links from other Web pages like online discussions or by personal invitations. These can be valuable in keeping up with friends and relatives and are a good way to disseminate information ("John is in remission!") quickly.

Another resource is the weblog, also called "blog," which is like a personal journal put online for the world to read. Many of these are indeed very public, but some are distributed only to a small designated list of people, who can respond if they wish. These can be among either the good or the bad, depending on the content and who's doing the writing. With the Internet, there's always something new.

The U.S. National Cancer Institute is funding grants to study various ways to communicate with different audiences, from researchers to patients in disadvantaged communities. Preliminary results show that a better understanding by everyone on the team can lead to a better outcome, longer survival, decreased sickness (morbidity), and therefore saved funds. The Internet plays a major role in this wide dissemination of information.

The Web is also home to uncounted discussion groups and chat sites. In the former, interested people register in advance and then receive regular messages to which they can reply. The best of these provide a wonderful source of remote support for families, who often develop a loving relationship with other list members and who genuinely care and understand the situation better than anyone could who has not experienced it.

Rarely, discussions are moderated, which means the list owners (often but not always professionals in the field) prescreen the messages ("posts") for appropriateness. Other discussion lists have "owners" who keep a close eye on the posts and put a halt to questionable, too-heated, or done-to-death topics. Some lists are not monitored and, as with any organization, all should be approached with caution because some discussions can veer quickly into the unacceptable—for example, pressure to try a specific type of therapy or a certain doctor or cancer center. At best, however, these groups (called "lists") validate personal experience, suggest courses of action or research, and offer a gratifying level of caring support. Some groups are more public than others, with nonmembers being able to look up and read your comments; the best and safest allow only members to search the archives.

Chat groups are online, real-time discussions of virtually any topic, are usually not moderated, and can be somewhat free-for-all. It's rather like taking part in a conference call with strangers. Chatting in real time with other cancer patients would be especially useful for teens, for example, as long as the group was carefully limited to include only actual patients.

MySpace, Facebook, and similar social sites, used with care and caution, can provide opportunities to connect with other cancer patients and their families.

Many hospitals and clinics are creating patient "portals," dedicated Web sites used to exchange patient information. Portals can be used to record and share patient information and allow communication between patient and doctor or other medical staff. Some portals are strictly for staff use; others are open to registered patient users. These sites can be used to post medical records and test results, renew prescriptions, and update personal information. With this technology comes a concern for privacy, a fear that unscrupulous hackers will access the data. Portal communications are encrypted (coded) and password-protected, but as with compromised financial and credit card sites, the potential exists for unauthorized access. The quarterly magazine *Cure* had an excellent article on patient portals, referenced at the end of this chapter.

Whether using a portal or just regular e-mail, never send critical questions or timely comments to the doctor by e-mail. Use the phone, where you have a reasonable certainty that someone will answer quickly.

Some of the information even on good sites can be either questionable or inaccurate, not to mention impenetrable, due to typos, misinformation, or the rampant use of acronyms. The latter seems to be an especially common feature of the disease-specific lists I sampled online for several months. If you are confused, by all means ask. Look, too, for the FAQs—frequently asked questions—about most lists; these FAQs are essential for newcomers to the list and valuable for everyone.

Another good feature of the Web is the abundance of research sites. Medline and PubMed, for example, the U.S. National Library of Medicine's periodical databases, can be searched for free from any-where in the world, yielding a great deal of information. Some online databases are fee-based but can often be accessed through subscribing libraries, both public and health-related special institutions. Your public library may provide a rich array of such resources.

The advice and guidance of a professional librarian (sometimes called an "information specialist") is extremely helpful, particularly for your first searches on the Web. He or she can steer users to reputable sites while bypassing most of the dreck.

I have spent years both using the Internet and training others in its wonders and foibles. From my experience I have identified and cited appropriate Web sites among the chapter-end references throughout this book. Be advised, though, that especially for beginners, there is no ally more valuable than a trained librarian to help find information both on the Web and elsewhere.

Internet 101

A little basic information about the Internet for those who have little experience using it. First, material found on the Internet, no matter how accurate and timely, is no substitute for a strong relationship with your health care team.

Use the Internet to find:

- Technical articles
- Cutting-edge/experimental therapies
- Support groups of fellow travelers along the cancer highway
- Pro and con facts regarding various treatments, including unproven methods

There is no quality control department. There is no assurance that what you find today, no matter how valid, will be there tomorrow. Don't expect privacy or confidentiality. While reputable Web discussion groups ask that postings remain confidential, in truth there is no way to enforce it.

The Web can be frustrating. Web addresses must be entered exactly or you can't access them—right down to the punctuation. The addresses (URL, or uniform resource locators) may be case-sensitive; that is, if you enter a capital letter and it expects lower case, you may not be connected.

In the United States, Web addresses often indicate broadly what sort of site to expect:

- .edu has an educational sponsor
- .gov is a government site
- .com is commercial
- .org is used by nonprofit organizations
- .net indicates Internet-based site, often part of an email address

"Search engines" abound to plumb the World Wide Web for information. These are somewhat like the index in a book (put very basically); they poke around trying to match the terms you enter with terms found in various Web sites. Each search engine "searches" a little differently, although there will be a huge overlap in search results. I recommend that library patrons learn how to use one or two and stick with them. My personal favorite (as mentioned earlier) is www.google.com, but there are others probably equally user-friendly. Don't be alarmed if your search returns many thousands or even millions of "hits." The first few usually have just what you're looking for, or will at least get you started, assuming your search terms are on target. The very first listings, though, may be advertisements, so learn to recognize the beginning of your real "hit list"; the formatting is varied to make it easier to identify the different types of "hits."

Web sites may leave out significant information, medical or otherwise, whether through bias or simple error. Expect most sites to be incomplete. Be skeptical if the site is sponsored or supported by a commercial enterprise—the ads that pop up may be simply annoying but at worst they can offer misleading or inappropriate products for sale.

Occasionally sites will require payment to fully access the information. Sometimes you have to pay to read the entire article in some periodicals. Other sites may provide a tease of information and then offer a book for sale. In these cases, your local library may be able to provide the materials for free or at a cheaper price. (On the other hand, in the case of articles, an instantly available publication may be worth a charge on your credit card, if time is of the essence.)

Don't rely on a single site—cross-check everything. A Web page from a scientific institution like a hospital or cancer center is more likely to be thorough than one created by an individual. The more people who stand behind the information, the more balanced it is likely to be. Pro's and con's should both be addressed where appropriate. Remember, as with investments and the like, if it sounds too good to be true, it probably is. Miracle cures sound so attractive—but being wary is essential for your child's well-being.

Don't expect to find all the information you need in a few minutes. Be prepared to take the time needed to search and evaluate—or enlist trusted friends to do it for you. Ask the following questions when evaluating Internet resources:

- Who put the information online? A pharmaceutical manufacturer eager to improve sales, for example, might not be as neutral as a government agency or a respected health-related association. Even former U.S. Surgeon General Dr. Koop (www.DrKoop.com) was revealed to be taking payment from commercial sources mentioned on his site, although reportedly that is no longer the case.
- Beyond the list owner, who actually wrote the materials on the site? A commercial site might have sections or articles written by reputable experts.
- When was the information last updated? The date should be somewhere on the Web page; you can often find it by scrolling down to the bottom. Information that was valid when posted 2 or 3 years ago might no longer be true.
- Be wary when using links to click from one Web site to another. While the first might well be highly respected and up to date, subsequent links may not be. All sources should be evaluated carefully.
- Is there a way to contact the owners of the Web site offline, whether by e-mail, phone, or "snail mail"? Do they have a physical address?
- Do the site owners explain who they are, and their qualifications? Often there is a "who we are" link at the beginning of the page; it's worth checking out.
- Are some of the links on the page "dead"? If so, it's likely that the page has not been kept current.
- How attractive and how easy is the site to navigate? A Web page that is a balance between text and graphics is generally easier to read and helps people who find graphically presented information easier to understand.

- Is there a search function within the page to look for terms or phrases? Being taken directly to the information or data you are looking for is a real boon.
- Beware of personal opinions stated as fact.
- Is there a privacy policy?
- The best Web pages state clearly and often, "See your doctor for details."

The Internet is constantly changing, growing, and improving. By the time this book appears, no doubt there will be several "great new things" to learn about. Maybe it will be wikis, software that simplifies the linkages between Web sites. Whatever the future may hold, the Internet will certainly take a lead in communications. Like it or not (and I generally do like it), the World Wide Web is a vast ocean of fast-moving information. Use it with respect and a touch of skepticism.

I'd like to offer my special heartfelt thanks to Patty Feist, an experienced list administrator and Web page author, whose thoughtful comments kept me from making some embarrassing blunders in this chapter.

The section on further resources that follows is extremely selective. The sites mentioned here are general, broad-based sources for online information. Of course, there are many more sites, many equally valuable and valid, but these are a few of the best. Sites geared to specific diseases are cited at the end of the appropriate chapters.

Further Resources

READING

Silver, Marc. Portal authority—patients log on to access medical records and talk with doctors. *Cure*, vol. 6 (4) (Summer 2007), pp. 22. Available at www.curetoday.com

ORGANIZATIONS/WEB SITES

Association of Cancer Online Resources (www.acor.org; 173 Duane St., Suite 3A, New York, NY 100013; 212-226-5525; Interactive Pediatric Oncology Center: www.acor.org/ped-onc)

General information and links. A gateway to trustworthy links—by parents, for parents. An award-winning site. The best of the Web: solid information; an authoritative, up-to-date source for connecting with other patients. For parents and friends, too. Also suggestions for handling the holidays and end-of-life issues. Fosters many online discussion groups related to specific cancers. One of the best cancer information sites today.

Association of Pediatric Hematology Oncology Nurses (www.aphon.org; 4700 West Lake Avenue, Glenview, IL 60025; 847-375-4724)

Professional organization for nurses but with helpful links for others as well.

Cancer Index (www.cancerindex.org)

This Web site provides a rich array (over a thousand) links to reputable information, terminology, anatomy, and more. Maintained by a professional researcher in the United Kingdom (check his amusing home page).

CancerCare (www.cancercare.org)

This national nonprofit organization's mission is to provide free professional help to people with all cancers through counseling, education, information, and referrals and direct financial assistance. Also in Spanish. Offers online, telephone, or onsite help (four locations in Greater New York) free to individuals or groups. Offers the booklet "Caregiving for your Loved One with Cancer" by Diane Blum, MSW, free to download.

Cancernet (www.cancer.gov)

This service of the U.S. National Cancer Institute is, as promised, "credible, current, comprehensive." A huge amount of recent research is located at this site. A particularly valuable feature is the PDQ (Physician Data Query) articles with explanations of various forms of cancer and related treatments presented on two levels—one for health professionals and, thankfully, one for laypeople like parents.

CaringBridge (www.caringbridge.org; 1715 Yankee Doodle Road, Suite 301, Eagan, MN 55121; 651-452-7940)

Provides free Web sites to help patients and families keep in touch with friends and others during significant life events—like cancer. Many families have their own sites here—an excellent way to keep far-flung (and nearby) loved ones up to date.

Cure Search (www.curesearch.org)

Primo! Sponsored by the National Childhood Cancer Foundation and the Children's Oncology Group. Approach from your current situation: newly diagnosed, off therapy, etc.

Kids Health (http://kidshealth.org)

This is a comprehensive Web site for parents, kids, and teens on a wide range of medical issues—much more than cancer is covered. Sponsored by Nemours, one of the largest health care organizations in the United States.

MedLine and PubMed (www.medlineplus.gov)

These National Cancer Institute Web sites provide access to medical information across the board, not just cancer. If you have trouble searching, a librarian can help you.

Patient-Centered Guides (O'Reilly & Associates, Inc., 1005 Gravenstein Hwy North, Sebastopol, CA 95472; 800-998-9938; 707-827-7000, Ext. 7118; e-mail: health@oreilly.com)

Another good general site sponsored by the American Cancer Society and the U.S. National Cancer Institute. Rich resource of links to free fact sheets and more. One of their subsites, OncoNurse (www.onconurse.com) is packed with trustworthy information about the medical and emotional as well as practical aspects of cancer, including pediatric.

Virtual Hospital from the University of Iowa (www.uihealthcare.com/vh)

Gateway resource for an impressive array of children's health concerns. Descriptions of tests (e.g., spinal tap); information for and by kids; games, puzzles, and activity sheets. Not just cancer—general pediatric health issues.

WebMD (www.webmd.com, www.medscape.com, and http://emedicine. medscape.com)

This is one of the best and most highly rated medical sources online. Includes eMedicine, written by health experts, and MedScape, with free information on a huge range of medical issues, not just cancer. Registration is required to get to some content, but the process is simple.

Clinics and Local Organizations in the United States and Canada

At the time of diagnosis, most families react with shock, disbelief, and denial. It is too much to bear. There must be some mistake. Not my son. Not my daughter. The tests are wrong.

While parents are still in this state, they must begin to make decisions. Where will the child be treated? Whom should they tell? How? Even families whose children eventually die remember diagnosis as the worst time.

Earlier sections of this book have repeatedly emphasized the importance of having the child evaluated at a major pediatric cancer center, where medical specialists and staff provide the most current treatments. These professionals are also aware of the special problems facing young cancer patients and their families, and they offer warmth, compassion, and a climate of hope. These centers have special facilities so that parents can stay with their hospitalized child and help with his care. When desirable, these clinics plan a course of therapy that can be carried out to some extent in the child's local hospital.

These clinics are located across the United States and in many other countries. Most of them are in close contact with other clinics through an international network of specialists called the Children's Oncology Group (COG), which has recently been formed by the merger of several similar organizations. Many of the centers are affiliated with medical schools. Some have all these ties, some have none, but the most important thing is that each has a staff of pediatricians with special training in hematology or oncology.

The final diagnosis for most children with cancer is made at a major center, so most readers will already be in contact with at least one such facility. Yet occasionally, perhaps when relationships between the staff and the family do not seem to be working, a parent might want to explore alternative arrangements.

This is not intended as a comprehensive list of every single clinic in these countries qualified to care for pediatric cancer patients. Rather, it represents a cross-section of institutions, expanded from lists created by the Candlelighters and the COG. Addresses and Web site URLs are accurate at the time of publication. Clinics outside the United States and Canada are included in Appendix C.

COG comprises 5,000 pediatric oncology specialists in most states of the United States, across Canada, and around the world. They share research results and common goals (to cure childhood cancer while easing the therapies and their side effects). These physicians and their support staff provide the best available current treatments. Notes indicate which centers have long-term survivor (LTS) clinics. For current lists of LTS clinics, see www.patientcenters.com. Most now offer bone and peripheral stem cell transplants.

Recent articles in the popular press rated some of the hospitals as "the best." *Parents* magazine named St. Jude as the number one, followed by Children's Hospital of Philadelphia; Children's Hospital, Boston; Children's Hospital, Los Angeles; and Children's Hospital and Regional Medical Center, Seattle.

Another article published in *U.S. News and World Report* and enhanced on their Web site (www.usnews.com) lists the top 30 institutions in the United States for treating childhood cancers. Their top five were Children's Hospital of Philadelphia; Children's Hospital, Boston; Texas Children's Hospital, Houston; Cincinnati Children's Hospital; and Seattle Children's Hospital.

These articles and ratings are included here to make two points. First, experts do not agree on what's "best." And second, there are many fine institutions caring for our children with expertise and loving care that are not on either of these lists. The highly regarded, internationally renowned hospital where Lisa was treated is not even listed in the top 30.

This appendix has a state-by-state list of organizations, clinics, and other sources of help. If more than one state is involved, complete information is provided under the home state, with cross references to other states served. Some organizations like the Candlelighters and the American Cancer Society have too many local groups to include. To find a nearby chapter, contact the national headquarters or call the Cancer Information Service at 1-800-4-CANCER, a toll-free number that can be used throughout the United States.

The U.S. National Cancer Institute selects more than 50 hospitals around the country as Comprehensive Cancer Centers; those are designated here with CCC.

The Ronald McDonald House Charities and the American Cancer Society Hope Lodge programs provide low-cost or free housing for patients and families. Their locations are noted. For updated information on these programs, go to www.cancer.org (ACS) or www.rmhc.org (Ronald McDonald).

Web site URLs are listed as often as possible. Many of these sites have excellent information about not only their services but also disease- and therapy-specific links. Many provide the information in more languages than just English.

Alaska

Susan Butcher Family Center
    Providence Cancer Center
    3851 Piper St., Suite U220
    Anchorage, AK 99508
    (907) 212-6876
    www.providence.org

Although final diagnosis is made and treatment plans designed in the Lower 48 for Alaskan children, this center (named for the beloved Iditarod dog sled racer who died of cancer) provides a variety of support systems and continues close-to-home therapy over time.

Alabama

University of Alabama (CCC, LTS)
    Pediatric Hematology Oncology
    The Children's Hospital
    1600 Seventh Avenue South
    Birmingham, AL 35233
    (205) 939-9100
    www.chsys.org

University of South Alabama
    Children's and Women's Hospital
    Pediatric Hematology/Oncology
    1504 Springhill Avenue, Suite 5230

Mobile, AL 36604
(251) 405-1361
www.southalabama.edu/usacwh/usshope.html

There are Ronald McDonald Houses in Birmingham and Mobile. There is an
ACS Hope Lodge in Birmingham.

Arizona

Banner Children's Hospital
    1400 South Dobson Road, Suite 108
    Mesa, AZ 85202
    (480) 512-3000
    www.bannerhealth.com

Phoenix Children's Hospital
    Hematology/Oncology
    1919 East Thomas Road
    Phoenix, AZ 85016
    (602) 546-1000
    www.phoenixchildrens.com

University of Arizona Health Sciences Center (CCC)
    Pediatric Hematology/Oncology
    1501 North Campbell Avenue
    Tucson, AZ 85724
    (520) 694-0111
    www.umcza.org

Ronald McDonald Houses (2) are in Phoenix and Tucson. There is a Hope
Lodge in Phoenix.

Arkansas

University of Arkansas
    Arkansas Children's Hospital
    Pediatric Hematology/Oncology
    One Children's Way
    Little Rock, AR 72202
    (501) 364-1100
    www.archildrens.org

There is a Ronald McDonald House in Little Rock.

California

Southern California Permanente Medical Group
4700 Sunset Blvd, 3B
Downey, CA 90027
(562) 657-2479

City of Hope National Medical Center (LTS, CCC)
Division of Pediatrics
Medical Office Building Fourth Floor
1500 East Duarte Road
Duarte, CA 91010
(626) 256-4673
www.cityofhope.org

Loma Linda University Medical Center
Children's Hospital
Oncology Clinical Research
11234 Anderson St.
Loma Linda, CA 92354
(909) 558-8000
www.lomalindahealth.org/childrens-hospital

Miller Children's Hospital/Harbor-UCLA
Jonathan Jacques Cancer Center
2801 Atlantic Ave.
Long Beach, CA 90801
(562) 933-8600
www.jjccc.com

Children's Hospital Los Angeles (LTS)
Division of Hematology-Oncology
4650 Sunset Blvd.
Los Angeles, CA 90027
(323) 660-2450
www.childrenshospitalla.org

Cedars-Sinai Medical Center
Department of Pediatric Hematology/Oncology
Ahmanson Pediatrics Center
8700 Beverly Blvd., Suite 4221
Los Angeles, CA 90048
(800) CEDARS1 (233-2771)
www.csmc.edu

UCLA School of Medicine (CCC)
Pediatric Hematology/Oncology
Mattel Children's Hospital
757 Westwood Plaza
Los Angeles, CA 90095
(310) 825-9111
www.uclahealth.org

Children's Hospital Central California
Craycroft Cancer Center
9300 Valley Children's Place F13
Madera, CA 93636
(559) 353-3000
www.childrenscentralcal.org

Children's Hospital Oakland
Department of Hematology/Oncology
747 52nd St.
Oakland, CA 94609
(510) 428-3372
www.childrenshospitaloakland.org

Children's Hospital of Orange County
Hematology-Oncology
455 South Main St.
Orange, CA 92868
(714) 997-3000
www.choc.org

Stanford Medical Center
Lucile Packard Children's Hospital
Pediatric Hematology/Oncology
725 Welch Rd.
Palo Alto, CA 94304
(650) 497-8953
www.pch.org

Sutter Medical Center
Sutter Children's Center
5151 F Street
Sacramento, CA 95819
(916) 733-1757
www.sutterhealth.org

University of California, Davis
UC Davis Children's Hospital
Department of Pediatrics
2315 Stockton Blvd.
TICON II
Sacramento, CA 95817
(916) 734-2782
www.ucdmc.ucd.edu/children

Rady Children's Hospital San Diego
Hematology/Oncology
3020 Children's Way
San Diego, CA 92123
(858) 576-1700

UCSF School of Medicine (CCC)
Moffit Hospital
Department of Pediatrics
505 Parnassus Avenue
San Francisco, CA 94143
(415) 502-7816
www.pediatrics.medschool.ucsf.edu/hemonc

Sutter Medical Center, Sacramento
California Pacific Medical Center
Pediatric Hematology/Oncology
2340 Clay St., 3d Floor
San Francisco, CA 94115
(415) 600-3268
www.cpmc.org

Santa Barbara Cottage Children's Hospital
P. O. Box 689
Pueblo at Bath St.
Santa Barbara, CA 93105
(805) 682-7111
www.sbch.org

There are Ronald McDonald Houses in Bakersfield, Madera, Loma Linda, Los Angeles (2), Orange, Palo Alto, San Diego, San Francisco, Sacramento, and Pasadena.

Colorado

The Children's Hospital (LTS)
    Division of Pediatrics
    13123 East 16th Avenue, B115
    Aurora, CO 80045
    (720) 777-1234
    www.thechildrenshospital.org

Presbyterian/St. Luke's Medical Center
    Rocky Mountain Hospital for Children
    1719 East 19th St.
    Denver, CO 80218
    (303) 839-6000
    www.pslmc.com

There are Ronald McDonald Houses in Colorado Springs, Aurora, and Denver.

Connecticut

Connecticut Children's Medical Center
    Hematology-Oncology Department
    282 Washington St.
    Hartford, CT 06106
    (860) 545-9000
    www.ccmckids.org

Yale University School of Medicine (CCC)
    Pediatric Hematology/Oncology
    20 York St.
    New Haven, CT 06510
    (203) 785-4081
    www.ynhh.org

There is a Ronald McDonald House in New Haven.

Delaware

Alfred I. DuPont Hospital for Children
    Pediatric Hematology-Oncology
    1600 Rockland Rd.

P. O. Box 269
Wilmington, DE 19803
(302) 651-4000
www.nemours.org

There is a Ronald McDonald House in Wilmington.

District of Columbia

Children's National Medical Center
Department of Pediatric Hematology-Oncology
111 Michigan Ave NW
Washington, DC 20010
(202) 476-5000
www.childrensnational.org

Georgetown University Medical Center (CCC)
Division of Pediatric Hematology/Oncology
Lombardi Cancer Center
3800 Reservoir Rd., NW
Washington, DC 20007
(202) 444-7599
www.lombardi.georgetown.edu

Walter Reed Army Medical Center, USOC
Pediatric Hematology/Oncology Service, Building 2, Ward 52
6900 Georgia Ave., NW
Washington, DC 20307
(202) 782-9453
www.wramc.amedd.army.mil

There is a Ronald McDonald House in DC.

Florida

Broward General Medical Center
Cancer Center—Pediatrics
1600 S. Andrews Ave.
Ft. Lauderdale, FL 33316
(954) 355-4400
www.browardhealth.org

The Children's Hospital of Southwest Florida
Lee Memorial Health
Pediatric Oncology/Hematology
9981 South Healthpark Drive
Fort Myers, FL 33908
(239) 433-7799
www.leememorial.org

University of Florida
Pediatric Hematology/Oncology
Shands Teaching Hospital
1600 Southwest Archer Rd.
P. O. Box 100296
Gainesville, FL 32610
(352) 392-5633
www.peds.ufl.edu

Joe DiMaggio Children's Hospital at Memorial
Pediatric Hematology/Oncology
1150 North 35th Ave., Suite 520
Hollywood, FL 33021
(954) 265-2234
www.jdch.com

Mayo Clinic
4500 San Pablo Road
Jacksonville, FL 32224
(904) 953-2000
www.mayoclinic.org/jacksonville

Nemours Children's Clinic—Jacksonville (LTS)
Hematology/Oncology
807 Children's Way
Jacksonville, FL 32207
(904) 697-3600
www.nemours.org

Baptist Children's Hospital
Pediatric Oncology/Hematology
8900 N. Kendall Drive
Miami, FL 33176
(786) 596-1960
www.baptisthealth.net

Miami Children's Hospital
    Hematology/Oncology
    3100 S.W. 62nd Ave
    Miami, FL 33155
    (305) 666-6511
    (800) 432-6837
    www.mch.com

University of Miami School of Medicine
    Sylvester CCC
    Pediatric Hematology/Oncology
    1601 NW 12th Ave.
    Miami, FL 33136
    (305) 585-5635
    www.pediatrics.med.miami.edu

Nemours Children's Clinic—Orlando
    Pediatric Hematology Oncology
    1717 South Orange Avenue
    Orlando, FL 32806
    (407) 650-7000
    www.nemours.org

Disney Children's Hospital at
    Florida Hospital Cancer Institute
    Pediatric Hematology/Oncology
    601 East Rolling St.
    Orlando, FL 32803
    (407) 303-2080
    www.disneychildrenshospital.com

M. D. Anderson Cancer Center
    1400 South Orange Avenue
    Orlando, FL 32806
    (407) 648-3800
    www.mdandersonorlando.org

Sacred Heart Hospital
    Pediatrics
    5153 North 9th Ave.
    Pensacola, FL 32504
    (850) 416-7000
    www.sacred-heart.org/childrenshospital

All Children's Hospital
Pediatric Hematology/Oncology
801 6th Ave. So., Suite 140
St. Petersburg, FL 33701
(727) 898-7451
www.allkids.org

H. Lee Moffitt Cancer Center and Research Institute (CCC)
University of South Florida
12902 Magnolia Drive
Tampa, FL 33612
(813) 745-4673
(800) 456-3434
www.moffitt.org

Tampa Children's Hospital
Pediatric Hematology/Oncology
3001 W. M. L. King Jr. Blvd.
Tampa, FL 33607
(813) 870-4252
www.stjosephchildrens.com

Nicklaus St. Mary's Children's Hospital
Pediatric Hematology Oncology
901 45th St.
West Palm Beach, FL 33407
(561) 844-6300
www.stmarysmc.com

There are Ronald McDonald Houses in Gainesville, Fort Myers, Jacksonville, Miami, Orlando (2), Pensacola, St. Petersburg, Tallahassee, Tampa, and Fort Lauderdale. There are Hope Lodges in Gainesville and Tampa.

Georgia

Children's Healthcare of Atlanta, Emory University (LTS)
Aflac Cancer Center
Division of Hematology/Oncology
1405 Clifton Road, NE, 3d floor
Atlanta, GA 30322
(404) 785-1200
www.choa.org
www.aflaccancercenter.org

Medical College of Georgia Children's Medical Center
  Pediatric Hematology/Oncology
  BG-2011
  1120 15th St.
  Augusta, GA 30912
  (706) 721-3626
  www.mcghealth.org

Backus Children's Hospital at MHUMC
  Pediatric Oncology
  4700 Waters Ave.
  Savannah, GA 31443
  (912) 350-8000
  www.memorialhealth.com

There are Ronald McDonald Houses in Atlanta (2), Augusta, Columbus, Savannah, and Macon. There is a Hope Lodge in Atlanta.

Hawaii

Cancer Research Center of Hawaii (CCC)
  University of Hawaii
  1236 Lauhala St.
  Honolulu, HI 96813
  (808) 586-3010
  www.crch.org

Kapi'olani Medical Center for Women and Children
  1319 Punahou St.
  Honolulu, HI 96826
  (808) 983-6000
  www.kapiolani.org

Tripler Army Medical Center (USOC)
  MCKH-PE
  1 Jarrett White Road
  Honolulu, HI 96859
  (808) 433-6057
  www.tamc.amedd.army.mil

There is a Ronald McDonald House in Honolulu.

Idaho

St. Luke's Mountain States Tumor Institute
190 East Bannock St.
Boise, ID 83712
(208) 381-2711
www.slrmc.org

There is a Ronald McDonald House in Boise.

Illinois

University of Chicago Comer Children's Hospital (CCC)
5721 S. Maryland Ave.
Chicago, IL 60637
(773) 702-1000
www.uchicagokidshospital.org

University of Illinois
Department of Pediatrics
MC 856
840 S. Wood St.
Chicago, IL 60612
(312) 996-6143
www.hospital.uic.edu

Children's Memorial Medical Center at Chicago (LTS)
Hematology/Oncology
2300 Children's Plaza
Box 30
Chicago, IL 60614
(773) 880-4000
www.childmmc.edu

Rush-Presbyterian St. Luke's Medical Center
Pediatric Hematology/Oncology
1725 W. Harrison, Suite 710
Chicago, IL 60612
(312) 942-5000
www.rush.edu

Loyola University Medical Center
Ronald McDonald Children's Hospital
Department of Pediatrics, B-105, Room 3315

Maguire Center 3d Floor
2160 South First Ave.
Maywood, Il 60153
(877) 216-KIDS
www.luhs.org/rmch

Advocate Hope Children's Hospital
Pediatric/Hematology-Oncology
4440 West 95th St.
Oak Lawn, IL 60453
(708) 684-8000
www.advocatehealth.com/hope

Lutheran General Children's Medical Center
Department of Pediatric Hematology-Oncology
1775 Dempster St.
Park Ridge, IL 60068
(847) 723-5437
www.advoccatehealth.com/lgch

Southern Illinois University School of Medicine
Department of Pediatrics
415 North 9th St., 2Wa06
P. O. Box 19678
Springfield, IL 62794
(217) 545-5817

There are Ronald McDonald Houses in Chicago (2), Hines, Oak Lawn, and
Springfield.

Indiana

Peyton Manning Children's Hospital
St. Vincent Children's Hospital
Children's Center for Cancer and Blood Diseases
2001 West 86th St.
Indianapolis, IN 46260
(317) 338-4673
www.stvincent.org

Indiana University, Riley Children's Hospital (CCC)
Pediatric Hematology-Oncology
702 Barnhill Drive

Indianapolis, IN 46202
(317) 274-8784
www.rileychildrenshospital.com

There are Ronald McDonald Houses in Fort Wayne and Indianapolis

Iowa

Raymond Blank Children's Hospital
  Pediatric Hematology/Oncology
  1212 Pleasant St., Suite 300
  Des Moines, IO 50309
  (515) 241-6500
  www.blankchildrens.org

University of Iowa Children's Hospital (CCC)
  Department of Pediatrics/Hematology-Oncology
  200 Hawkins Drive
  Iowa City, IO 52242
  (319) 365-2229
  www.uihealth.com

There are Ronald McDonald Houses in Des Moines, Iowa City, and Sioux City. There is a Hope Lodge in Iowa City.

Kansas

University of Kansas Medical Center
  Pediatric Oncology
  3901 Rainbow Blvd., MS 4004
  Kansas City, KS 66160
  (913) 588-6301
  www2.kumc.edu/kids/specialty_HemOnc.htm

Via Christi Regional Medical Center
  929 North St. Francis St.
  Wichita, KS 67214
  (316) 268-5000
  www.via-christi.org

There are Ronald McDonald Houses in Topeka and Wichita (2).

Kentucky

A.B. Chandler Medical Center, University of Kentucky
  Pediatric Hematology Oncology
  2d Floor, Room L230
  740 South Limestone St.
  Lexington, KY 40536
  (859) 257-4554
  www.ukhealthcare.uky.edu

Kosair Children's Hospital
  Pediatric Hematology/Oncology
  Department of Pediatrics
  231 E. Chestnut St.
  Louisville, KY 40202
  (502) 629-KIDS
  www.KosaircChildrens.com

There are Ronald McDonald Houses in Lexington and Louisville and a Hope Lodge in Lexington.

Louisiana

Children's Hospital of New Orleans
  Pediatrics Hematology/Oncology
  200 Henry Clay Ave.
  New Orleans, LA 70118
  (504) 896-9740
  www.chnola.org

Tulane University Medical Center
  Pediatric Hematology/Oncology
  Department of Pediatrics SL-37
  1430 Tulane Avenue
  New Orleans, LA 70112
  (504) 988-5456
  www.tulane.edu/som

Ochsner Clinic
  Pediatrics
  Pediatric Hematology/Oncology
  1514 Jefferson Highway

New Orleans, LA 70121
(866) OCHSNER
www.ochsner.org

There are Ronald McDonald Houses in Monroe and New Orleans and a Hope Lodge in New Orleans.

Maine

Eastern Maine Medical Center
Hematology/Oncology
489 State St., 305
Bangor, ME 04401
(207) 973-7520
www.emmc.org

Maine Children's Cancer Program
Pediatric Hematology-Oncology
100 U.S. Route One, Unit 107
Scarborough, ME 04074
(207) 885-7565
www.mmc.org

There are Ronald McDonald Houses in Bangor and Portland.

Maryland

University of Maryland at Baltimore
Division of Pediatric Hematology/Oncology
22 South Greene St., Suite N5E16
Baltimore, MD 21201
(410) 328-2808
www.umm.edu/pediatrics

Sinai Hospital of Baltimore
Department of Pediatrics
2401 W. Belvedere Ave.
Baltimore, MD 21215
(410) 601-5864
www.sinai-balt.com

Johns Hopkins Hospital (LTS, CCC)
  Pediatric Oncology
  600 North Wolfe St.
  CMSC 800
  Baltimore, MD 21287
  (410) 955-7385
  www.hopkinskimmelcancercenter.org
  Hopkins has its own housing for pediatric patients and families.

National Cancer Institute—Pediatric Branch
  Building 10, CRC, Room 1W-3750
  9000 Rockville Pike
  Bethesda, MD 20892
  (301) 496-4256
  http://home.ccr.cancer.gov/
  They have their own housing across the street at Children's Inn at NIH
    (www.childrensinn.org).

There are a Ronald McDonald House and a Hope Lodge in Baltimore.

Massachusetts

Dana-Farber Cancer Institute and Children's Hospital (LTS, CCC)
  Pediatric Oncology
  44 Binney St., Room SW-350
  Boston, MA 02115
  (617) 632-3971
  www.dana-farber.org
  Home of the Jimmy Fund Clinic, this was the first cancer center in the
    United States designed specifically for children (1951).

Boston Floating Hospital for Infants and Children
  Tufts-New England Medical Center
  Pediatric Hematology-Oncology
  800 Washington St., Box 14
  NEMC 14
  Boston, MA 02111
  (617) 636-5535
  www.floatinghospital.org

Massachusetts General Hospital
    Pediatric Hematology-Oncology
    55 Fruit St., Yawkey 8B
    Boston, MA 02114
    (617) 724-3315
    www.massgeneral.org

Baystate Medical Center
    Division of Pediatric Oncology
    759 Chestnut St.
    Springfield, MA 01199
    (413) 794-5316
    www.baystatehealth.com/bmch

University of Massachusetts Medical School
    U Mass Memorial Children's Medical Center
    Pediatric Hematology/Oncology
    55 Lake Avenue N.
    Worcester, MA 01655
    (508) 856-4225 ext. 6219
    www/umassmed.edu

There are Ronald McDonald Houses in Brookline and Springfield. There are Hope Lodges in Boston and Worcester.

Michigan

Bay Health
    (517) 667-6642
    Provides patients and supporters cancer retreat nights at a nominal cost.

C.S. Mott Children's Hospital (CCC)
    1500 E. Medical Center Dr.
    CCGC-B1-207
    Ann Arbor, MI 48109
    (734) 936-8785
    www.mcancer.org

Children's Hospital of Michigan
    Hematology/Oncology
    3901 Beaubien Blvd.
    Detroit, MI 48201
    (313) 745-5649
    www.childrensmc.org

Michigan State University
Pediatrics/Human Development
B220 Clinical Center
138 Service Road
East Lansing, MI 48824
(517) 355-8998
www.phd.msu.edu

Hurley Medical Center
Pediatric Hematology/Oncology Clinic
One Hurley Plaza
Flint, MI 48503
(810) 762-7304
www.hurleymc.com

DeVos Children's Hospital
Division of Pediatric Hematology/Oncology
100 Michigan St., NE
NEMC MC 85
Grand Rapids, MI 49503
(616) 391-2086
www.devoschildrens.org

St. John Hospital and Medical Center
Pediatric Hematology/Oncology
19229 Mack Ave., Suite 28
Gross Pointe Woods, MI 48236
(313) 647-3200
www.stjohn.org

Kalamazoo Center for Medical Studies
Bronson Methodist Hospital
Pediatric Hematology/Oncology
601 John St., Suite E-300
Kalamazoo, MI 49007
(606) 341-6350
www.kcms.msu.edu/pho

William Beaumont Hospital
Division of Pediatric Hematology/Oncology
3601 West 13 Mile Rd.
Royal Oak, MI 48073
(248) 551-0360
www.beaumonthospitals.com

There are Ronald McDonald Houses in Ann Arbor, Detroit, Grand Rapids, and Lansing and a Hope Lodge in Grand Rapids.

Minnesota

Duluth Clinic
   400 East Third St.
   Duluth, MN 55805
   (218) 786-8364
   www.smdc.org

University of Minnesota Cancer Center (CCC)
   Division of Pediatric Hematology/Oncology
   Room D557, Mayo Building MMC 484
   420 Delaware St., SE
   Minneapolis, MN 55455
   (612) 626-2778
   (888) 601-0787
   www.cancer.umn.edu

Children's Hospitals and Clinics-Minneapolis (LTS)
   Hematology Oncology Clinic
   2525 Chicago Ave., SO, Suite 4150
   Minneapolis, MN 55404
   (612) 813-5940
   www.chldrenshc.org

Mayo Clinic and Foundation (CCC)
   Pediatric Hematology-Oncology, E-12A
   200 First St. SW
   Rochester, MN 55905
   (507) 284-4822
   www.mayoclinic.org

Children's Hospitals and Clinics-St. Paul
   Hematology/Oncology
   345 North Smith Avenue
   Mail Stop 70-301
   St. Paul, MN 55102
   (651) 220-6733
   www.childrensmn.org

There are Ronald McDonald Houses in Minneapolis and Rochester. There are Hope Lodges in Rochester and Minneapolis.

Mississippi

University of Mississippi Medical Center Children's Hospital
  Pediatric Hematology/Oncology
  2500 North State St.
  Jackson, MS 39216
  (610) 984-5220
  www.umc.edu/healthcare/children.html

Madigan Army Medical Center (USOC)
  Pediatric Hematology/Oncology
  81st MDG/SGOC
  301 Fisher St., Rm. 1A132
  Keesler AFB, MS 39534-2511
  (228) 377-6631

There is a Ronald McDonald House in Jackson.

Missouri

University of Missouri-Columbia
  Department of Child Health
  Room 7W-12
  One Hospital Drive
  Columbia, MO 65212
  (573) 882-3961
  http://www.muhealth.org/default_ch.cfm?id=72

The Children's Mercy Hospital
  Department of Hematology-Oncology
  2401 Gillham Rd.
  Kansas City, MO 64108
  (816) 234-3265
  www.childrens-mercy.org

Washington University Medical Center (LTS)
  Pediatric Hematology/Oncology
  One Children's Place, Box 8116
  St. Louis, MO 63110
  (314) 454-4132
  (800) 635-2317
  www.stlouischildrens.org

Cardinal Glennon Children's Hospital
  Department of Pediatrics—Division of Hematology/Oncology
  1465 South Grand Blvd.
  St. Louis, MO 63104
  (314) 577-5644
  www.cardinalglennon.com

There are Ronald McDonald Houses in Columbia, Kansas City, Springfield, Saint Louis (2), and Joplin. There are Hope Lodges in Kansas City and Saint Louis.

Nebraska

Children's Memorial Hospital of Omaha
  Pediatric Hematology/Oncology
  8200 Dodge St.
  Omaha, NE 68114
  (402) 955-3950
  www.chsomaha.org

University of Nebraska Medical Center
  982168 Nebraska Medical Center
  Omaha, NE 68198
  (402) 559-7257
  www.unmc.edu

There is a Ronald McDonald House in Omaha.

Nevada

Sunrise Children's Hospital
  Sunrise Hospital and Medical Center, Pediatrics
  3920 S. Eastern, Suite 200
  Las Vegas, NV 89119
  (702) 737-0117
  www.sunrisehospital.com

There are Ronald McDonald Houses in Las Vegas and Reno.

New Hampshire

Dartmouth-Hitchcock Medical Center (CCC)
    Children's Hospital at Dartmouth
    Norris Cotton Cancer Center
    Pediatric Oncology
    One Medical Center Drive
    Lebanon, NH 03756
    (603) 650-5541
    www.hitchcock.org
    www.cancer.dartmouth.edu/pediatric

New Jersey

Hackensack University Medical Center (LTS)
    Pediatric Hematology/Oncology
    Tomorrow's Children's Institute
    30 Prospect Avenue
    Hackensack, NJ 07601
    (201) 996-5437
    www.tcikids.com

St. Barnabas Medical Center (Valerie Fund)
    Pediatric Hematology-Oncology
    94 Old Short Hills Road
    East Wing, First Floor, Suite 182
    Livingston, NJ 07039
    (973) 322-2800
    www.saintbarnabas.com/hospitals/childrens_hospital

Atlantic Health System (Valerie Fund)
    Goryeb Children's Hospital
    Morristown Memorial Hospital
    100 Madison Ave., Second Floor
    Morristown, NJ 07962
    (973) 971-6720
    www.atlantichealth.org

University of Medicine and Dentistry of New Jersey (CCC)
    Cancer and Blood Disorders
    The Cancer Institute of New Jersey

195 Little Albany St.
New Brunswick, NJ 08901
(732) 235-7898
www.cinj.umdjn.edu

Saint Peter's University Hospital
Pediatric Hematology/Oncology
254 Easton Ave.
New Brunswick, NJ 08901
(732) 565-5437
www.childrenshospitalspuh.com

Newark Beth Israel Medical Center (Valerie Fund Center)
Department of Pediatrics
201 Lyons Avenue
Newark, NJ 07112
(973) 926-7000
www.saintbarnabas.com

St. Joseph's Hospital and Medical Center
Pediatric Hematology/Oncology
703 Main St., Xavier 7
Paterson, NJ 07503
(973) 754-3230
www.stjosephshealth.org

There are Ronald McDonald Houses in Camden, Long Branch, and New Brunswick.

New Mexico

University of New Mexico School of Medicine (CCC)
Pediatrics/Pediatric Oncology
ACC Third Floor MSC10 5590
2211 Lomas Blvd.
Albuquerque, NM 87131
(505) 272-4461
http://hsc.unm.edu

There is a Ronald McDonald House in Albuquerque.

New York

Albany Medical Center
Department of Pediatrics
47 New Scotland Ave. Mail Code MC-24
Albany, NY 12208
(518) 262-5513
www.amc.edu

Montefiore Medical Center
111 E 210th St.
Bronx, NY 10467
(718) 920-7844
www.montekids.org

Maimonides Medical Center
Department of Pediatrics
4802 Tenth Ave.
Brooklyn, NY 11219
(718) 283-8173
www.maimonidesmed.org

SUNY Health Science Center at Brooklyn
Department of Pediatrics
450 Clarkson Ave.
Brooklyn, NY 11203
(718) 270-1625
www.biomedcom.downstate.edu

Brookdale Hospital Medical Center
Room 346 CHC
One Brookdale Plaza
Brooklyn, NY 11212
(718) 240-5904
www.brookdale.edu

Brooklyn Hospital Center
Department of Pediatrics
121 DeKalb Ave.
Brooklyn, NY 11201
(718) 250-6074
www.tbh.org

Roswell Park Cancer Center WCHOB (LTS, CCC)
Pediatrics
Elm and Carlton Streets
Buffalo, NY 14263
(718) 845-2333
(800) 685-6825
www.roswellpark.org

Winthrop University Hospital
Cancer Center for Kids
259 First St.
Mineola, NY 11501
(516) 663-0333
www.winthrop.org

Schneider Children's Hospital
Pediatric Hematology/Oncology
269-01 76th Avenue, Room 255
New Hyde Park, NY 11040
(718) 470-3460
www.schneiderchildrenshospital.org

New York Hospital—Cornell University Medical Center
Department of Pediatric Hematology-Oncology
525 East 68th St.
Payson Blg 695
New York, NY 10021
(212) 746-3415
http://nyp.org

New York University Medical Center (CCC)
Department of Pediatrics
317 E. 34th St. 8th Floor
New York, NY 10016
(212) 263-7144
http://hassenfeld.med.nyu.edu

Memorial Sloan Kettering Cancer Center (LTS, CCC)
Department of Pediatrics
1275 York Ave.
Box 411
New York, NY 10021
(212) 639-7951
www.mskcc.org

Columbia Presbyterian College of Physicians and Surgeons (Valerie Fund Center)
> Division of Pediatric Oncology
> 161 Fort Washington Ave., I-7
> New York, NY 10032
> (212) 305-9770
> http://nyp.org

Mount Sinai Medical Center
> Division of Pediatric Hematology-Oncology
> 1 Gustave L. Levy Place, Box 1208
> New York, NY 10029
> (212) 241-6031
> www.mountsinai.org

University of Rochester Medical Center (LTS)
> Strong Memorial Hospital
> Pediatric Hematology-Oncology
> 601 Elmwood Ave., Box 777
> Rochester, NY 14642
> (585) 275-2981
> www.urmc-rochester.edu/pediatrics

State University of New York at Stony Brook
> Pediatric Hematology/Oncology
> HSC T-11 Room 029
> Stony Brook, NY 11794
> (631) 444-7720
> www.stonybrookmedicalcener.org
> www.schoolreentry.com

SUNY Upstate Medical University (LTS)
> Pediatric Hematology/Oncology
> 750 East Adams St.
> Syracuse, NY 13210
> (315) 464-5294
> www.upstate.edu/pediatrics

New York Medical College
> Department of Pediatrics, Section of Hematology/Oncology
> Children's Hospital at Westchester Medical Center
> Munger Pavillion, Room 110
> Valhalla, NY 10595
> (914) 493-7997
> www.worldclassmedicine.com

There are Ronald McDonald Houses in Albany, Buffalo, New Hyde Park, New York City, Rochester, Syracuse, and Valhalla. There are Hope Lodges in Buffalo, New York City, and Rochester.

North Carolina

Ruth and Billy Graham Children's Health Center
    Mission Hospitals
    50 Doctors Drive, Suite M105
    Asheville, NC 28801
    (828) 213-1740
    www.missionhospitals.org

University of North Carolina at Chapel Hill (CCC)
    Department of Pediatric Hematology-Oncology
    CB 7220
    Burnett-Womack Building
    Chapel Hill, NC 27599
    (919) 966-0985
    www.ncchildrenshospital.org

Presbyterian Hospital
    Blume Children's Cancer Clinic
    Center for Cancer Research
    301 Hawthorne Lane
    Charlotte, NC 28204
    (704) 384-1900
    www.presbyterianblume.com

Carolinas Medical Center
    Pediatric Hematology Oncology
    1000 Blythe Blvd.
    Charlotte, NC 28203
    (704) 355-2000
    www.carolinashealthcare.org

Duke University Medical Center (LTS, CCC)
    Pediatric Hematology-Oncology
    228 Baker House
    Box 2916
    Durham, NC 27710
    (919) 684-3401
    www.dukechildrens.org

East Carolina University School of Medicine
   Department of Pediatric Hematology/Oncology
   PCMH-288W
   200 Stantonsburg Road
   Greenville, NC 27854
   (252) 816-4676
   www.ecu.edu/pediatrics

Wake Forest University School of Medicine (CCC)
   Pediatric Hematology/Oncology
   Medical Center Blvd.
   Winston-Salem, NC 27157
   (336) 716-2356
   www.ecu.edu/pediatrics

There are Ronald McDonald Houses in Durham, Chapel Hill, Charlotte, Greenville, and Winston-Salem. There is a Hope Lodge in Greenville.

North Dakota

Dakota Clinic
   Department of Pediatric Hematology-Oncology
   1702 South University Drive
   Fargo, ND 58103
   (701) 364-3000
   www.innovishealth.com/

MeritCare Medical Care Group
   Roger Maris Cancer Center
   820 4th St. N
   Fargo, ND 58122
   (701) 234-7544
   www.meritcare.com

There are Ronald McDonald Houses in Fargo and Bismarck.

Ohio

Children's Hospital Medical Center
   Pediatric Hematology/Oncology
   One Perkins Square

Akron, OH 44308
(330) 543-8580
www.akronchildrens.org

Children's Hospital Medical Center (LTS)
Department of Hematology and Oncology
3333 Burnet Ave.
Cincinnati, OH 45229
(513) 636-4266
www.cincinattichildrens.org

The Children's Hospital at The Cleveland Clinic
Department of Pediatric Hematology/Oncology
9500 Euclid Ave., Desk S35
Cleveland, OH 44195
(216) 444-8407
www.clevelandclinic.org

Rainbow Babies' and Children's Hospital (CCC)
Division of Pediatric Hematology/Oncology
11100 Euclid Ave.
Mail Stop RBC 6054
Cleveland, OH 44106
(216) 844-3345
www.rainbowbabies.org/hemonc

Nationwide Children's Hospital
Department of Pediatric Hematology-Oncology
700 Children's Drive
Columbus, OH 43205
(614) 722-3564
www.nationwidechildren.org

Children's Medical Center Dayton
Hematology/Oncology Department
One Children's Plaza
Dayton, OH 45404
(937) 641-3111
www.childrensdayton.org

Mercy Children's Hospital
Department of Pediatric Hematology-Oncology
2222 Cherry St., Suite 2800
Toledo, OH 43608
(419) 251-8215
www.mercyweb.org/childrens

Toledo Children's Hospital
    Pediatric Oncology
    2142 N. Cove Blvd., 5 SW
    Toledo, OH 43606
    (419) 291-7815
    www.promedica.org

Tod Children's Hospital
    Western Reserve Care System
    Pediatric & Adolescent Hematology/Oncology
    Medical Education Center
    500 Gypsy Lane
    Youngstown, OH 44501
    (330) 740-3955
    www.forumhealth.com

There are Ronald McDonald Houses in Akron, Cincinnati, Cleveland, Columbus, Dayton, and Toledo. There are Hope Lodges in Cincinnati and Cleveland.

Fernside
    4380 Malsbary Road
    Cincinnati, OH 45242
    (513) 745-0111
    www.fernside.org

This nonprofit organization helps Ohio families in grief and also has school programs.

Oklahoma

University of Oklahoma Health Sciences Center
    Children's Hospital of Oklahoma
    Hematology/Oncology
    940 NE 13th St., Room 3308
    Oklahoma City, OK 73104
    (405) 271-5311
    www.oumedicine.com

Warren Clinic, Inc.
    Pediatric Hematology Oncology
    Saint Francis Hospital, Level A
    6161 South Yale Ave.

Tulsa, OK 74136
(918) 494-2525
www.sfh-childrenshospital.com

There are Ronald McDonald Houses in Oklahoma City and Tulsa.

Oregon

Doernbecher Children's Hospital (CCC)
 Oregon Health Sciences University
 Department of Pediatric Hematology-Oncology
 3181 SW Sam Jackson Park Rd.
 Portland, OR 97201
 (503) 494-1543
 www.ohsu.edu

Emanuel Hospital Health Center
 Legacy Emanuel Children's Cancer Program
 501 North Graham, Suite 355
 Portland, OR 97227
 (503) 413-2560
 www.legacyhealth.org

There are Ronald McDonald Houses in Bend and Portland (2).

Pennsylvania

Lehigh Valley Hospital—Muhlenberg
 3545 Schoenersville Road
 Bethlehem, PA 18017
 (484) 884-3333

Geisinger Medical Center
 Pediatric Hematology-Oncology
 100 N. Academy Ave.
 Danville, PA 17822
 (570) 271-6848
 www.geisinger.org

Penn State Children's Hospital

Hershey Medical Center
Department of Pediatrics
500 University Ave., Room C7830
Hershey, PA 17033
(717) 531-6012
www/pennstatehershey.org

Children's Hospital of Philadelphia (LTS)
Division of Oncology
324 South 34th St.
Philadelphia, PA 19104
(215) 590-1000
www.chop.edu

St. Christopher's Hospital for Children
Pediatrics–Oncology
Erie Avenue at Front St.
Philadelphia. PA 19134
(215) 427-5000
www.stchristohershospital.com

Children's Hospital of Pittsburgh
Department of Pediatric Hematology-Oncology
3705 Fifth Ave.
Pittsburgh, PA 15213
(412) 692-5947
www.chp.edu

There are Ronald McDonald Houses in Danville, Hershey, Philadelphia (2), Pittsburgh, and Scranton. There are Hope Lodges in Hershey and Philadelphia.

Puerto Rico

San Jorge Children's Hospital
Pediatric Hematology/Oncology
258 San Jorge St., Suite 504
Santurce, PR 00912
(787) 727-1000
www.metropaviahealth.com/

There is a Hope Lodge in San Juan.

Rhode Island

Rhode Island Hospital
Pediatric Hematology/Oncology
593 Eddy St.
Providence, RI 02903
(401) 444-5241
www.lifespan.org/hch

There is a Ronald McDonald House in Providence.

South Carolina

Medical University of South Carolina (LTS)
Pediatric Hematology/Oncology
135 Rutledge Ave., Room 480
P. O. Box 250558
Charleston, SC 29425
(843) 792-2957
www.musckids.com

South Carolina Cancer Center
Suite 203
7 Richland Medical Park
Columbia, SC 29203
(803) 434-3533
www.palmettohealth.org

Children's Hospital of the Greenville Hospital System
Pediatric Hematology/Oncology
900 West Faris Rd.
Greenville, SC 29605
(864) 455-8898
www.ghs.org

There are Ronald McDonald Houses in Columbia, Charleston, and Greenville.
There is a Hope Lodge in Charleston.

South Dakota

Dakota Midwest Cancer Institute
1001 East 21st St., Suite 3100
Sioux Falls, SD 57105
(605) 322-7595
www.averamckennan.org

Sanford Children's Specialty Clinics
USD Department of Pediatrics
1305 West 18th St.
Sioux Falls, SD 57117
(605) 333-7171
www.sanfordhealth.org

There is a Ronald McDonald House in Sioux Falls.

Tennessee

T. C. Thompson Children's Hospital
910 Blackford St.
Chattanooga, TN 37403
(423) 778-7289
www.erlanger.org/childrens

East Tennessee State University
Pediatric Hematology/Oncology
ETSU Cancer Center at JCMC
400 N. State of Franklin Rd.
Johnson City, TN 37604
(423) 433-6200

East Tennessee Children's Hospital
Pediatric Hematology Oncology
2018 Clinch Ave., SW
P. O. Box 15010
Knoxville, TN 37901
(865) 541-8266
www.etch.com

St. Jude Children's Research Hospital Memphis (CCC)
Hematology/Oncology
262 Danny Thomas Place

Memphis, TN 38105
(901) 495-3335
www.stjude.org

Vanderbilt Children's Hospital (CCC)
Pediatric Hematology/Oncology
2220 Pierce Ave., Room 397 PRB
Nashville, TN 37232
(615) 936-1762
www.vanderbiltchildrens.com/cancer

There are Ronald McDonald Houses in Chattanooga, Johnson City, Memphis, Nashville, and Knoxville. There is a Hope Lodge in Nashville.

Texas

Texas Tech UHSC
Pediatrics
1400 S. Coulter Rd.
Amarillo, TX 79106
(806) 354-5434
www.ttuhsc.edu

Children's Hospital of Austin
Specialty for Children Pediatrics Hematology/Oncology
1301 Barbara Jordan Blvd., Suite 401
Austin, TX 78723
(512) 628-1901
www.dellchildrens.net

Driscoll Children's Hospital
Hematology/Oncology
3533 S. Alameda
Corpus Christi, TX 78411
(512) 694-5311
www.driscollchildrens.org/

Children's Medical Center of Dallas
1935 Medial Dist. Drive
Dallas, TX 75235
(214) 456-7000
www.childrens.com

Medical City Children's Hospital (LTS)
  Pediatric Hematology/Oncology
  7777 Forest Lane, Suite D400
  Dallas, TX 75230
  (972) 566-6647
  www.mcchildrenshospital.com

UT Southwestern Medical Center
  Pediatric Hematology/Oncology
  5323 Harry Hines Blvd.
  Dallas, TX 75390
  (214) 456-2382
  www.utsouthwestern.edu

Cook Children's Medical Center (LTS)
  Hematology/Oncology
  801 Seventh Ave., Suite 220
  Fort Worth, TX 76104
  (682) 885-4000
  www.cookchildrens.org

University of Texas Medical Branch
  Pediatrics
  801 University Blvd. Rm. 3.270
  Galveston, TX 77555
  (409) 772-3695
  www.utmb.org

Children's Cancer Hospital at the University of Texas
  M. D. Anderson Cancer Center (LTS, CCC)
  Division of Pediatrics Box 87
  1515 Holcombe Blvd.
  Houston, TX 77030
  (713) 792-5410
  www.mdanderson.org/children

Texas Children's Cancer Center at Baylor College of Medicine (LTS)
  Pediatric Oncology
  6621 Fannin St. CC1410.00
  Houston, TX 77030
  (832) 824-4200
  www.txccc.org

San Antonio Military Pediatric Cancer and Blood Disorders Center
Wilford Hall Medical Center
2200 Bergquist Dr., Suite 1
Lackland AFB, TX 78236
(210) 292-5684

Children's Hematology/Oncology Team
Covenant Children's Hospital
3606 21st Place, Suite 106
Lubbock, TX 79410
(806) 725-0400
www.covenanthealth.org

Texas Tech University Medical Center
Children's Hospital
602 Indiana Avenue
Lubbock, TX 79415
(806) 775-8200
www.umchealthsystem.com/childrenshospital

Southwest Texas Methodist Hospital
Pediatric Hematology/Oncology
7711 Louis Pasteur, Suite 306
San Antonio, TX 78229
(210) 614-4011
www.sahealth.com

University of Texas Health Science Center at San Antonio
Pediatric Hematology Oncology
333 N. Santa Rosa St., 8th Floor, Mail Code 7810
San Antonio, TX 78207
(210) 704-2187
www.uthscsa.edu/hem

Scott & White Memorial Hospital
Texas A&M Medical School
Pediatric Hematology/Oncology
2401 S. 31 St.
Temple, TX 76508
(254) 724-2006
www.sw.org

There are Ronald McDonald Houses in Fort Worth, Amarillo, Austin, Corpus Christi, Dallas, El Paso, Galveston, Harlingen, Houston (2), Lubbock, and San Antonio (2). There is a Hope Lodge in Lubbock.

Utah

Primary Children's Medical Center
    Department of Pediatric Hematology-Oncology
    100 N. Mario Capecci Drive
    Salt Lake City, UT 84113
    (801) 588-2680
    www.intermountainhealthcare.org

There are two Ronald McDonald Houses in Salt Lake City.

Vermont

University of Vermont College of Medicine (CCC)
    Pediatrics
    Given Medical Bldg.
    111 Colchester Avenue
    UVM College of Medicine
    Burlington, VT 05401
    (802) 847-2850
    www.fahc.org/Childrens_Hospital

Burlington has a Ronald McDonald House and a Hope Lodge.

Virginia

University of Virginia Health Sciences Center (CCC)
    Pediatric Hematology Oncology
    University of Virginia Hospital
    Box 386
    Charlottesville, VA 22908
    (434) 982-4361
    www.healthsystem.virginia.edu/inernet/pediatrics

INOVA Fairfax Hospital
    Pediatric Hematology/Oncology
    8301 Arlington Blvd., Suite 209
    Fairfax, VA 22031
    (703) 876-9111
    www.inova.org

Children's Hospital—King's Daughters
Department of Hematology/Oncology
601 Children's Lane
Norfolk, VA 23507
(757) 668-7000
www.chkd.org

Naval Medical Center Portsmouth (USOC)
620 John Paul Jones Circle
Portsmouth, VA 23708
(757) 953-4529

Virginia Commonwealth University Health System—MCV (CCC)
Pediatric Hematology/Oncology
250 East Marshall St.
Richmond, VA 23298
(804) 828-9000
www.vcuchildrens.org

Carilion Medical Center for Children at Roanoke Community Hospital
Pediatric Hematology/Oncology
1906 Belleview Ave.
Roanoke, VA 24014
(540) 981-7376
www.carilionclinic.org

There are Ronald McDonald Houses in Charlottesville, Norfolk, Richmond, Roanoke, and Falls Church.

Washington

Seattle Children's Hospital (LTS)
Department of Hematology/Oncology
4800 Sand Point Way NE
Seattle, WA 98105
(206) 987-2106
www.seattlechildren.org

Affiliated through Seattle Cancer Alliance with:

Fred Hutchinson Cancer Research Center
1100 Fairview Avenue, NW
P O Box 1902

Seattle, WA 98109
(800) 804-8824
www.fhcrc.org

Deaconess Medical Center
Pediatric Oncology Office
800 West 5th Avenue
Spokane, WA 99204
(509) 473-7230
www.deaconess-spokane.org

Sacred Heart Children's Hospital
Pediatric Hematology/Oncology
101 W. 8th Ave.
P. O. Box 2555
Spokane, WA 99204
(509) 474-2777
www.shmcchildren.org

Madigan Army Medical Center (USOC)
Building 9040 Fitzsimmons Drive
Tacoma, WA 98431
(253) 968-1980
www.mamc.amedd.army.mil

Mary Bridge Children's Hospital
Pediatric Hematology-Oncology
311 South L St.
P. O. Box 5299
Tacoma, WA 98405
(253) 403-3481
www.mulitcare.org

There are Ronald McDonald Houses in Seattle (2) and Spokane.

West Virginia

West Virginia University HSC
Department of Pediatric Hematology/Oncology
830 Pennsylvania Ave., Suite 104
Charleston, WV 25302
3(04) 388-1540
www.hsc.wvu.edu

Edwards Comprehensive Cancer Center
  Department of Pediatrics
  1400 Hal Greer Blvd.
  Huntington, WV 25701
  (304) 399-6503www.edwardssccc.org/pediatric_oncology

Children's Hospital
  West Virginia University
  Pediatric Hematology/Oncology
  Health Sciences N
  Robert C. Byrd HSC
  P. O. Box 9100
  Morgantown, WV 26506
  (304) 293-1217
  www.hsc.wva.edu

There are Ronald McDonald Houses in Charleston, Huntington, and Morgantown.

Wisconsin

St. Vincent Hospital
  Wisconsin Regional Cancer Center
  835 S. Van Buren St.
  P. O. Box 13508
  Green Bay, WI 54307
  (920) 433-8670
  www.stvincenthospital.org

Gundersen Lutheran
  Department of Pediatric Specialties
  1900 South Avenue
  East Building, 2d floor
  La Crosse, WI 54601
  (608) 775-2208
  www.gundersonlutheran.com

University of Wisconsin
  Children's Hospital Madison (CCC, LTS)
  Department of Pediatrics
  600 Highland Ave.
  Madison WI 53792

(608) 263-4200
www.uwhealth.org

www.outlook-life.org is an excellent Web site for patients and especially survivors of childhood cancer, although the links and information would be helpful for almost anybody.

Marshfield Clinic
    Pediatric Hematology-Oncology 1A4
    1000 N. Oak Ave.
    Marshfield, WI 54449
    (715) 387-5511
    www.marshfieldclinic.org

Midwest Children's Cancer Center
    Pediatric Hematology-Oncology
    8701 Watertown Plank Rd.
    Milwaukee, WI 53226
    (414) 607-5280

There are Ronald McDonald Houses in Madison, Marshfield, and Wauwatosa. There is a Hope Lodge in Marshfield.

Canada

Canadian Cancer Society's Cancer Information Service (UICC)
    10 Alcorn Avenue, Suite 200
    Toronto, ON, M4V 3B1
    Tel: +1 416 934 5636
    Fax: +1 416 961 4189
    For Canada only: +1 888 939 3333 (Monday to Friday
        9 a.m.–6 p.m.)
    E-mail: info@cis.cancer.ca
    Web site: www.cancer.ca

Alberta

Alberta Children's Hospital
    2888 Shagnappi Trail, NW
    Calgary, AB T3B 6A8
    (403) 955-7211

Stollery Children's Hospital
  Pediatric Oncology
  11560 University Avenue
  University of Alberta
  Edmonton, AB T6G 1Z2
  (780) 407-8829
  www.pediatrics.ualberta.ca

British Colombia

British Colombia's Children's Hospital
  Division of Pediatric Hematology/Oncology
  4480 Oak St., Room A119
  Vancouver, BC V6H 3V4
  (604) 875-2345
  www.bcchildren.ca
  www.kidscancer.bc.ca

There is a Ronald McDonald House in Vancouver.

Manitoba

CancerCare Manitoba
  Pediatric Hematology/Oncology
  100 Olivia St.
  Winnipeg, MB R3E OV9
  (204) 787-2197
  www.cancercare.mb.ca
There is a Ronald McDonald House in Winnipeg.

Newfoundland

Janeway Child Health Center
  Section of Pediatric Hematology/Oncology
  710 Janeway Place
  St. John's, NL A1B 1R8
  (709) 777-6300
  www.easternhealth.ca

Nova Scotia

IWK Health Center
  Department of Pediatric Hematology-Oncology
  5850 University Ave.
  Box 9700
  Halifax, NS B3J 3G9
  (902) 470-8888
  www.iwk.nshealth.ca

There is a Ronald McDonald House in Halifax.

Ontario

McMaster Children's Hospital
  Pediatric Hematology/Oncology
  1200 Main St. West
  Hamilton, ON L8N 3Z5
  (905) 521-2100
  www.mcmasterchildrenshospital.ca

Kingston General Hospital/Kingston Regional Cancer
  76 Stuart St.
  Burr Wing 1, Room 21-1058
  Kingston, ON K7L 2V7
  (613) 549-6666 ext. 3831
  www.kgh.on.ca

Children's Hospital of Western Ontario
  800 Commissioners Rd. E, Room E6-302
  P O Box 5010
  London, ON N6A 5W9
  (519) 685-8500
  www.chwo.org

Children's Hospital of Eastern Ontario
  Medical Director of Oncology
  401 Smyth Rd.
  Ottawa, ON K1H 8L1
  (613) 737-7600 X2370
  www.cheo.on.ca

Hospital for Sick Children
  Pediatrics, Division of Hematology/Oncology
  555 University Avenue
  Toronto, ON M5G 1X8
  (416) 813-1391
  www.sickkids.on.ca

There are Ronald McDonald Houses in Hamilton, London, Ottawa, and Toronto.

Quebec

Hopital Sainte-Justine
  Pediatric Hematology/Oncology
  3175 Côte Sainte-Catherine
  Montreal, PQ H3T 1C5
  (514) 345-4931
  www.hsj.qu.ca

McGill University Health Center/Montreal Children's Hospital
  Hematology/Oncology
  2300 Tupper St., C-402
  Montreal, PQ H3H 1P3
  (514) 412-4400
  www.mcgill.ca/peds

Centre Hospitalier Universitaire de Sherbrooke
  3001 12th Ave. North
  Sherbrooke, PQ J1H 5N4
  (819) 346-1110
  www.chus.qc.ca (French only)

Centre Hospitalier Universitaire de Quebec
  Pediatrics
  2705 Boul. Laurier
  Sainte-Foy, Quebec City, PQ G1V 4G2
  (418) 656-4141
  www.chuq.qc.ca (French only)

Saskatchewan

Allan Blair Cancer Centre
Saskatchewan Cancer Agency
4101 Dewdney Ave.
Regina, SK S4T 7T1
(306) 766-2213
www.saskcancer.ca

Saskatoon Cancer Centre
20 Campus Drive
Saskatoon, SK S7N 4H4
(306) 655-2662
www.saskcancer.ca
There is a Ronald McDonald House in Saskatoon.

Further Resources

READING

Baldauf, Sarah and Lyon, Lindsay, "America's Best Hospitals," *U S News and World Report*, vol. 145 (2) (July 31, 2008), p. 32.
Cicero, Karen, "10 best children's hospitals.". *Parents Magazine*, vol. 84 (2) (February 2009), p. 105.

Organizations in the United States and Canada

M aybe one reason that it becomes easier to cope as time passes is the discovery that there is a surprisingly strong network of support to help children and parents facing cancer and other life-threatening diseases. There are local and national parents' groups, age-appropriate support groups for the children and their siblings, organizations working to improve health care, and even some that help with expenses. The Internet and the World Wide Web have spread that support net so wide that they are addressed in a separate chapter (Chapter 33).

This is intended as a generous sampling of clinics and organizations that help families who are dealing with childhood cancer. A scattering of associations not specializing in cancer exclusively have been included as examples of others who might be able to help in a particular way.

This appendix has a list of organizations that serve more than one state. Many are national in scope, others regional, but addresses are given for headquarters. Note, too, that some dedicated organizations are listed instead in the Internet chapter, since they provide excellent online resources.

Many organizations or resources target a specific form of cancer (e.g., brain tumors) or therapy (e.g., bone marrow transplant). To avoid repetition, these will be listed only in the appropriate chapter rather than twice.

Air Charity Network

4620 Haygood Road, Suite 1
   Virginia Beach, VA 23455
   (800) 549-9980
   (877) 621-7177 to request flights
   www.aircharitynetwork.org

Network of private pilots. Need-based transport to therapy, transplant location, and other destinations in cases of family crisis.

Alliance for Childhood Cancer

www.allianceforchildhoodcancer.org

An umbrella organization for patient advocacy groups, professional medical and scientific organizations to increase awareness of childhood cancer, advocate for research, and promote quality care for pediatric patients.

American Cancer Society

1599 Clifton Road NE
   Atlanta, GA 30329-4251
   (404) 320-3333
   (800) 227-2345
   www.cancer.org

Voluntary organization with many regional and local units. Check the phone book for the closest group. Provides help with transportation. Loans some equipment like wheelchairs and hospital beds. Sponsors seminars and support groups for the professional medical and dental community as well as for the patient and the family. Issues many publications on the various forms of cancer and treatments.

American Society of Pediatric Hematology/Oncology

4700 West Lake Avenue
Glenview, IL 60025-1485
(847) 375-4716, (847) 375-4700
www.aspho.org

Clinical and scholarly organization founded in 1981; has over 650 member-physicians living in the United States and abroad. Aims to improve the care of children with cancer and fosters clinical and basic research.

Believe in Tomorrow Children's Foundation

6601 Frederick Road
Baltimore, MD 21228
(800) 933-5470
www.believeintomorrow.org

For over 20 years this organization has provided overnight accommodations designed to keep families together while the child is treated. Besides a residence at Johns Hopkins, they have respite housing, Hands-on Adventures, and an initiative for military families with sick children.

Canadian Cancer Society

National Office
10 Alcorn Ave, Suite 200
Toronto, Ontario, Canada M4V 3B1
(416) 961-7223
www.cancer.ca

With chapters across the country, this Canadian organization leads the fight against cancer through fund-raising, public service announcements, research, and support for patients and caregivers.

CancerCare, Inc.

275 Seventh Avenue
New York, NY 10001
(212) 712-8400
(800) 813-4673
www.cancercare.org

Practical and financial aid and support through oncology social workers.

Cancer Fund of America

2901 Breazewood Lane
Knoxville, TN 37921
(800) 578-5284
www.cfoa.org

Provides free products to hospices and other nonprofit health care providers.

Candlelighters Childhood Cancer Foundation

P.O. Box 498
10400 Connecticut Avenue, Suite 205
Kensington, MD 20895
(800) 366-2223
(301) 962-3250
www.candlelighters.org

This is the oldest international organization for the families of children who have or have had cancer. Candlelighters (named after the old quotation, "It is better to light one candle than to curse the darkness") has hundreds of chapters in virtually every state and in many foreign countries. Wig banks and transportation referrals are just two of the varying services of local chapters. Meetings provide education, entertainment, and support from people who truly understand the family's problems, fears, and hopes. The national office lobbies lawmakers on related legislation and helps set up chapters. Information on available publications, professionally staffed summer camps for patients and siblings, and a forum for local groups to communicate.

Candlelighters CCF Canada

1300 Yonge St., Suite 405
　　Toronto, Ontario, Canada 4MT 1X3
　　(416) 489-6440
　　(800) 363-1062
　　www.candlelighters.ca

Canuck Place

1690 Mathews Avenue
　　Vancouver, BC V6J 2T2
　　(604) 731-4847
　　www.canuckplace.org

The first free-standing hospice for children in North America. Respite, palliative, and bereavement services. Serves British Columbia.

CorStone

33 Buchanan Drive
　　Sausalito, CA 94965
　　(415) 331-6161
　　www.corstone.org

Formerly the Center for Attitudinal Healing, this organization works with children or adults facing a catastrophic illness. Supplements traditional health care. Advocates inner peace through conquest of fear. The organization prepares audiovisual materials and books like the excellent *There is a Rainbow Behind Every Dark Cloud* and *Another Look at the Rainbow.*

Children's Hospice International

1101 King Street, Suite 360
　　Alexandria, VA 22314
　　(703) 684-0330
　　(800) 242-4453
　　www.chionline.org

Promotes hospice support through pediatric care facilities. Information clearinghouse. Sponsors seminars and lectures for professionals. Issues publications and cassette tapes. Backs legislation to fund better care for children, whether seeking a cure or at the end of their lives.

Children's Oncology Camping Association International

P.O. Box 41433
　　Des Moines, Iowa 50311
　　(515) 669-4580
　　www.coca-intl.org
　　Serves US, Canada, and Europe. The list of camps seems incomplete, at least in New England.

Children's Oncology Group (COG) / National Children's Cancer Foundation (NCCF)

CureSearch
　　National Childhood Cancer Foundation
　　4600 East West Highway, Suite 600
　　Bethesda, MD 20814-3457

　　and
　　CureSearch
　　Children's Oncology Group
　　Research Operations Center
　　440 E. Huntington Drive, Suite 400
　　Arcadia, CA 91006
　　(800) 458-6223
　　www.curesearch.org

COG is a National Cancer Institute-funded research organization, formed by the merger of several earlier groups like the Pediatric Oncology Group and the Children's Cancer Group. "Dedicated to Discovery, Committed to Care." Clinical trial information. Worldwide partnership with similar groups. COG is the largest cooperative clinical research group, including more than 250 institutions (clinics and hospitals) in the United States and abroad. Aims to increase the number of children treated on clinical trials. The merged

CureSearch Web site is a strong resource; click on "resources" for a list of COG members by location.

Children's Wish Foundation, International

8615 Roswell Road
    Atlanta, GA 30350
    (770) 393-WISH
    (800) 323-WISH

Has filled wishes for children under the age of 18 in 53 countries.

Compassionate Friends, Inc.

P. O. Box 3696
    900 Jorie Blvd., Suite 78
    Oak Brook, IL 60522
    (630) 990-0010
    (877) 969-0010
    www.compassionatefriends.org

Organization for grieving parents. Many chapters across the United States. Prints bibliographies, publishes pamphlets for bereaved parents and other relatives. Nonsectarian "Suggestions for Clergy" pamphlet. "Suggestions for Doctors and Nurses" pamphlet is well done. Chapters hold supportive meetings.

Corporate Angel Network, Inc.

Westchester County Airport, Building 1
    One Loop Road
    White Plains, NY 10604
    (914) 328-1313
    (866) 328-1313
    www.corpangelnetwork.com

Clearinghouse that matches flights of corporate aircraft with patients needing transportation to medical treatment. Covers entire United States, including

Alaska and Hawaii, plus Puerto Rico. Patients must be able to climb steps and sit for flight. Cannot accommodate patients on stretchers, life-support systems, IVs, or oxygen, but chemotherapy pumps are acceptable. Patient needs medical authorization in writing from doctor, specific date and time of appointment, to match flight. Organ donors and accompanying parent eligible, too.

First Descents

P.O. Box 2193
  Vail, CO 81658
  (970) 845-8400
  www.firstdescents.org

A Vail, Colorado-based nonprofit providing outdoor adventures for young cancer patients.

Gold Ribbons for Childhood Cancer

P.O. Box 542
  Yamhill, OR 97148
  (503) 724-4166
  www.goldribbons.com

Official ribbon of childhood cancer awareness. Endorsed by major organizations. Sells pins, holiday items, etc. Supports an annual Childhood Cancer Awareness Tree on Capitol Hill in Washington, DC. Very reasonable prices.

Heavenly Hats Foundation

c/o Anthony D. Leanna
  2325 Pamperin Rd., Suite 3
  Green Bay, WI 54313
  (920) 434-4151 ext. 1400
  (920) 362-2668
  www.heavenlyhats.com
Donates cool new hats to cancer patients who have lost their hair.

International Confederation of Childhood Cancer Parent Organizations

www.icccpo.org

A rich resource representing 118 member organizations in 73 countries. Contact information is provided for each country on the Web site. A worldwide network of parent organizations. Many of the non-North American sites provide translation into English.

Kids Cancer Network

P. O. Box 4545
Santa Barbara, CA 93140
(805) 693-1017
www.kidscancernetwork.org

Links to online childhood cancer resources. "A dose of hope for children and their families isolated by...cancer treatment." Distributes *Funletter* activity magazine. Information and "cool stuff."

Locks of Love

234 Southern Blvd.
West Palm Beach, FL 33405
(516) 833-7332
(888) 896-1588
www.locksoflove.org

This organization accepts donations of human hair and gives the resulting wigs to financially disadvantaged children with long-term hair loss. Donation guidelines are on their Web site.

Make-a-Wish Foundation of America

3550 North Central Avenue, Suite 300
Phoenix, AZ 85012
(602) 279-9474

(800) 722-WISH
www.wish.org

Helps seriously ill children's wishes come true—like trips or meeting with celebrities. Has 66 chapters in the United States and its territories, with affiliates worldwide.

Make Today Count, Inc.

c/o Mid-America Cancer Center
   1235 East Cherokee
   Springfield, MO 65804
   (417) 885-3324
   (800) 432-2273

Has a number of chapters that meet as support groups. Some have separate meetings for parents of children with cancer and for the youngsters themselves.

National Association of Hospital Hospitality Houses (NAHHH Inc.)

P.O. Box 18087
   Asheville, NC 28814
   (828) 253-1188
   (800) 542-9730
   www.nahhh.org

Source of information on free or reduced-rate houses near hospitals around the United States. Search for resources by state and city. Also provides access to individuals who open their homes to patients and families.

National Cancer Institute

www.cancer.gov

This federal agency, a branch of the Public Health Service, is charged with research into the causes and treatments of all forms of cancer. American citizens referred to NCI clinics by their physicians are treated free of charge.

Their Cancer Information Clearinghouse is affiliated with the Cancer Information Service, which can be reached by calling 800-4-CANCER from anywhere in the United States. They can provide publications and tell you where you may find other help. If finances are a problem, they will suggest specific funding sources. Many of their publications are available full-text online and are kept admirably up to date. Live help via Internet chat enhances this service.

National Children's Cancer Society

Patient and Family Services
    One South Memorial Drive, Suite 800
    St. Louis, MO 63102
    (314) 241-1600
    (800) 532-6459
    www.nationalchildrenscancersocity.com

Direct financial support to children with cancer and their families. Fundraising help, financial assistance for bone marrow transplants. International in scope, distributing drugs and supplies to pediatric cancer centers in less privileged nations. Many corporate partners. Peer support. U.S. and global outreach. Download "Sammie's New Mask: a Coloring Book for Friends of Children with Cancer" for grades K–3, or a nifty bookmark-format list of ways to help such children ("Friend-O-Meter Ruler").

National Coalition for Cancer Survivorship

1010 Wayne Avenue, Suite 770
    Silver Spring, MD 20910
    (301) 650-9127
    (888) 650-9127
    www.canceradvocacy.org

Works on behalf of people with cancer, families, caregivers. Advocates for quality. The organization defines "survivor" as anyone surviving a cancer diagnosis, whether yesterday or 10 years ago. Their Web site has links to breaking news on the oncology front. Their "Cancer Survival Toolbox" is a free self-learning audio program teaching basic skills like problem solving and special topics such as caregiver care. Corporate sponsors fund publications to accompany the audio program. Also in Spanish.

National Patient Travel Center

4620 Haygood Road, Suite 1
  Virginia Beach, VA 23455
  (800) 296-1217
  www.patienttravel.org

See also Air Charity Network earlier in this list. 24-hour referrals for transportation services.

  Mercy Medical Airlift (www.mercymedicalairlift.org) has up-to-date information on available flights. Provides assistance for patients who can't afford long-distance travel for medical care, diagnosis, and treatment.

Padres Contra el Cáncer

http://iamhope.org

The only Latino organization to focus on childhood cancer. Provides links (in English and Spanish) throughout the United States.

Re-Mission The Game

Hope Lab
  1991 Broadway St., Suite 136
  Redwood City, CA 94063
  (650) 569-5900
  www.re-mission.net

From a nonprofit organization, this is a fast-paced, fun, yet educational way to "conquer cancer" with Roxxi, the cancer- and infection-fighting nanobot. Download or order a free CD in English, Spanish, or French.

Ronald McDonald House Charities

One Kroc Drive
  Oak Brook, IL 605213 (630) 623-7048
  www.rmhc.com

Temporary residential facilities for the families of children being treated for a serious illness. There is a small charge but it can be waived in cases of need. There are houses throughout the United States, in Canada, and as far away as Australia, each created by a community effort. Most but not all are located adjacent to a cancer center. They also give grants to non-profit organizations that serve children and scholarships (students need not be cancer patients or survivors).

Special Love for Children With Cancer

117 Youth Development Center
　　Winchester, VA 22602
　　(888) 930-2707
　　www.SpecialLove.org

Provides educational and recreational programs for children with cancer and their families. Scholarships for college students with cancer. Their Web site has many links to appropriate resources for children and families. Serves the Tidewater region of Virginia and Maryland.

Starlight Foundation

5757 Wilshire Blvd., Suite M100
　　Los Angeles, CA 90036
　　(310) 479-1212
　　www.starlight.org

Free videos for teen patients. Virtual online playground where hospitalized children can "meet," etc. Materials to help children and adolescents cope. Educational AV materials including CD-ROM. Online story "webisodes" on coping with cancer as well as game-like programs to learn about bone marrow, medical tests, and much more.

Sunshine Foundation

1041 Mill Creek Drive
　　Feasterville, PA 19053
　　(215) 396-4770

(800) 767-1976
www.sunshinefoundation.org

A nonprofit organization founded by a police officer to grant special wishes for child victims of disease and accidents, the terminally and critically ill. There are no geographic qualifiers for the children, thousands of whom have been treated to trips to Disneyland, the seashore, and other places. Accepts referrals from anyone. Also serves abused children. They have a "Dream Village" in central Florida for those visiting Disney World or Sea World. All expenses paid for the entire family living in the child's household.

Ulman Cancer Fund for Young Adults

10440 Little Patuxent Parkway, Suite G1
   Columbia, MD 21044
   (410) 964-0202
   (888) 393-FUND (3863)
   www.ulmanfund.org

Their Web site is a nice gateway to several teen-oriented sites that facilitate communication among patients, raise awareness, and just plain have fun.

United Ostomy Association

P.O. Box 66
   Fairview, TN 37062
   (800) 826-0826

Some cancer patients may have a stoma (surgical opening) on the abdominal wall through which body wastes are collected. This organization helps these "ostomates" return to normal living. Many chapters in every state plus in Canada. Publishes books and pamphlets on various aspects of ostomy.

The Wellness Community (Group Loop)

919 18th St. NW, Suite 54
   Washington, DC 20006
   (202) 888-WELL
   www.grouploop.org

This is a great site for ages 13 to 19, with support, resources, and information. Connect with other teens fighting cancer.

Wigs for Kids

21330 Center Ridge Road, Suite 26
Rocky River, OH 44116
(440) 333-4433
www.wigsforkids.org

"Helping Kids Look Themselves." Lists of participating hair salons around the United States. Need-based services.

World Child Cancer Foundation

www.worldccf.org

An international organization to extend diagnosis and treatment advances for childhood cancer to developing countries, where the prognosis is often grim.

Organizations and Clinics Outside the United States

This appendix lists resources beyond the United States and Canada. A few clinics are briefly mentioned, but contacts are provided for many countries around the world. Web site addresses have been provided where possible for further, up-to-date information.

This listing does not include every single source in every country. After I spent hours and days trying to fact-check the chapters on organizations and clinics/hospitals in the United States and Canada, it was obvious, given rapid changes in Web sites, not to mention frequently changing telephone numbers and the like, that keeping these lists current would be an impossible task. With the permission of the International Cancer Information Service Group, I am using their membership list, which was current as of January 2009. An up-to-date version is available at their website, www.icisg. org. The clinics listed are taken from the Children's Oncology Group membership list, accessed at www.curesearch.org in March 2009.

Africa

A new Oxford, UK-based organization is dedicated to improving cancer awareness and therapy throughout Africa; it is general in scope, not specific to pediatric malignancies. www.afrox.org.

Argentina

Centro Oncológico Buenos Aires
Hipolito Yrigoyen 4221
Buenos Aires, Argentina C1212ACA
Tel: 541149811128
Fax: 541149816623
www.coba.org.ar

Red Oncologica
E-mail: info@redoncologica.com.ar
Tel: 011 15 5154 1940
www.redoncologica.com.ar

Australia

The Cancer Council Victoria
Cancer Information and Support Service
1 Rathdowne Street
Carlton VIC 3053, Australia
Tel: +61 3 9635 5129
Fax: +61 3 9635 5290
www.cancervic.org.au

The Cancer Council South Australia
Cancer Helpline & Cancer Connect
202 Greenhill Road
Eastwood SA 5063
Tel: +61 8 8291 4161
Fax: +61 8 8291 4122
www.cancersa.org.au/

Cancer Foundation of Western Australia
Cancer Helpline
A.H. Crawford Lodge
55 Monash Ave.
Nedlands, WA 6009, Australia
Tel: +61 89489 7300
Fax: +61 89381 8616
E-mail: inquiries@cancerwa.asn.au

Cancer Council New South Wales
P.O. Box 572
Kings Cross NSW, Australia
Tel: +61 2 9334 1829
Fax: +61 2 9334 1741
http://www.cancercouncil.com.au/

COG Institutions in Australia
Children's Hospital at Westmead,
Crn Hawkesbury Rd & Hainsworth Street
Westmead, NSW 2145
Tel: 011 612 9845 0000

Royal Children's Hospital, Brisbane
Herston Road
Brisbane, QLD 4029
Tel: 0011 61 7 3636 1357
http://www.gheps.health.gld.gov.au.rch/

Women's and Children's Hospital, Adelaide
72 King William Road
North Adelaide, SA 5006
Tel: 61 8 8161 7000
http://www.wch.sa.gov.au

Royal Children's Hospital, University of Melbourne
Flemington Road
Parkville, VIC 3052
Tel: 03 9345-5522
http://www.rch.org.au/ccc

Princess Margaret Hospital for Children
GPO Box D 184
Roberts Rd., SUBIACO
Perth, WA 6001
Tel: 61 8 934 08234

Additional clinics in Australia are located at:
John Hunter Children's Hospital, Newcastle, NSW
Sydney Children's Hospital, Randwick, NSW
Royal Children's Hospital, Brisbane, QLD

Bangladesh

Khwaja Yunus Ali Medical College & Hospital
   73 Green Road, Dhaka
   Bandladesh Khwaja Yunus Ali Medical College & Hospital Village
     Enayetpur
   Thana chouhali, District Sirajgon
   Bangladesh, 1205
   E-mail: infor@kyamch.org
   Tel: 880 751 63761-3, 0176 291681
   Fax: 880 751 62853
   www.kyamch.org

Bermuda

Bermuda Cancer & Health Centre
   P.O. Box HM 1562
   Hamilton HM FX Bermuda, HMFX
   E-mail: Pr@Chc.Bm
   Tel: 1-441-236-1001
   Fax: 1-441-236-0880
   www.cancer.bm

Brazil

Associação Nacional de Informação e Apoio sobre Câncer de Mama
   Alameda Lorena, 1336 cj. 13
   São Paulo – SP – Brazil, 01424-001
   E-mail: mamainfo@mamainfo.org.br
   Tel: 55 11 38912531
   Fax: 55 11 38912531
   www.mamainfo.org.br

Another clinic is located at the Centro ce Hematologia e Oncologic Pediátrica (CEHOPE) in Rua Dos Coelhos.

Bulgaria

International Medical Association Bulgaria (IMAB)
    55 M. Drinov str.
    Varna, Bulgaria, BG-9002
    Tel: +359-52-634107
    Fax: +359-52-634107
    www.imab-bg.org

Canada

Canadian Cancer Society's Cancer Information Service
    10 Alcorn Avenue, Suite 200
    Toronto, ON, M4V 3B1
    Contact: Heather Logan
    E-mail: hlogan@cancer.ca
    Tel: +1 416 934 5636
    Fax: +1 416 961 4189
    For Canada only: +1 888 939 3333 (Monday to Friday,
      9 a.m.—6 p.m.)
    info@cis.cancer.ca
    www.cancer.ca

Chile

A Chilean clinic is located at Hospital Luis Calvo MacKenna in Santiago.

China

Clinics in China are located at the Beijing Children's Hospital and the Shanghai Children's Medical Center.

Commonwealth of Independent States (CIS)

Moscow Cancer Relief Society
    Korneychuka Street 39-59
    Moscow, Russia 127543
    Tel: +7 095 405 8094

There are clinics at the Research Institute of Pediatric Hematology in Moscow and the Ivano-Matryoninskaya Children's Clinical Hospital in Irkutsk.

Costa Rica

A clinic is located at the Hospital Nacional de Niños in San Jose.

Czech Republic

League Against Cancer Prague
    Na Slupi 6
    Prague 2 - 12842, Czech Republic
    E-mail: lpr@lpr.cz
    Tel: +420 2 24919732
    Fax: +420 2 24919732

Denmark

Kraeftens Bekaempelse Danish Cancer Society
    Strandboulevarden 49
    DK-2100 Kobenhavn O.Denmark
    E-mail: avs@cancer.dk
    Tel: +45 35 25 75 00
    Fax: +45 35 25 77 01

Dubai

The Mayo Clinic has a branch in Dubai, UAE. There is a pediatric oncology institute.

Egypt

Egyptian Cancer Information Service for Young People
4 Masjed Al-Eman St.
Alexandria, Egypt
Tel: (+2) 0181657000
http://www.mans.eun.eg

Association of the Friends of the National Cancer Institute
33 Kasr el Aini, 9th Floor, Suite 36
Cairo, Egypt
202 362 3350

El Salvador

There is a clinic at Hospital de Niños Benjamin Bloom in San Salvador.

Finland

CancerContact: Cancer Society of Finland
Liisankatu 21 B
FIN 00170
Helsinki
Tel: +358 9 1353 3268
Fax: +358 9 2609210
or
Tel: +358 9 1353 3236
Fax: +358 9 2609210
Care Tel: +358 9 135331
www.cancer.fi

France

Ligue nationale contre le cancer
14 rue de Corvisart,
Paris, 75013
Tel: +33 1 53 55 24 18

Fax: + 33 1 43 36 91 49
www.ligue-cancer.net

Information des publics,
   Institut national du cancer
   52, avenue André Morizet
   Boulogne-Billancourt Cedex, 92513
   Tel: +33 (0) 1 41 10 15 31
   www.e-cancer.fr

Germany

Deutsches Krebsforschungszentrum
   (German Cancer Research Centre)
   Krebsinformationsdienst (Cancer Information Service)
   Im Neuenheimer Feld 280,
   D 69120 Heidelberg, Germany
   Tel: +49 6221 422 898
   Fax: +49 6221 401 806
   www.krebsinformation.de

There are pediatric hematology clinics at University Children's Hospital in Essen and at Phillips Universität in Marburg.

Greece

Hellenic Cancer Society
   18 - 20 Tsoha Street
   Athens 11521, Greece
   E-mail: hellas-cancer@ath.forthnet.gr
   Tel: +30210-6456713-5
   Fax: +30210-6410011
   http://www.addgr.com/org/hc/grinfo.htm

Guatemala

There is a clinic at Unidad Nacional De Oncologia Pediatrica in Guatemala City.

Honduras

There is a clinic at Hospital Escuela Bloque Materno Infantil in Tegucigalpa.

Hong Kong

Hong Kong Cancer Fund
    Suite 1301, Kilnwick Centre
    32 Hollywood Road
    Central, Hong Kong
    Tel: +852 2868 0780
    Fax: +852 2524 9023

Hungary

Hungarian League Against Cancer
    P.O. Box 7
    1507 Budapest, Hungary
    Tel: +36 1 225 1621
    Fax: +36 1 202 4017

India

Agra Cancer Society
    37, Bansal Nagar Fatehabad Road
    Agra, India
    E-mail: Sandeepcancer@rediffmail.com
    Tel: +915622331271
    Fax: +915622855060

Cancer Aid & Research Foundation
    Byculla Municipal School Bldg.
    Ground Floor, Room 15-18
    N.M. Joshi Marg, near 'S' Bridge
    Byculla (W), Mumbai 400-011, India
    E-mail: cancerarfoundation@yahoo.com

Tel: 23007000 / 23008000 / 39538800 / 39538801
Fax: 23008000
www.cancerarfoundation.org

VCare Foundation
132 Maker Tower 'A'
Cuffe Parade
Mumbai, India, 4000 005
Tel: +91 22 218 8828
Fax: +91 22 218 4457

South Asian Inst. of Oncology & Cancer Research
CK 103
Salt Lake
Kolkutta 700 091, India
Tel: +91 33 359 0713
Fax: +91 33 217 2456

Tata Memorial Hospital
Mumbai, India 400 012
Tel: +91 22 415 4002
Fax: +91 22 414 6937

Gujarat Cancer & Research Institute
M.P. Shah Cancer Hospital
Medical Oncology Department
Civil Hospital Campus Asarwa
Ahmedabad - 380 016
Tel: +91 79 268 1451/268 5555
Fax: +91 79 268 5490

Ireland

Irish Cancer Society
5 Northumberland Road
Dublin 4, Ireland
Tel: +353 1 231 0500/0519
Fax: +353 1 231 0555
http://www.cancer.ie/

Ulster Cancer Foundation
40-44 Eglantine Avenue
Belfast, Northern Ireland, BT15 3LB

Tel: 028 9066 3281
Fax: 028 9066 8715
www.ulstercancer.org

Israel

Israel Cancer Association
  Revivim 7
  Givatayim, Israel 53104
  Tel: +972 3 571 9584
  Fax: +972 3 571 9578

Italy

Associazione Italian Malati di Cancro
  Parenti e Amici - AIMaC
  Via Barberini 11 - 00187 Roma, Italy
  Email: info@aimac.it or aimac@tin.it
  http://www.aimac.it/
  Tel: +39 06 4825107
  Fax: +39 06 42011216

Japan

Center for Cancer Control & Information Services
  National Cancer Center
  5-1-1, Tsukiji
  Chuo-ku, Tokyo, Japan, 104-0045
  Tel: 03-3547-5293
  Fax: 03-3547-6074
  http://ganjoho.jp/

Jordan

There is a clinic at King Hussein Cancer Center (formerly Al-Amal Cancer Center) in Amman.

Kenya

Nairobi Cancer Registry
Centre for Clinical Research
Kenya Medical Research Institute (KEMI)
P.O. Box 20778
Nairobi, 0020, Kenya
Tel: 254 020 2722541/27133498
Fax: 252 020 2720030
E-mail: glcc@asia.com
www.kemri.org

Lebanon

There is a children's cancer clinic at American University of Beirut.

Malaysia

National Cancer Society of Malaysia
66 Jalan Raja Muda Abdul Aziz
Kuala Lumpur, Malaysia 50300
Tel: 60 3 2698 7300
Fax: 60 3 2698 4300
www.cancer.org.my

Cancer Information and Support Centre
Department of Radiotherapy & Oncology
Hospital Kuala Lumpur
Jalan Pahang
50586 Kuala Lumpur, Malaysia
Tel: +60 3 2615 5810
Fax: +60 3 2692 5713

Mexico

COG Institution in Mexico
Hospital Infantil de Mexico Federico Gomez
Calle Dr. Marguez Num 162 Colonia Doctores

Mexico City, 06720
Tel: 525 55 228-9917
http://www.himfg.edu.mx

There are other clinics at Hospital Pediatrico de Sinaloa, Hospital Miguel Hidalgo in Aguascalientes, the Institute Nacional de Pediatria in Mexico City, and the Dr. Jose E. Gonzalez University Hospital in Monterey.

Morocco

There are clinics at the Hospital d'Engants Rabat-Maroc in Rabat and the Service d'Hematologie et d'Oncologie Pediatrique in Casablanca.

Netherlands

Dutch Cancer Society
Sophialaan 8
1075 BR Amsterdam, Netherlands
Tel: +31 20 570 0551/0542
Fax: +31 20 675 0302
www.kwfkankerbestrijding.nl

COG Institution in Netherlands
Radboud University Nijmegen Medical Centre
921/KOC P.O. Box 1901
Nijmegen, 6500 HB
Tel: 31 24 361-7489
www.umcn.nl

There is a clinic at the Beatrixkliniek in Groningen.

New Zealand

Cancer Society of New Zealand Ltd.
Level 6, Wakefield House
90 The Terrace
P.O. Box 10 847
Wellington, New Zealand

Tel: +64 4 494 7270
Fax: +64 4 494 7271
http://www.cancernz.org.nz

Cancer Society of New Zealand
Canterbury West Coast Division
246 Manchester Street
PO Box 13 - 450
Christchurch 8001, New Zealand
Tel: +64 3 379 5835
Fax: +64 3 377 2804
http://www.cancernz.org.nz/divisions/canterbury-westcoast/about/

Cancer Society of New Zealand
Wellington Division
52 Riddiford Street
Newtown
Wellington, New Zealand
http://www.cancernz.org.nz/divisions/wellington/about/

Cancer Information Service
Auckland Cancer Society
P.O. Box 1724
Auckland, New Zealand
Tel: +64 9 308 0173
Fax: +64 9 308 0175
or
Tel: 0800 800 426 or (09) 308 0162

COG Institutions in New Zealand
Starship Children's Hospital
Private Bag 92-024
Auckland, 1
Tel: 64 9 307 4949 ext. 6295
http://www.starship.org.nz/cg/Home

South Island Child Cancer Service
Private Bag 4710
Christchurch, 8140
Tel: 64 3 364 0740

Nigeria

The Bloom Cancer Care & Support Centre
    8 Merrett Road
    Yaba, Lagos, Nigeria
    E-mail: thebloom@hotmail.com or thebloomcancercare@yahoo.com
    Tel: +234 (0) 1 8043413

Children Living with Cancer Foundation
    23 Ayoola Olatunde St.
    Anthony Village, Lagos, Nigeria
    Tel: 234 1 4723559 or 234 8033156908
    www.clwcf.org

C.O.P.E. Breast Cancer
    34, Adeniyi Jones Avenue,
    Ikeja Lagos, Nigeria, 01234
    Tel: 08023121883
    E-mail: copebc@yahoo.com
    www.copebreastcancer.com

Radiotherapy and Oncology Centre
    Roc Aumadu Bello University Teaching Hospital
    P.O. Box 06
    Shika, Zaria, Kudune State, Nigeria
    Contact: Dr. T.A. Olasinde, Department Head
    Tel: +2348024771779
    E-mail: abuthroc@yahoo.com

Society of Clinical Oncology & Cancer Research
    Division of Oncology, Department of Surgery
    University Hospital
    Ibadan, Nigeria 20000
    Tel: 234-2-2410995
    Fax: 234-2-2410995
    www.westafricanbioethics.net

Norway

Norwegian Cancer Society
    P.O. Box 4, Sentrum
    0101 OSLO

Norway
Tel: +47 947 91 317
Tel: Operator +47 815704777
Fax: +47 22 86 66 10
www.kreftforeningen.no

Romania

There are clinics at Maria Sklodowska-Curie Children's Hospital in Bucharest and the Children's Hospital "St. Mary" in Iasi.

Saudi Arabia

There is a children's cancer center at the King Faisal Specialist Hospital and Resource Centre near Riyadh.

Serbia

Ecumenical Humanitarian Organization
"Rakinfo"
Cara Dusana 31,
21000 Novi Sad,
Serbia & Montenegro
Tel: 381 21 469 616
Fax: 381 21 469 588
www.rakinfo.ehons.org

There is a clinic at the Mother and Child Care Institute in Belgrade.

Singapore

Cancer Education & Information Service
National Cancer Centre
11 Hospital Drive
Singapore, 169610
Division of Medical Affairs

E-mail: nccypy@nccs.com.sg
Tel: (65) 6 236 9438
Fax: (65) 6 324 5664
www.nccs.com.sg

Slovakia

League Against Cancer in Slovakia
Spitalska 21
812 32 Bratislava, Slovakia
Tel: +42 7 321735
Fax: +42 7 321735

South Korea

Cancer Information Branch
National Cancer Center Research Institute
809 Madu-dong, Ilsan-gu, Goyang-si
Gyeonggi-do, 410-769
Korea (South)
E-mail: info@cancer.go.kr
Tel: +82 31 920 2161
Fax: +32 31 920 2032
Call center: +82 1577 8899
www.cancer.go.kr

South Africa

Cancer Association of South Africa
26 Concorde Road W,
Bedfordview 2007
Tel: +27 21 616 7662
Fax: +27 21 622 3424
www.cansa.org.za

Spain

Asociación Española Contra el Cáncer
c/ Amador de los Ríos,
5 Madrid, 28010
Tel: 0034913108221
Fax: 0034913190966
www.todocancer.org; www.muchoxvivir.org; www.aeccjunior.org

Sweden

Cancer Information Service
Radiumhemmet
Karolinska Hospital
S-171 76
Stockholm, Sweden
E-mail: cancerinfo@ks.se
Tel: +46 8 517 766 00 (helpline); +46 8 517 755 25 (office)
Fax: +46 8 318 204

Swedish Cancer Society
10155 Stockholm
Sweden
Tel: +4686771000
Fax: +4686771001
www.cancerfonden.se

Switzerland

Swiss Cancer League Krebstelefon
Effingerstrasse 40
3001 Bern, Switzerland
Tel: +41 31 389 9167
Fax: +41 31 389 9160
www.swisscancer.ch

COG Institutions in Switzerland
Swiss Pediatric Oncology Group Bern
Inselspital

Universitats-Kinderklinik
Bern, 3010
Tel: 41 31 6329372

Swiss Pediatric Oncology Group Geneva
6 Rue Willy Donze/1205 Geneva
Clinique De Pediatrie
Geneva, 1205
Tel: 41223823311 ext. 2458

Swiss Pediatric Oncology Group Lausanne
Rue DuBugnon 46
Centre Hosp. Univ. Vaudois, CHUV
Lausanne, 1011
Tel: 41 21 3143567
http://www.chuv.ch

Turkey

Turkish Association for Cancer Research and Control
Atac Sokak No:21/1 Yenisehir-Ankara
Turkey, 06410
Tel: +90-312 431 2950
Fax: +90-312 431 3958
www.turkcancer.org

United Kingdom

Macmillan Cancer Support
89 Albert Embankment
London, SE1 7UQ
Contact: S. Willis
E-mail: SWillis@macmillan.org.uk
Tel: +44 (0) 20 7840 7840
Fax: +44 (0) 20 7840 7841
For UK only: Cancerline 0808 808 2020 (Monday to Friday
9 a.m.–6 p.m.)
http://www.macmillan.org.uk/

Cancer Research UK
P.O. Box 123
London, WC2A 3PX
Tel: +44 (0) 20 7061 6017
Fax: +44 (0) 20 7061 6086
Helpline: (0) 207 061 8355
www.cancerhelp.org.uk
www.cancerresearchuk.org

There are clinics at the Great Ormond Street Hospital for Children in London, the Royal Marsden Pediatric Oncology units in London and Surrey, and the North of England Children's Cancer Research Unit at the Royal Victoria Infirmary in Newcastle, among others.

Venezuela

There are clinics at the Hospital de Ninos J.M. de los Rios in Caracas and the Hospital de Especialidades Pediatricas in Maracaibo.

Zambia

Zambian Cancer Society
P.O. Box 51127
Lusaka, Zambia, 1001
E-mail: info@zambiancancersociety.org
Tel: +2601 293574
http://zambiancancersociety.cfsites.org/

Medical Tests

Note: Throughout this section two terms are used to describe substances that help the physician or technician distinguish various body tissues and make cells clearer for study. A *dye* is a coloring matter used in tests like a lymphangiogram. (A *stain* is also a material used to color tissues on slides for microscopic study; the specific stain used in each instance depends on what the doctor is looking for.) A *contrast medium*, like the barium used in a GI series, shows up opaque in x-rays.

AFP (Alpha-fetoprotein) assay Blood test to detect a specific antigen in the blood. Normal in the fetus, but when AFP is found in older infants and children, it may be an indication of primary liver cancer, testicular or ovarian tumors, germ cell tumors, perhaps Hodgkin disease, lymphoma, some kidney tumors, or malignant teratoma. It is never found in benign teratoma. Patients in remission have a negative test for AFP and those relapsing either locally or through metastases again have a positive reading. Not used as much for diagnosing cancer as for monitoring a patient's response to therapy.

Angiogram Also called *arteriogram* if an artery (blood vessel carrying blood from the heart to body tissues) is used, or *venogram* if a vein (carrying the blood to the heart on the return trip) is used. An angiogram studies these blood vessels using an injected contrast medium that helps doctors differentiate tissues. After the injection the patient is x-rayed to follow the track of the contrast medium. The test is performed to locate tumors before surgery or radiation and to follow the progress of therapy. Some angiograms are now replaced by CT scans, but if the surgeon needs information on the blood supply to and from a tumor or organ, a CT scan is inadequate. The patient is usually not allowed food or, less often, drink for several hours before the test and may be asked to empty his bladder. Any metal jewelry will need to be removed. If the area to be studied is in the lower abdomen, the patient may have an enema or a laxative before the test is begun. Sometimes the contrast medium can be given by a needle directly into a blood vessel, but in other cases a catheter (thin tube) must be inserted into the blood vessel, in which case a local anesthetic deadens the pain at the site. After the contrast medium is introduced, a series of x-rays is taken in rapid succession. The test, which usually takes from an hour up to half a day, may require hospitalization. It is hard for the child to be still, but the only pain is from the contrast medium, which may cause a burning sensation. If a catheter is used, the patient may feel cramps in the artery as it is slipped into place, but they don't last long. Some patients can taste the contrast medium and others have headaches or nausea afterwards. If the injection site hurts or is developing a black-and-blue mark, ask for an ice pack. Serious side effects, including allergic reactions, are rare but catheters have been known to rupture blood vessels or to inject air bubbles to block the vessels.

Barium enema   Also called *lower GI series* or *colon x-ray*. Barium is a contrast medium that shows up clearly on x-rays. In children the test is used most often to locate pelvic tumors by identifying displacement, unusual compression, or other abnormalities of the colon or rectum. For this test barium is introduced into the colon and rectum by an enema. If a complete GI series is performed, this part is done first. The preparation is unpleasant, with the bowel cleansed through food restrictions, laxatives, and enemas. After the barium is introduced into the body, the child is moved to allow all areas of the large intestine to be coated with the substance. The technician takes pictures, then the child goes to the bathroom to eliminate as much of the contrast medium as possible, after which more x-rays are taken. Air may be blown into the colon to distend it for further study. The test is performed at the hospital, either as an inpatient or outpatient procedure, and in some doctors' offices. It takes up to an hour. The enemas are unpleasant and there may be cramps. Many patients are embarrassed to "dribble" the barium before they reach the bathroom; reassure your child that this is a typical, unavoidable occurrence. The child's stools may be white for several days after the test, and he may need extra fluid to keep from getting dehydrated and a laxative to get rid of the barium.

Barium meal   Also called *upper GI series, barium swallow,* or *esophagography.* This is not used as often in children, because stomach cancers are rare in this age group, but it may be performed to look for an esophagus pushed aside by a tumor or to check for a tumor in the small bowel. The patient may not be allowed to eat for several hours before the procedure. He is given a small amount of barium to swallow, and then the table he is lying on may be tilted to allow the material to spread throughout the upper gastrointestinal system. This is done on an outpatient basis at the hospital. It is not painful, but the barium, despite flavorings like chocolate and strawberry, is chalky and sure to produce a "Yuck!" from the patient. The stool will be white for a couple of days unless the doctor follows the test with an enema to clean out the barium more quickly. After the test, diarrhea may occur but constipation is a much more likely problem. Ask your doctor for a laxative.

Biopsy   A procedure to remove a sample of body tissue for close examination to determine if abnormal cells are present. The term is also used to describe the examination of the tissue itself. In some cases there is a risk that biopsy, in breaking into the tumor, will allow malignant cells to spread. Despite anesthesia, there may be bleeding or pain after the test, depending on the site and the procedure used, and scars may be left. Biopsies are done on either an inpatient or outpatient basis in the hospital or office. A final report on the biopsy results may not be available for a few days. Tissue for a biopsy is obtained in several ways:

- By surgical removal of part or all of a growth (incisional biopsy removes part of a tumor and excisional biopsy takes the whole thing)
- By a needle or aspiration biopsy, with a fine needle pushed into the suspected tissue and a tiny sample withdrawn, somewhat like a reverse injection (a bone marrow biopsy is an example)
- By a punch biopsy, which is like a needle biopsy but with an instrument to make a larger opening
- By scraping body cavities and linings, like a Papanicolaou (Pap) smear

Two biopsy procedures for solid tissue are commonly used. Either a frozen section is done on thin sheets of frozen materials—if this is definitive, results can be obtained within hours—or a fixed section is prepared, embedding tissue in paraffin and then making thin slices. Unless special stains and tests are used that take even longer, this usually takes 24 hours. Non-solid tissue is smeared on a slide.

A pathologist examines the sample under a microscope to determine what cells are present and, if malignant cells are found, to identify the type. Biopsy is a definitive step in diagnosis, preceded by tests like x-rays and other laboratory tests.

Preparation for a biopsy depends on the procedure. If general anesthesia is involved, the patient won't be able to eat or drink for some time, but if a needle biopsy is planned perhaps no advance preparation at all will be needed.

Blood count   Also called *CBC* or *complete blood count and smear.* A blood sample is drawn either by poking a little hole in the fingertip (a finger stick) or by taking larger amounts through a needle inserted in a vein or an indwelling catheter. The blood is smeared on a glass plate (slide), stained for greater contrast, and put under a microscope to assess normal cells and blasts. The laboratory technician looks at the size, shape, and appearance of red blood cells and the distribution of various white blood cells and estimates the number of platelets and whether they stick together. On the slide the smear may show either abnormal leukemic cells or an abnormal proportion of normal cell types. A CBC is performed routinely on all chemotherapy patients, whether they have leukemia or not, to watch for side effects of the medications. A low white cell count can indicate a predisposition to infection. A low platelet count may lead to easy bruising or bleeding, even internally. A low red cell count indicates anemia, resulting in tiredness and weakness in the child. The technician counts the number of white cells per cubic centimeter; the differential ("diff"), or proportion of different kinds of white blood cells; the number of platelets; and the shape, size, and color of red blood cells.

Bone marrow aspiration   Also called a *bone tap* or *bone marrow biopsy.* A form of biopsy used at regular intervals during leukemia therapy to check the percentage of blasts in the marrow, the spongy material at the middle of some bones where blood cells are made. This is a test to diagnose the specific form of leukemia, to stage lymphomas, to assess the child's progress during therapy, and to determine if it is necessary or possible to modify treatment. The doctor can spot a relapse early in the bone marrow and change the treatments before the child has any symptoms of illness. It is also used to find out if solid tumors have spread to the marrow and to evaluate a patient's response to therapy. The procedure can be frightening and painful, although the discomfort is eased some through local anesthesia or conscious sedation. The procedure can be performed almost anywhere. It takes about 5 minutes, but the most painful part, the actual drawing of the marrow, lasts only a few seconds. Sites used most often for the procedure are at the rear of the pelvis (ilium) or vertebrae; bones closest to the surface are best. The skin above the bone is cleansed and a local anesthetic injected. After allowing time for it to deaden the nerves, the needle is inserted into the bone cavity, the marrow sample is withdrawn, and the needle is removed. The child may feel pressure or brief pain when the needle is pushed through the bone, because it isn't possible to deaden the membrane around the bone itself. The site may be sore afterwards or marked by a bruise. There is a small risk of continued bleeding and infection at the injection site. Mild pain relievers may be appropriate for a couple of days after the procedure for pain at the puncture site.

Bone scan   (See *Scan*)

Brain scan   (See *Scan*)

Bronchoscopy   A lighted instrument is slipped into the trachea (windpipe) and moved along until the doctor can take a direct look at the bronchial branches (passages leading to the lungs). During the procedure the doctor can remove foreign bodies and take cell samples with a brush to examine under the microscope. The patient can't eat or drink anything before the procedure. General or local anesthesia is used, the latter perhaps sprayed or dripped into the mouth or throat. The test is done in the hospital, and although there is no danger that the patient will be unable to breathe, it is uncomfortable. Relaxing helps, perhaps with the aid of a sedative or guided imagery. Occasionally the throat, gums, teeth, or bronchi are damaged by the instrument but this is a minor risk factor. Any blood brought up after the test should be reported to the doctor.

BUN (Blood urea nitrogen)   (See *Kidney function tests*)

CAT or CT scan   (See *Computed tomography*)

Cerebral arteriography   Angiography of the brain, using contrast medium injected into a blood vessel in the neck, via a catheter inserted in an arm or leg and then threaded to the appropriate vessel in the neck. Brain x-rays follow. (See *Angiogram*)

Cisternal tap   An alternative test to a spinal tap, used to draw cerebrospinal fluid (CSF) from near the base of the brain. It may be done instead of or in addition to the spinal tap, perhaps to locate a blockage. The nape of the neck is shaved and the fluid is withdrawn through a needle inserted between the base of the skull and the top vertebrae of the neck. A local anesthetic is used. Usually done by neurosurgeons, it takes about 15 minutes but is usually an inpatient procedure to allow the hospital staff to watch for abnormal fluctuations in heartbeat and respiration. The patient will feel the usual needle pain from the anesthetic, pressure when the CSF is drawn, and maybe discomfort from the tucked chin position he must hold. A severe headache is less likely after a cisternal tap than after a lumbar puncture.

Computed tomography   Also called *CAT scan, computerized axial transverse tomography,* or *CT scan.* A special form of x-ray that provides a very detailed picture of a cross-section of the body. An outpatient procedure at the hospital, there are no preparations unless a contrast medium is used, for example barium for an abdominal scan. The patient lies down and the machine that takes the pictures rotates around him, passing radiation through a thin cross-section of the body. The resulting signals are analyzed by a computer on a television-type screen. The equipment may be frightening to children, and sedation or anesthesia may be used to ensure immobility since movement results in blurred images. The test actually measures the densities of the tissue in question; the resulting cross-section is like a three-dimensional image showing the body organs and tissues, how they relate to one another in shape and size, and differences in soft tissue and bones. The scans may be brain scans or whole-body scans, and the subsequent need for arteriographs may be eliminated. Exploratory surgery may even be avoided in some cases. CT scanning, often used to guide needle biopsy of a tumor or organ, is especially useful for studying eyes, chest, limbs, brain, and abdomen. It is generally painless and without after-effects. Because the process is so fast, there is far less exposure to radiation than with a single ordinary x-ray. Quicker than MRI, these scans provide images many times sharper and clearer than ordinary x-rays.

Creatinine   Creatinine levels are measured to determine how well the kidneys are filtering waste products from the blood. Creatinine can be measured through blood tests but is most commonly tested by collecting all urine passed for 24 hours (called, naturally, a "24-hour urine" creatinine clearance). It is sometimes possible to measure creatinine with urine collections over 2, 5, 6, or 12 hours. If you are collecting urine at home, you will have to be alert to ensure that all urine is collected and saved. If a child is hospitalized, a catheter or special bed may be used. Timing and accurate collection are important. See that the child drinks plenty of liquids during the test. When the test starts, the child urinates, that urine is discarded, and the clock starts running. Refrigerate the urine if you are collecting it at home.

Culture   The testing of body fluids, secretions, and tissues for the presence of disease-causing microbes (bacteria or germs, viruses, parasites and the like). Besides blood and urine, a culture may be made of secretions from the eyes, ears, nose, throat, stool, cervix, cerebrospinal fluid, or wounds. These microbes may be detectable under a microscope, but a culture is necessary to identify the exact type. Sterile specimens are obtained by taking a swab of the suspected area, or drawing blood from a vein or indwelling catheter, or collecting clean urine. The samples are then usually transferred to two or more dishes of "food" medium and left to grow, under carefully controlled temperature and oxygen conditions. The number and type of bacteria present are important. If microbes then grow, further tests are carried out to determine exactly what they are and which antibiotic will kill them. The whole process takes a day or two. Simple cultures can be carried out in doctors' offices, but others require sophisticated techniques and equipment found in laboratories and hospitals. In the case of urine cultures, you can collect the specimen at home.

Cystography   A contrast medium is instilled into the urinary bladder and x-rays are taken. The urologist or radiologist studies the bladder and the urethra, looking at the location, dislocation, or compression of the bladder and the bladder neck. It is most useful in children with pelvic tumors like rhabdomyosarcomas. Bladder function is also assessed by studying the rate at which it fills and empties.

Cystoscope   Also called *cystourethroscope*. The doctor inserts a lighted instrument through the urethra and into the bladder for a direct look. He can take a specimen for biopsy or remove small growths and stones at the same time. Expect eating and drinking restrictions before the test. For small children this is an inpatient procedure done under anesthesia, although some hospitals may perform cystoscopy as day surgery, allowing the child to go home after an observation period. It is often done as an outpatient procedure for older children, using local anesthesia. It may take only a few minutes or up to an hour. There may be nausea when the anesthesia wears off and perhaps some muscle stiffness. Cystoscopy is considered highly accurate and reliable because of the direct view it affords.

Cytology   Study of cells to detect abnormal (malignant) cells. Body materials tested include urine, cerebrospinal fluid, scrapings, sputum, and the like. Doctors use cytological techniques to make very early cancer diagnoses. It also shows the effects of radiation and infection. The cells in question are stained for greater contrast and then examined under the microscope. A Papanicolaou (Pap) smear is a form of cytological study.

Echogram   (See *Ultrasonography*)

Electroencephalogram (EEG)   Used to diagnose epilepsy and diseases of the brain. An EEG shows the electrical activity of the brain (brain waves) on a graph. In combination with other tests, it diagnoses brain tumors. The test is safe but the child may have to be sedated in preparation for it. It isn't as good as a scan or contrast ventriculography. One to two dozen electrodes are attached to the scalp with adhesive, and the child must remain still while the needle forms the graph. There should be no pain, however, providing the needle-less electrode is used.

Endoscopy   Direct examination of internal body structures by a lighted instrument. May be gastroscopy (examination of esophagus, stomach, and part of the small intestine) or colonoscopy (examination of the rectum and bowel). Not generally painful, although there may be temporary cramping or a feeling of pressure. May replace exploratory surgery and therefore avoid anesthesia, hospitalization, and recovery. May be safely repeated. In the case of a colonoscopy, the preparation to clean the bowel is often more unpleasant than the test itself.

Fluoroscopy A form of x-ray recorded on a fluorescent screen to study organs in motion. May include an examination of the esophagus, stomach, and the first part of the small intestine after a barium meal, or of the lower digestive tract after a barium enema. Used to outline or locate a tumor in the area behind the abdomen as well.

GI series (See *Barium enema and Barium meal*)

Gonadotropin level One of the tests used to determine if the testicles are functioning properly. Also used to test women for pregnancy. It checks the level of human chorionic gonadotropin (hCG), a hormone in the urine and blood. Used when tumors of the testes, ovaries, adrenal glands, hypothalamus, or pituitary are suspected.

Intravenous pyelogram (IVP) Also called *excretory urography*. Examination of the urinary tract by x-rays after injection of a contrast medium into a vein. Studies the kidneys, ureters, bladder, and urethra. Films are taken over a period of time to show how the system is working and the position of the organs. Preparation may require cleaning the bowel through laxatives or an enema, to avoid confusing images on the screen. Check this with your doctor, because children on chemotherapy don't get routine enemas. Don't assume the x-ray department and the oncology clinic each knows what the other is doing. The child will have to forego food and drink for a few hours before the test. The first x-ray is taken a short time after the injection and then a series are taken over a period of time, perhaps as long as 24 hours, depending on how efficiently the urinary system is working. It hurts when the IV is started but otherwise there is little discomfort.

Kidney function tests A series of urine tests to assess how the kidneys and urinary tract are working. They include, but are not limited to, a test for BUN and creatinine.

Laryngoscopy Also called *larynx test*. A laryngoscope, or hollow lighted tube, is inserted into the throat so the doctor can take a look. The patient can't eat or drink for a few hours before the test. Painkillers, a sedative, and perhaps a drug to cut down on throat secretions may be given, as well as general or local (sprayed or dripped) anesthetic. The doctor can take a specimen for biopsy, remove small growths, or apply medicine directly to the larynx (voice box). This is a half-hour outpatient procedure, although the doctor may observe the child for some time after. This is an uncomfortable test because of the position and the gag reflex but it isn't actually painful.

Risks are low, but do report bleeding or any pain beyond a few days' sore throat to the doctor.

Liver function tests   Blood or urine samples are tested for the following substances to assess function of the liver:

- Bilirubin—a waste product consisting mostly of broken-down red blood cells (blood and urine tested)
- Albumin/globulin—proteins that indicate kidney and liver function (blood is tested)
- Alkaline phosphatase—an enzyme tied to bone growth and liver function (blood is tested)
- Alanine aminotransferase (ALT, SGOT), aspartate aminotransferase (AST)—enzymes in the heart and liver, released into the blood when there is liver damage (blood is tested)
- Lactic acid dehydrogenase (LDH)—an enzyme (blood and spinal fluid are tested)

Lumbar puncture   Also called *spinal tap*. Used to check for abnormal cells in the cerebrospinal fluid (CSF; fluid in the spinal column and brain). This is more frightening than painful. A needle is inserted into the spinal canal between two vertebrae in the lower back and the fluid drawn is studied for cell content and color, to diagnose infection and central nervous system extension of leukemia. The fluid should be clear. The patient usually lies on his side in a tucked position and is given a local anesthetic. A young child might cooperate better if he practices the position ahead of time in a place where he feels safe. Spinal taps are sometimes done in the hospital but may be performed on outpatients in the clinic, too. The procedure takes up to half an hour. There is pain from the anesthetic injection and pressure from the needle. Scar tissue may build up as the test is repeated over a period of time. If a headache develops, the child should find relief by lying flat. There may also be a stiff neck or low-grade fever afterward.

Lymphangiography   Also called *lymphography*. A special technique used to look at the lymph system. After a local anesthetic is given, a blue dye is injected to color the lymphatic vessels. Then the skin is opened and a thin tube is slipped into a lymph channel in the foot, usually between the toes. It's tested to ensure proper placement, and a contrast medium is injected. X-rays are taken as the contrast medium spreads through the body. This is an outpatient procedure that takes from a couple of hours to a day; it is boring, so take along toys or reading material. There isn't much pain involved in lymphangiography except the sting of the anesthetic needle. It is tedious, technically difficult, and often unsuccessful, especially in small children.

The risks are small; the child's urine or stool might be blue after the test or, rarely, oil drops from the dye get in the lungs and complicate matters if the youngster is already having respiratory difficulties. It can lead to blood clots in lung blood vessels and shortness of breath. The test provides an x-ray of the lymph vessels and nodes, including tumors and metastases, which often disseminate via the lymph system. Its major pediatric uses are in Hodgkin disease and sarcomas in the lower body.

Lymphography   (See *Lymphangiography*)

Magnetic resonance imaging   Also called *MRI, nuclear magnetic resonance,* or *NMR,* this procedure allows doctors to look inside the body without surgery. It produces images sharper than those of ultrasound, and it studies soft tissues and organs invisible on x-rays to find tumors without biopsy and to watch chemical changes without a blood sample. MRI takes advantage of the varying chemical structures of different tissues and cells to create these images. The procedure works because different types of cells have nuclei (the core or "brain" of the cell) that spin or wobble at different speeds. MRI employs a powerful magnetic field to align the nuclei, and then a cross-field is turned on and off, causing the atoms to flip-flop at a predetermined frequency. The resulting motion is picked up by a computer, which creates a three-dimensional picture of the tissue or organ. Most commonly studied by MRI, the hydrogen atom is of course found in the body in water cells. MRI can find chemical changes in the body caused by drugs in just a few days. Because cancerous tissue, even at very early stages, responds to magnetic forces differently from normal tissue, MRI can distinguish between them. It shows the extent of cancer within a diseased organ and finds spread beyond the organ of origin earlier than other procedures can. While CT scans image slices of the body, MRI can study an entire vertical structure like the spine all at once. The patient is placed in a chamber inside a huge magnet. There is no pain involved and, unlike the radiation associated with CT scans or nuclear medicine scans, there is no known danger from magnetic fields. MRI is especially useful in studying muscles, fat, and internal organs in the abdomen, pelvis, and brain, but bone is not "seen" because of its low water content. MRI is slower than CT but much more sensitive and sharp and can be repeated without risk. With new equipment, even total body MRI can be performed quickly with high-quality images and is increasingly preferred over CT scanning. The equipment can be frightening, especially for patients who tend toward claustrophobia, but newer "open" MRIs address this problem effectively.

Nuclear medicine   A medical specialty that uses radioactive materials with an affinity for particular organs. (See *Scan*)

Ophthalmoscope   Not a "test" per se, an ophthalmoscope is an instrument used to examine the eyeball, especially the retina. A small beam of light is directed through the pupil onto the back of the eyeball. This is part of a routine physical examination and of an eye examination. It is also used to check for certain tumors or for early evidence of leukemia in the central nervous system. There is usually no preparation required and no risk or pain involved. It is also called *funduscopy*. To diagnose retinoblastoma, the specialist puts drops in the child's eyes and uses a binocular ophthalmoscope, which allows a better view. The instrument, which has a bright light, is worn on the doctor's head and can locate tumors less than a quarter-inch in diameter. It helps if the test is done by the same person who will be assessing the results of treatment later. It takes about 15 minutes to examine both eyes. The procedure may have to be done under general anesthesia to ensure that all areas of the retina are visualized, especially with retinoblastoma.

Positron emission tomography (PET)   PET is a diagnostic tool to detect and stage some cancers. It looks at the body's chemistry, finding abnormalities that might not be detected by CT or MRI scans alone. PET can show if some tumors are benign or malignant. Follow-up scans check the efficacy of therapy. PET scans are based on a radioactive form of glucose. The patient is usually not allowed to eat or drink for several hours before the test. A radioactive substance is injected by IV, and after a brief wait, the scans begin. The test takes between 90 minutes and 3 hours, with generally no after-effects.

Retrograde pyelogram   Also called *urethrography*. Performed by injecting a contrast medium directly into the urethra by a catheter or cystoscope, then up into the ureters and kidneys. This is used when the doctor thinks there is a problem in the urinary tract somewhere below the kidneys and needs to outline the bladder and ureters.

Scan   A test using a radioactive contrast medium to study specific tissues or organ systems. Different tissues take up the contrast medium differently, and the scan works by detecting radiation given off by the medium, noting where the material collects. The test outlines the shape, size, and precise location of the organ in question, assessing the function as well. If excess radioactive material is taken up, or if part of the organ doesn't take up the material at all, a defect or malfunction may be suspected. The contrast medium may be given orally or by IV, possibly preceded by another material (a blocker) that stops other organs from absorbing the material. Scanners then detect the radiation emitting from the target area, creating a visual image. Scans are also used to follow tagged blood cells to see where they go. Some older scanners move back and forth, but newer cameras are fixed. Scans are performed in nuclear medicine departments, usually on an outpatient basis.

The time needed to complete the test varies, but be prepared to wait; it is possible that pictures will be taken for hours, or there might be a lengthy delay after the contrast medium is injected before it moves into the system sufficiently to begin scanning. The large machines may frighten some children, and it is hard for them to lie still. You will probably be allowed to stay with your child, because, unlike x-rays, there is no danger of radiation. There is no need to fear the small amount of radioactive material used, which will be gone from the body in a day or so. Nor are the scanners dangerous. The injection of the contrast medium is the major discomfort from the test.

Bone scan   Used to look for bone tumors and metastases to bone, and to check the effects of therapy. Usually performed with radioactive technetium. A "hot spot" of increased contrast medium uptake most often means a tumor is present but can also mean a fracture, arthritis, or infection.

Gallium scan   A total body scan using radioactive gallium, which seeks inflamed tissue or accumulations of white blood cells, so it is used to check for suspected bone infections or lymphoma. Preparation includes an enema or laxative but no restriction of food or drink. The contrast medium is picked up by rapidly dividing cells like tumors. Usually 48 hours lapse between the injection and the scan, which may be repeated over a few days. The only pain is the injection of the contrast medium, and there are no side effects.

Kidney scan   Used to evaluate kidney function as well as to identify structural abnormalities. Distinguishes between Wilms tumor and neuroblastoma because the latter pushes the kidney aside without invading it, whereas the former replaces actual kidney tissue.

Liver scan   Used to check for primary tumors and metastases. When repeated, can follow the course of the disease and its therapy. Combined as a liver–spleen scan, it sorts out cysts (benign tumors) from malignancies. Lymphoma is, for all practical purposes, the only spleen malignancy, but there are numerous causes of an enlarged spleen.

Sed rate   Also called *ESR* or *erythrocyte sedimentation rate*. Tests certain activities of red blood cells taken in a blood sample. A raised sed rate indicates that an infection or inflammation is present somewhere in the body. (See *Liver function tests*)

Serum electrolytes   Analysis of chemical substances in the blood and urine to evaluate the balance of the body's fluids. Sodium, potassium, calcium, and magnesium are all positively charged; chloride, bicarbonate, phosphate, sulfate, protein, and organic acids are negatively charged. In a healthy body the positively charged ions and the negatively charged ions equal each other.

Spinal tap   (See *Lumbar puncture*)

Thoracentesis *(pleural tap)* Drawing fluid from the space around the lungs. A healthy chest does not contain any fluid, so when the pools are detected during x-rays or ultrasound, a needle is inserted and a sample drawn for study. In other words, the test seeks the cause of the fluid accumulation and searches for tumor or inflammatory cells. The doctor may give the patient medicine to suppress coughing during the test. A large amount of fluid may be withdrawn through thoracentesis to ease breathing difficulties. Follow-up x-rays may be taken to ensure the lung didn't collapse during the procedure.

24-hour urine Used to determine urine proteins and electrolytes. If you are collecting urine at home, use sterile containers and keep the specimen refrigerated until you deliver it to the doctor or the laboratory. (See *Creatinine*)

Ultrasonography Also called *ultrasound*; used especially to diagnose and locate tumors and blood clots in the body's trunk. Employs the principles of sonar: sound waves are bounced off tissues, echoes are picked up, and the results are recorded visually. The technician uses a handheld probe passed over the abdomen to find abnormal lymph nodes and primary or metastatic tumors. It can distinguish between solid masses and cysts. There is no radiation exposure and the doctor can study entire areas, unlike scans, which are specific to a single organ system. Ultrasound can locate growths an inch in diameter. The test is not painful and there is no preparation. The slippery-feeling substance spread on the target area to facilitate the test is easily wiped off.

Urinalysis Study of a urine specimen by chemical tests and under the microscope, checking acidity and waste materials content and looking for albumin (a protein), sugar, blood, and bacteria. Composition of the urine is an excellent indicator of general health as well as of kidney function. The lab prefers about 2 ounces or a quarter-cup of urine to test, but when that's impossible they can test smaller amounts. Some urine tests are performed by dipping specially treated paper strips into the urine. For very small children who are not yet toilet-trained, a clear plastic bag may be glued in place after the child is carefully cleansed to eliminate surface bacteria. The nurse may train you in this procedure. You should know how to do the special skin cleansing anyway, because you will surely have to collect a "clean voided specimen" someday if the urine has to be cultured, although it is not part of routine urinalysis. The trick to making the bag stick is ensuring that the skin is absolutely dry—but don't use a towel, which will contaminate your cleaning job. Even skilled nurses have trouble making the bags stick. Rip a hole in the diaper for the bag to drop through—then you can watch and remove it as soon as urine is collected and before it can leak. If the child doesn't urinate, running water may help, but having him play in lukewarm water with boats or syringes is better, as well as distracting.

Urogram   (See *Intravenous pyelogram and VCUG*)

VCUG   Also called *voiding cystourethrogram, voiding urethrogram, cystourethrogram, excretory urography,* this is an x-ray study of the bladder and urethra while the child urinates. The bladder is drained. A contrast medium is introduced into the bladder by a catheter through the urethra, monitored by a fluoroscope. More x-rays are taken while the child urinates onto a pad. The test takes only a few minutes and isn't painful, although the insertion of the catheter is uncomfortable. It may be embarrassing or inhibiting, especially for older children, and younger ones may not cooperate.

Venipuncture   Blood draw, the procedure used to withdraw a blood sample for testing in the laboratory. A needle is inserted into a vein, often inside one elbow, although almost any vein can be used. There is a sharp pain when the needle is inserted, continuing as it is moved into place, but otherwise there is no discomfort. Pressure is applied after the needle is pulled out to stop the bleeding, a process that may take a while if platelets are low. There may be a black-and-blue mark afterward. Children with indwelling catheters and ports are spared most of the venipunctures that earlier patients had to endure.

Venography   Angiography with contrast medium injected into a vein (blood vessel leading toward the heart). Useful in Wilms tumor to check for extension of disease along the renal vein and into the inferior vena cava, which may show a shifted location, compression, or a blockage.

VMA (vanillylmandelic acid) and catecholamines   A 24-hour urine test that is more accurate than a blood test to determine the level of certain substances. An elevated VMA level could indicate the presence of neuroblastoma. This is a noninvasive screening test. Not all neuroblastomas will respond to this test. There is a paper filter version of the VMA test. Some foods can skew the test results.

X-rays   Diagnostic x-rays are "pictures" taken of various areas of the body, like the chest or a limb, to look for abnormalities. They do not hurt, but the child must sit or lie still. Takes only a couple of minutes. Radiation builds up in the body over a period of time and can be dangerous, so doctors use the smallest dose possible to avoid injury to the patient. Special therapeutic x-rays are also used to treat some forms of cancer (radiation therapy). Special pediatric clinics have staff trained in taking and reading children's x-rays. A stool shaped like an animal or seasonal decorations help relax an apprehensive child. You may be able to stay with your child for some x-rays but you will be asked to wear a protective apron. If there is any possibility you may be pregnant, wait outside, because the fetus can be harmed by x-rays.

Further Information

These descriptions are minimal, but there are a number of good books and Web sites devoted entirely to medical tests.

"Lab Tests Online" by the professionals who perform them (American Association for Clinical Chemistry) (www.labtestsonline.org)

Information is given in several languages, including Australian and British forms of English. Has quick and longer versions of hundreds of tests. Excellent site.

Medical tests sourcebook: Basic consumer health information about medical tests.

Detroit: Omnigraphics, 3d ed., 2008.

A huge compendium of medical test information, most likely to be found in a library's reference section.

Pagana, Kathleen Deska, and Timothy J. Pagana. *Mosby's diagnosis and laboratory tests reference.* St. Louis, MO: Mosby, 2007.

Segen, Joseph C., MD, and Joseph Stauffer, PhD. *The patient's guide to medical tests: Everything you need to know about the tests your doctor prescribes.* New York: Facts on File, 1998.

www.bloodbook.com
This Web site has an extensive discussion of normal blood counts and ranges that seems very complete.

http://childhoodcancerguides.org/c-bld-mean.html
On the Childhood Cancer Guides Web site, mounted by a nonprofit organization, this page has a list of normal blood counts and values, followed by a clear description of the meaning of each. Clearly written and highly recommended.

Bibliography

Over the course of updating *Children with Cancer: A Reference Guide for Parents,* I consulted thousands of sources: books, articles, Web sites, other online resources, and more. Some of the items I cite are old, but they are the foundation on which the new material is built. I consulted many of the Web sites repeatedly, but I cite only enough dates here to recognize the value of the sites and their owners to this book and to the childhood cancer community. Additional sources are listed at the ends of some chapters.

5 suggestions for evaluating a healthcare web site. *Messageline,* vol. 33 (1) (Spring 2006), p. 1.

Ablin, Arthur. *Supportive Care of Children with Cancer (Series in Hematology Oncology).* Baltimore, MD: Johns Hopkins University Press, 2d ed., 1999.

Abrahms, Sally. How I got through it. *Parade Magazine,* October 19, 2008, pp. 2–3. Available at www.parade.com/inspiration

Abrams A N., et al. Psychosocial issues in adolescents with cancer. *Cancer Treatment Reviews,* vol. 33 (2007), pp. 622–630.

Accessing implanted venous access ports. *CareNotes* [Thomson Healthcare Inc.], December 2001.

Acute Lymphocytic Leukemia: A Guide for Patients and Families. White Plains, NY: Leukemia & Lymphoma Society, 2006.

Adams, David W. When a brother or sister is dying of cancer: the vulnerability of the adolescent sibling. *Death Studies,* vol. 11 (4) (1987), pp. 391–395.

Adams, Patch, with Maureen Mylander. *Gesundheit: Bringing Good Health to You.* Rochester, VT: Healing Arts Press, 1993, 1998.

Ahlbom, Anders, and Maria Feychting. Current thinking about risks from currents. *Lancet,* vol. 357 (9263) (April 14, 2001), p. 1143.

Akyüz, C., et al. Medulloblastoma in children: a 32-year experience from a single institution. *Journal of Neuro-Oncology*, vol. 90 (1) (October 2008), pp. 99–103.

Albritton, Karen. Age matters: The problems with teen cancer care. *Quarterly Journal of the National Office, Candlelighters Childhood Cancer Foundation,* Spring 2005, pp. 1.

Alexander, Freda A. Clusters and clustering of childhood cancer: a review. *European Journal of Epidemiology*, vol. 15 (9) (October 1, 1999), pp. 847–852.

Allen, Scott. New marrow brings hope for kidney recipients. *Boston Globe,* January 12, 2004, p. A1.

Alternative drugs may cause trouble for cancer patients. *Reuters Health Information.* Retrieved on July 21, 2001, from www.medformation.com

Altman, Arnold J., et al. The Management of Pain. Chapter 11 in *The Supportive Care of Children with Cancer,* edited by Arthur Ablin. Baltimore, MD: Johns Hopkins University Press, 2d ed., 1999, pp. 155–173.

Altman, Roberta, and Michael J. Sarg, MD. *The Cancer Dictionary*. New York: Facts on File, Inc., 1992.

American Cancer Society. Web exclusive: Types of non-Hodgkin lymphoma. *Cure Today*. Retrieved on November 21, 2009, from www.curetoday.com

American Cancer Society's Guide to Complementary and Alternative Cancer Methods. Atlanta, GA: American Cancer Society, 2000.

Anderson, Patricia. *Affairs in Order: A Complete Resource Guide to Death and Dying.* New York: Macmillan Publishing Company, 1991.

Anderson, W.A. EST of the vagina—the role of primary chemotherapy. *Cancer,* vol. 56 (5) (September 1, 1985), pp. 1025–1027.

Andreae, Christine. *When Evening Comes: The Education of a Hospice Volunteer.* New York: St. Martin's Press, 2000.

Angier, Natalie. Theory links clinic lights and a cancer. *New York Times* (July 29, 1992), p. C12.

Annual Report, National Childhood Cancer Foundation. Arcadia, CA: NCCF, 1999.

Are electric blankets safe? *Consumer Reports,* vol. 54 (11) (November 1989), pp. 715–716.

Arjona, David E. World without cancer: Simply the most successful cancer therapy available, vitamin B-17 cancer therapy. *World Without Cancer.* Retrieved on February 4, 1999, from www.vitaminb17.net

Arms Around Those Touched by Cancer. Center for Cancer Support and Education, nd.

Avoiding the charlatans. In *Web of Deception,* Anne P. Mintz, et al., eds. Medford, NJ: CyberAge Books, 2002, pp. 41–45.

Aydin, S., et al. Rituximab plus ASHAP for the treatment of patients with relapsed or refractory aggressive non-Hodgkin's lymphoma. *Annals of Hematology,* vol. 86 (4) (April 2007), pp. 271–276.

Back to School: IEPs and legal rights of cancer patients in the public education system. Ped-Onc Resource Center. Retrieved on December 8, 2009, from www.acor.org/ped-onc

Baertlein, Lisa. Video game maker targets teens with cancer. *PC World.* Retrieved on June 4, 2007, from www.reuters.com

Bain, Lisa J. *A Parent's Guide to Childhood Cancer [The Children's Hospital of Philadelphia].* New York: Dell Publishing, 1995.

Baker, P. J., and D. G. Hoel. Meta-analysis of standardized incidence and morality rates of childhood leukaemia in proximity to nuclear facilities. *European Journal of Cancer Care*, vol. 16 (4) (July 2007), pp. 355–363.

Balancing Act: Tips for the Cancer Caregiver. Washington, DC: The Wellness Community, nd.

Balen, R., et al. An activity week for children with cancer: who wants to go and why? *Child: Care Health & Development*, vol. 24 (2) (March 1, 1998), pp. 169–177.

Balter, Michael. Chernobyl's thyroid cancer toll. *Science*, vol. 270 (5243) (December 15, 1995), pp. 1758.

Band-Aids & blackboards. *Chronic Illness, Adults, Health Education.* Retrieved on November 23, 2002, from www.faculty.fairfield.edu

Barnard, Anne. New cancer type identified. *Boston Globe*, August 31, 2001, p. A8.

Barrera, Maru, et al. Educational and social late effects of childhood cancer and related clinical, personal, and familial characteristics. *Cancer* vol. 104 (8) (2005), pp. 1751–1760.

Barrett, Stephen, and Victor Herbert. More ploys that may fool you. Retrieved on July 16, 2001, from www.quackwatch.com

Barrow, Karen. Re-Mission impossible: Teaching kids how to make cancer self-destruct. Retrieved on May 26, 2006, from http://attworldnet.healthology.com

"Baywatch" beauty had a bout with cancer as a child. *Childhood Cancerline*, vol. 7 (1) (2001?), pp. 1.

Because…Someone I Love Has Cancer…Kids' Activity Book. Atlanta, GA: American Cancer Society Health Content Products, 2003.

Bell, Laura. A different kind of caring. *Cure*, vol. 5 (4) (Winter 2006), pp. 66–69.

Bennett, Amanda, and Terence B. Foley. *In Memoriam, a Practical Guide to Planning a Memorial Service.* New York: Simon & Schuster, 1997.

Berglund, Rita. *An Alphabet About Kids with Cancer.* Denver, CO: Children's Legacy, 1994.

Bessell, A. G. Children surviving cancer: psychosocial adjustment, quality of life & school experience. *Exceptional Children*, vol. 67 (3) (Spring 2001), pp. 345.

Betty Crocker's Living With Cancer Cookbook. New York: Hungry Minds, 2002.

Bhatnagar, Ajay, and Melvin Deutsch. The role for intensity modulated radiation therapy (IMRT) in pediatric population. *Technology in Cancer Research*, vol. 5 (6) (2006), pp. 591–595.

Bickels, Jacob, et al. The role and biology of cryosurgery in the treatment of bone tumors. *Acta Orthopaedica Scandinavica*, vol. 70 (3) (June 1999), pp. 308–315.

Biggar, Robert J., et al. Risk of cancer in children with AIDS. *Journal of the American Medical Association*, vol. 284 (2) (July 12, 2000), pp. 205–209.

Bird, Hector R., et al. Stresses and traumas of childhood. In: *The Columbia University College of Physicians and Surgeons Complete Home Guide to Mental Health.* New York: Henry Holt and Company, 1992, pp. 290.

Bleyer, Archie, MD. Clinical trials debate. *U.S. News and World Report* (November 29, 1999), p. 6.

Blood counts. Childhood Cancer Resource Center. Retrieved on February 8, 2005, from www.childhoodcancerguides.org

Blood test results: Normal ranges. Retrieved January 21, 2005, from www.bloodbook.com

Blood Transfusion. White Plains, NY: Leukemia & Lymphoma Society, 2006.

Board game helps kids cope with cancer. *USA Today (Magazine)*, vol. 121 (2575) (April 1993), p. 16.

Bognar, David. *Cancer: Increasing Your Odds for Survival*. Alameda, CA: Hunter House Publishers, 1998.

Bogo, Jennifer. Children at risk. *E Magazine* (September–October 2001), pp. 26.

Boman, K., and G. Bodegård. Long-term coping in childhood cancer survivors: influence of illness, treatment, and demographic background factors. *Acta Paediatrica*, vol. 89 (1) (January 12, 2000), pp. 105–111.

Bone and Marrow Stem Cell Transplantation. New York: Leukemia and Lymphoma Society, nd.

Bone cancer. *Clinical Reference Systems*. Annual 2000, p. 177. Retrieved on November 27, 2001, from http://galenet-galegroup.com

Bone tumors. *Merck Manual Home Edition*, chapter 49. Retrieved on November 30, 2001, from www.merckhomeedition.com

Book describes cancer experience from a child's point of view [Andrew's Story by Chris Bridge]. *Childhood Cancerline*, vol. 7 (3) (January 2002), p. 4.

Bozzone, Donna M. *Cancer Genetics*. Biology of Cancer Series. New York: Chelsea House, 2007.

Brennan, Bernadette, et al. On nutritional status and cancer in children. *Cancer Strategy*, vol. 1 (4) (December 1, 1999), pp. 195–202.

Brody, Jane. Cancer and childbirth: Mutually exclusive no longer. *New York Times*, May 28, 2002, pp. D5 (N), F5 (L).

Brody, Jane. Treating ills in childhood cancer survivors. *New York Times*, February 3, 1993, p. C13.

Brown, Harriet. My daughters are fine, but I'll never be the same. *New York Times*, April 8, 2008, p. F5.

Brain tumor advances, 2006. *Messageline* vol. 33 (2) (Summer 2006) pp. 1.

Broniscer, A., et al. Phase I trial of single-dose temozolomide and continuous administration… in brain tumors. *Clinical Cancer Research*, vol. 13 (November 15, 2007), pp. 6712–6718.

Broviac and Hickman catheters. *University of Michigan Section of Pediatric Surgery*. Retrieved on April 15, 2004, from http://pediatric.um-surgery.org

Broviac/Hickman catheter parent teaching handbook. University of Michigan Section of Pediatric Surgery. Retrieved on April 15, 2004, from http://pediatric. um-surgery.org

Brownlee, Shannon. Trials of a cancer doc. *U.S. News and World Report*, vol. 12 (13) (October 5, 1998), p. 28.

Buck, Jari Holland. *Hospital Stay Handbook: A Guide to Becoming a Patient Advocate for Your Loved One*. Woodbury, MN: Llewellyn Publications, 2007.

Buckley, J. D., et al. Epidemiology of osteosarcoma and Ewing's sarcoma in childhood: a study of 305 cases by the Children's Cancer Group. *Cancer*, vol. 83 (7) (October 1, 1998), pp. 1440.

Bunce, Marianne. Troubleshooting central lines. *RN*, vol. 66 (12) (December 2003), pp. 28.

Butler, R. W., et al. Brief report: the assessment of posttraumatic stress disorder in pediatric cancer patients and survivors. *Journal of Pediatric Psychology*, vol. 21 (4) (August 1996), pp. 499–504.

C is for cure. Retrieved on October 19, 2001, from www.childhoodcancerawareness.org

Cahill, Cheryl, et al. Pediatric cancer pain [Oncology Nursing Service Position Paper]. *Oncology Nursing Forum*, vol. 17 (6) (November–December 1990), pp. 39–42.

Caley, Beverly A. Hodgkin disease: the other side. *Cure*, vol. 4 (1) (Spring 2005), pp. 40–47 (www.curetoday.com).

Cancer. *World Almanac*. Retrieved on April 6, 2001, from www.2facts.com

Cancer treatment affects the lives of children and their families. Retrieved on April 5, 2005, from www.curesearch.org

Cancer treatments. *Encyclopedia of Technology and Applied Sciences*. New York: Marshall Cavendish, 2000, vol. 2, pp. 218–219.

Cancer treatments. *Newton's Apple: Teacher's Guides*. Retrieved on March 22, 2002, from www.pbs.org

Cancer trials provide best care for cancer patients. *National Childhood Cancer Foundation, Childhood Cancerline*, vol. 5 (3) (nd), p. 6.

Cardonick, Elyce. How does a history of cancer affect a subsequent pregnancy? *Cure*, vol. 4 (2) (Summer 2005), p. 21.

Cario, G., et al. High interleukin-15 expression characterizes childhood acute lymphoblastic leukemia with involvement of the CNS. *Journal of Clinical Oncology*, vol. 25 (30) (October 20, 2007), pp. 4813–4820.

Carlson, Thor. Five Wishes: A user-friendly living will. *Good Age Newspaper*, Amherst H. Wilder Foundation. Retrieved on October 14, 2003, from www.wilder.org

Carolyn Pryce Walker Conquer Childhood Cancer Act. *Cure*, vol. 7 (3) (Fall 2008), p. 14.

Castellino, Sharon M., and Thomas W. McLean. Pediatric genitourinary tumors. *Current Opinions in Oncology*, vol. 19 (3) (May 2007), pp. 248–253.

Castellow, Fran (February 23, 2005). Patient assistance programs: what every oncologist should know. Retrieved on March 18, 2005, from www.patientadwvocate.org

Catheters for children. *Help for Oncology Nurses*. Retrieved on March 3, 2002, from www.onconurse.com

Cavallo, Jo. Confronting death. *Cure*, vol. 5 (2) (Summer 2006), pp. 21–26.

Cavallo, Jo. The shadow survivors. *Cure*, vol. 5 (3) (Fall 2006), pp. 66–69.

Cefrey, Holly. *Coping With Cancer*. New York: Rosen Publishing Group Inc, 2000.

Center for Attitudinal Healing. *Advice to Doctors & Other Big People from Kids*. Berkeley, CA: Celestialarts, 1991.

Central venous catheters. Retrieved on August 6, 2001, from www.cancerq.org

Chamberlain, Shannin. *My ABC Book of Cancer*. San Francisco, CA: Synergistic Press, 1990.

Chan, Helen. *Understanding Cancer Therapies: A Practical and Helpful Guide to the Many Treatments Available*. Jackson, MS: University Press of Mississippi, 2007.

Chapman, Simon. Fear of frying: power lines and cancer. *British Medical Journal*, vol. 322 (7287) (March 17, 2001), p. 682.

Charlton, A., et al. Children's return to school after treatment for solid tumors. *Social Science & Medicine*, vol. 22 (12) (1986), pp. 1337–1346.

Chekryn, J., et al. Impact on teachers when a child with cancer returns to school. *Children's Health Care*, vol. 15 (3) (Winter 1987), pp. 161–165.

Chemotherapy and You: A Guide to Self-Help During Cancer Treatment. National Cancer Institute. Retrieved on July 21, 2001, from http://cancernet.nci.nih.gov

Chen, S. J., et al. Endodermal sinus (yolk sac) tumors of vagina and cervix in an infant. *Pediatric Radiology*, vol. 23 (1) (1993), pp. 57–58.

Chicken pox vaccine. (1999) American Academy of Pediatrics. Retrieved on November 12, 2009, at www.aap.org.

Childhood cancer survival study. Fairview Healthcare for Children. Retrieved on October 29, 2001, from www.fairview.org

Childhood Cancer Survivorship: Improving Care and Quality of Life. Washington, DC: The National Academies Press, 2003.

[Children's Cancer Group] puts fears to rest—power lines do not cause leukemia. *Childhood Cancerline, National Childhood Cancer Foundation*, vol. 3 (1) (nd), pp. 1.

Child's Bill of Rights. *Columbus Children's Hospital: Staying at Children's.* Retrieved on May 18, 2005, from www.columbuschildrens.com (now Nationwide Children's Hospital, www.nationwidechildrens.org)

Chin, Lawrence, and William Regine. *Principles and Practice of Stereotactic Radiosurgery.* New York: Springer Verlag, 2008.

Cincotta, Nancy F. *Childhood Cancer Survivorship: The Family's Journey Forward.* Leukemia & Lymphoma Society Telephone Education Program, May 29, 2009.

Clements, Mark. What we can learn from cancer. *Parade Magazine*, February 6, 2000, p. 12.

Clifford, Christine. *Not Now...I'm Having a No Hair Day; Humor and Healing for People with Cancer.* Duluth, MN: Pfeifer-Hamilton Publishers, 1996.

Cohn, Victor. When your child has cancer. *Washington Post*, April 5, 1998, pp. z8.

Coleman, C. Norman. *Understanding Cancer: A Patient's Guide to Diagnosis, Prognosis, and Treatment.* Baltimore, MD: The Johns Hopkins University Press, 1998.

Collins, Nancy. Architectural Digest visits Don Imus. *Architectural Digest*, vol. 58 (12) (December 2001), pp. 110.

Collins, H. S. EST of the infant vagina treated exclusively by chemotherapy. *Obstetrics and Gynecology*, vol. 73 (3) part 2 (March 1989), pp. 507–509.

Connolly, Harry. *Fighting Chance: Journey Through Childhood Cancer.* Baltimore, MD: Woodholme House, 1998.

Considering complementary and alternative medicine? *National Center for Complementary and Alternative Medicine.* Retrieved on July 21, 2001, from http://nccam.nih.gov

Controlling Cancer Pain [videocassette]. National Institutes of Health, National Cancer Institute and Johns Hopkins Oncology Center, 2000.

Copeland, L. J. EST of the vagina and cervix. *Cancer*, vol. 55 (11) (June 1, 1985), pp. 2558–2565.

Coppes, Max J., et al. Alternative therapies for the treatment of childhood cancer [letter to the editor]. *New England Journal of Medicine* (September 17, 1998), pp. 846.

Coping. White Plains, NY: Leukemia & Lymphoma Society, 2005?

Coradini, Patricia, et al. Ototoxicity from cisplatin therapy in childhood cancer. *Journal of Pediatric Hematology/Oncology*, vol. 29 (6) (June 2007), pp. 355–360.

Costly cancer treatment aimed at protecting kids' hearts offers no additional benefit. *Doctor's Guide Personal Edition.* Retrieved on March 19, 2002, from www.docguide.com.

Cozzens, Jeffrey. What are the recent advances for brain tumors? *Cure*, vol. 4 (4) (Winter 2006), p. 39.

Cromie, William J. Study: Children with cancer suffer needlessly. *Harvard University Gazette*, vol. XCV, (16) (February 3, 2000), pp. 1.

Cunningham, D. Scott. Role of oncogenes in stem cell division elucidated" *MDLinx Oncology*. Retrieved on November 20, 2007, from www.mdlinx.com

Curiel, David T., MD, and Casey Cunningham, JD. Gene therapy: a targeted therapeutic. *Cure*, vol. 3 (1) (Spring 2004), p. 53. Available at www.curetoday.com,

Dahlquist, Lynda M. The problem of discipline. *Candlelighters Quarterly Newsletter*, vol. 14 (2) (Summer 1990) pp. 1.

Daleo, Roxanne. How your mind can help you feel better. *CCCF Youth Newsletter*, vol. 19 (1) (Winter 1997), pp. 1.

Daniels, Julie L. Pesticides and childhood cancers. *Journal of the American Medical Association*, vol. 279 (6) (February 11, 1998), p. 414H.

De Backer, I. C., et al. High-intensity strength training improves quality of life in cancer survivors. *Acta Oncologica*, vol. 46 (8) (2007), pp. 1143–1151.

Debes, Anette, et al. Role of heat treatment in childhood cancers. *Pediatric Blood & Cancer*, published online May 31, 2005. Retrieved on June 9, 2005, from www3.interscience.wiley.com

De Roos, A. J., et al. Parental occupational exposures to chemicals and incidence of neuroblastoma in offspring. *American Journal of Epidemiology*, vol. 154 (2) (July 15, 2001), pp. 106.

Dickens, Monica. *Miracles of Courage: How Families Meet the Challenge of a Child's Critical Illness*. New York: Dodd, Mead, 1985.

Dixon-Woods, Mary, et al. Parents' accounts of obtaining a diagnosis of childhood cancer. *The Lancet*, vol. 357 (9257) (March 3, 2001), pp. 670.

Dockerty, John D., et al. Electromagnetic field exposures and childhood cancers in New Zealand. *Cancer Causes and Controls*, vol. 9 (3) (May 1, 1998), pp. 299–309.

Dodd, Michael. *Oliver's Story: For 'Sibs' of Kids with Cancer*. Candlelighters Childhood Cancer Foundation, 2004.

Dorfman, Elena. *The C Word: Teenagers and Their Families Living With Cancer*. Portland, OR: NewSage Press, 1994.

Dorfman, Elena, and Heidi Schultz Adams. *Here and Now—Inspiring Stories of Cancer Survivors*. New York: Marlowe & Co., 2002.

Dougherty, Catherine. Musculoskeletal transplant. *Critical Care Nursing Quarterly*, vol. 21 (2) (August 1998), pp. 55.

Druker, Brian J. Targeting cancer in the 21st century. *Candlelighters Childhood Cancer Foundation Quarterly Newsletter* (Spring 2002), pp. 1.

Drum, David. *Making the Chemotherapy Decision*. Los Angeles, CA: Lowell House, 3d ed., 2000.

Dunn, Cathy. On the mark: Targeted therapies for non-Hodgkin's lymphoma. *Cure*, vol. 1 (1) (2002). Retrieved on May 18, 2005, from www.curetoday.com

Each New Day: Ideas for Coping with Leukemia, Lymphoma or Myeloma. White Plains, NY: Leukemia & Lymphoma Society, 2006?

Earle, E. A. Building a new normality: mothers' experiences of caring for a child with acute lymphoblastic leukaemia. *Child: Care, Health and Development*, vol. 33 (2) (March 2007), pp. 155–160.

Eating Hints for Cancer Patients Before, During and After Treatment. National Institutes of Health, National Cancer Institute, 1999.

Eland, Jo. Current problems and new developments in pediatric pain control. *Candlelighters Progress Reports*, vol. 10 (1) (1993), pp. 1.

Eland, Jo. Myths about pain in children. *Candlelighters Childhood Cancer Foundation Progress Reports* vol. 5 (1) (1985).

Encyclopedia of Associations. 46th ed. Detroit, MI: Gale Research Company, 2008.

Epstein, Samuel S. The cancer establishment. *Washington Post* (March 10, 1992), op/ed, p. A17.

Epstein, Fred J., and Elaine Fantle Shimberg. *Gifts of Time*. New York: Morrow, 1993.

Escalating incidence of childhood cancer is ignored. *Cancer Weekly* (June 11, 2002), p. 22.

Ewing's sarcoma and PNET. Retrieved on November 28, 2009, from www.intelihealth.com

Extragonadal germ cell tumors. Retrieved on August 4, 2001, from www.intelihealth.com

Fackelmann, Kathy. A favor for kids with cancer. *Science News*, vol. 137 (14) (April 7, 1990), p. 221.

Facts 2006–2007. White Plains, NY: Leukemia & Lymphoma Society, 2006.

Fake cancer cures. Retrieved on January 26, 2009, from http://cancer.about.com

Fano, Alix. Environmental factors in the rise of children's cancer. *Green Guide*, June 1, 1998, pp. 1.

Farley, John W. Power lines and cancer: nothing to fear. Retrieved on July 16, 2001, from www.quackwatch.com

Farrell, Jocelyn. Central venous access devices versus peripheral intravenous catheters in the oncology setting. Retrieved on April 15, 2004, from www.n1hba.nf.ca

Feist, Patty. Chemotherapy vs. transplant as treatment for relapsed ALL. *CCCF Newsletter* (Fall/Winter 2007), pp. 2.

Feist, Patty. Relapsed ALL: questions for parents to ask. *Candlelighters National Journal*, (Spring–Summer 2007), pp. 2.

Fermé, C., et al. Chemotherapy plus involved-field radiation in early-stage Hodgkin's disease. *New England Journal of Medicine*, vol. 357 (19) (November 8, 2007), pp. 1916–1927.

Ferrari, S., et al. Predictive factors of histologic response to primary chemotherapy in patients with Ewing sarcoma. *Journal of Pediatric Hematology/Oncology*, vol. 29 (6) (June 2007), pp. 364–368.

Ferrell, Sue. Traveling a new road. *Candlelighters Quarterly Newsletter*, vol. 17 (4) (Winter 1994), p. 5.

Ferry, C., et al. Long-term outcomes after allogeneic stem cell transplantation for children with hematological malignancies. *Bone Marrow Transplantation* advance online publication retrieved May 28, 2007, from www.nature.com

Fertile Hope. *Childhood Cancer and Fertility: A Guide for Parents*, 2004. Retrieved on November 21, 2009, from www.fertilehope.org [now part of LiveStrong]

Fever and infections: Understanding the problem. *Hershey Home Medical Guide*. Retrieved on August 4, 2001, from www.hmc.psu.edu.

Feychting, Maria, et al. Parental occupational exposure to magnetic fields and childhood cancer. *Cancer Causes and Control*, vol. 11 (2) (February 1, 2000), pp. 151–156.

Fiduccia, Dan. ADA gives new rights to survivors and their families. *Candlelighters Childhood Cancer Foundation Quarterly Newsletter*, vol. 16 (4) (Winter 1992), pp. 1.

Filston, Howard C. What's new in pediatric surgery. *Pediatrics*, vol. 96 (4) (October 1995), p. 748.

Financial assistance. Retrieved on March 6, 2009, from www.nationalchildrens-cancersociety.org

Finger, Paul T. 2009 Eye Cancer Network. Retrieved on November 21, 2009, from www.eyecancer.com

Fischer, David S., et al. *The Cancer Chemotherapy Handbook*, 6th ed. St. Louis, MO: Mosby, 2003.

Fisher, Alan (as told to Ann M. Mayer). Dad and plate spinner. *Candlelighters Childhood Cancer Foundation Quarterly Newsletter*, vol. 17 (1) (Spring 1993), pp. 1.

Fisher, P. G., et al. Outcome analysis of childhood low-grade astrocytomas. *Pediatric Blood & Cancer*, vol. 51 (2) (2008), pp. 245–250.

FitzGerald, Susan. Children surviving cancer—only to face it again. *Philadelphia Inquirer*, July 21, 2001, np.

For research on risks, numbers are a challenge. *National Cancer Institute Bulletin*, vol. 5 (6), (March 18, 2008), p. 4.

Foreman, Judy. Helping someone you love to die. *Boston Globe*, March 7, 1994, p. 31.

Foreman, Judy. Medical marijuana—A cure or a curse? *Boston Globe*, October 7, 1991, pp. 25.

Foreman, Judy. New drugs fight sores from cancer treatment. *Boston Globe*, March 8, 1999, pp. c1.

Foreman, Judy. New guidelines stress cancer pain treatment. *Boston Globe*, March 3, 1993, pp. 1.

Frangoul, H., et al. A prospective study of G-CSF-primed bone marrow as a stem-cell source for allogeneic bone marrow transplantation in children. *Blood*, vol. 110 (13) (December 15, 2007), pp. 4584–4587.

Fredey, Maura. Surf sense. *Healthy Lifestyle* (Spring 2001), p. 11.

Friedman, Debra, et al. Keeping your heart healthy after treatment for childhood cancer. *CureSearch Health Link*. Retrieved on November 21, 2009, from www.survivorshipguidelines.org

Friedrich, M. J. Lowering risk of second malignancy in the survivors of childhood cancer. *Journal of the American Medical Association*, vol. 285 (19) (May 16, 2001), p. 2435.

Fry, Rae. *E-lixir of e-health: what to believe online*. Retrieved on August 17, 2001, from www.abc.net.au

Fryer, David R., and Laurence Brugieres. Adolescent and young adult oncology: transition of care. *Pediatric Blood and Cancer*, vol. 50 (S5) (May 2008), pp. 116–119.

Fryer, Lynn L., et al. Helping the child with cancer: what school personnel want to know. *Psychological Reports*, vol. 65 (1989), pp. 563–566.

Gardner, Laura. Does intercessory prayer for sick people actually heal them? *Medical News Today*, June 19, 2009. Retrieved from www.medicalnewstoday.com

Gershenson, D. M., et al. Treatment of malignant germ cell tumors of the ovary with bleomycin, etoposide and cisplatin. *Journal of Clinical Oncology*, vol. 8 (4) (April 1990), pp. 715–720.

Getz, Kenneth, and Deborah Borfitz. *Informed Consent: A Guide to the Risks and Benefits of Volunteering for Clinical Trials.* Boston, MA: CenterWatch, 2002.

Gift baskets for families in the hospital. Ped-Onc Resource Center. Retrieved on November 29, 2009, from www.acor.org

Gilchrist, Gerald, MD. Private correspondence, February 1985.

Giller, Cole A. Lessons learned. *Cure,* vol. 5 (3) (Fall 2006), p. 80.

Giobannini, Joseph. Newman's own: the movie star's camp for kids is built for hands-on fun. *House and Garden,* vol. 161 (June 1989), pp. 22.

Goldberg, Allan. Survivor's search for meaning. *Cure,* vol. 5 (special issue 2006), p. 80.

Goldberg, Debbie. Tide of fear: Cancer seems to stalk children in New Jersey seashore town. *Washington Post* (June 1, 1996), p. A3.

Goldman, Benjamin A. *The Truth About Where You Live: An Atlas for Action on Toxins and Mortality.* New York: Times Books/Random House, 1991.

Gootman, Marilyn. *When a Friend Dies: A Book for Teens about Healing.* Minneapolis, MN: Free Spirit Pub, rev. ed., 2005.

Gordon, James S., and Sharon Curtin. *Comprehensive Cancer Care: Integrating Alternative, Complementary and Conventional Therapies.* Cambridge, MA: Perseus Publishing, 2000.

Gordon, Melanie Apel. *Let's Talk About When Kids Have Cancer.* New York: The Rosen Publishing Group's PowerKids Press, 1999.

Gorfinkle, Kenneth. *Soothing Your Child's Pain.* Chicago: Contemporary Books, 1997.

Grady, Denise. For cancer patients, empathy goes a long way. *New York Times,* January 8, 2008, p. F5.

Granet, Roger. *Surviving Cancer Emotionally.* New York: John Wiley & Sons, 2001.

Green, Lila. *Making Sense of Humor.* Manchester, CT: Knowledge, Ideas & Trends, 1993.

Greer, Michael. Interleukin-16 is too toxic for use after pediatric chemotherapy. *Immunotherapy Weekly,* March 21, 2001, np.

Gribbon, M., et al. Pediatric malignant ovarian tumors: a 43-year review. *Journal of Pediatric Surgery,* vol. 27 (4) (April 1992), pp. 480–484.

"GriefNet—a community of persons dealing with grief." Retrieved on December 9, 2009, from www.rivendell.org

Grizzi, F., et al. Antiangiogenic strategies in medulloblastoma: reality or mystery. *Pediatric Research,* vol. 63 (5) (May 2008), pp. 584–590.

Grollman, Earl A., ed. *Bereaved Children and Teens: A Support Guide for Parents and Professionals.* Boston: Beacon Press, 1995.

Grollman, Earl A. *Caring and Coping When Your Loved One is Seriously Ill.* Boston, MA: Beacon Press, 1995.

Groopman, Jerome E. A Lottery. In: *Second Opinions: Stories of Intuition and Choice in the Changing World of Medicine.* New York: Viking, 2001, pp. 167–195.

Grootenhuis, M. A., and Bob F. Last. Adjustment and coping by parents of children with cancer: a review of the literature. *Supportive Care in Cancer,* vol. 5 (6) (November 3, 1997), pp. 466–484.

Growth hormone therapy does not increase cancer recurrence risk. *Journal of Clinical Endocrinology and Metabolism,* vol. 84 (2002), pp. 3136–3141.

Gruman, Jessie. 6 ways to help when someone has cancer. *Parade Magazine* (October 19, 2008) pp. 4.

Grundy, R. G., et al. Primary postoperative chemotherapy without radiotherapy for intracranial ependymoma in children. *Current Neurology and Neuroscience Reports*, vol. 9 (2) (2009), pp. 94–96.

Grundy, R. G., et al. Fertility preservation for children treated with cancer. *Archives of Disease in Childhood*, vol. 84 (4) (2001), pp. 355.

Guide for Families of Children with Cancer. Boston, MA: MassGeneral Hospital for Children, nd.

Guidelines for the pediatric cancer center and role of such centers in diagnosis and treatment. *Pediatrics* vol. 99 (1) (January 1997), pp. 139–141. Also online at www.aapp.org

Gutberlet, Manuela. Cancer main killer of Egyptian children. *Middle East Times*. Retrieved on March 24, 2002, from www.metimes.com

Gutierrez, Juan C., et al. Malignant breast cancer in children: a review of 75 patients. *Journal of Surgical Research*, vol. 147 (2) (June 15, 2008), pp. 182–188.

Hagen, Amy Erickson, Cryogenic Laboratories, Inc. Private e-mail, December 3, 2007.

Haggerty, Maureen. Sarcomas. *Gale Encyclopedia of Medicine*. Detroit, MI: Gale Research, 1999.

Hall, Stephen S. Cheating fate. *Health*, vol. 6 (2) (April 1992), pp. 38.

Hammer, M. R., and W. B. Jonas. Managing social conflict in complementary and alternative medicine research: the case of antineoplastons. *Integrated Cancer Therapies*, vol. 3 (1) (March 2004), pp. 59–65.

Halpern, Susan P. *The Etiquette of Illness: What to Say When You Can't Find the Words*. New York: Bloomsbury, 2004.

Hamilton, Virginia. *Bluish*. New York: Blue Sky Press, 1999.

Harris, Angela, editor-in-chief. *Cancer Rates and Risks*, 4th ed. National Institutes of Health, National Cancer Institute, U.S. Department of Health and Human Services, Public Health Service, 1996.

Hartley, S. (November 19, 2007). A pox on your cancer. Retrieved on November 20, 2007, from www.mdlinx.com/HemeOncLinx

Hashii, Y., et al. A case series of children with high-risk metastatic neuroblastoma treated with a novel treatment strategy consisting of postponed primary surgery until the end of systemic chemotherapy including high-dose chemotherapy. *Pediatric Hematology and Oncology*, vol. 25 (5) (June 2008), pp. 439–450.

Hatch, Maureen, et al. Cancer near the Three Mile Island nuclear plant: radiation emissions. *American Journal of Epidemiology*, vol. 132 (3) (1990) pp. 397–412.

Hawkes, Nigel. The power to kill? *Times of London*, 64920 (April 5, 1994), p. 15.

Health risks from exposure to low levels of ionizing radiation. *BEIR VII*, U. S. National Research Council, p. 173, nd.

Helmreich, M., and A. Eaton. Interacting with two treatment centers. *The Main Vein [CCCF]*, Winter 1997, p. 1.

Help for patients. *Cure*, vol. 4 (4) (Winter 2006), p. 49.

Helping brothers and sisters cope. Hershey Medical Center. Retrieved August 4, 2001, from www.hmc.psu.edu

Heritable proportion of childhood cancers. Cancer Genetics Web. Retrieved on November 20, 2003, from www.cancerindex.org

Herndon, Lucia. Children with cancer are tough and deserve respect and praise. *Knight-Ridder/Tribune News Service*, March 15, 1994.

Hero, B., et al. Localized infant neuroblastomas often show spontaneous regression. *Journal of Clinical Oncology*, vol. 26 (9) (March 20, 2008), pp. 1504–1510.

Hess, David J. *Evaluating Alternative Cancer Therapies: A Guide to the Science and Politics of an Emerging Medical Field*. New Brunswick, NJ: Rutgers University Press, 1999.

Hilden, Joanne, and Daniel R. Tobin with Karen Lindsay. *Shelter From the Storm: Caring for a Child with a Life-Threatening Condition*. Cambridge, MA: Perseus Publishing, 2003.

Hilden, Joanne, and Sarah Friebert. Palliative or hospice care: Does my child need this service? *Candlelighters National Journal*, Fall 2001, pp. 2.

Hirschfeld, Steven. Clinical Trials Part I. *Candlelighters National Journal*, Fall 2002, pp. 6.

Hobbie, Wendy, et al. Symptoms of posttraumatic stress in young adult survivors of childhood cancer. *Journal of Clinical Oncology*, vol. 18 (24) (December 2000), pp. 4060–4066.

Hodder-Janes, Honna, and Nancy Keene. *Childhood Cancer: A Parent's Guide to Solid Tumor Cancers*. Sebastapol, CA: O'Reilly, 1999.

Hodgson, David, et al. Pediatric Hodgkin lymphoma: Maximizing efficacy and minimizing toxicity. *Seminars in Radiation Oncology*, vol. 17 (3) (July 2007), pp. 230–242.

Hoffman, Barbara. Cancer survivors' employment and insurance rights: a primer for oncologists. *Oncology*, vol. 13 (6) (June 1999), pp. 841–846.

Hoffman, Ruth. Four Thousand gold ribbons adorn rotunda. *Candlelighters National Journal*, Fall 2001, p. 2.

Holcomb, George W. III, et al. Minimally invasive surgery in children with cancer. *Cancer*, vol. 76 (1) (July 1, 1995), pp. 121.

Holley, Michael. At 12, he won't stop for cancer. *Boston Globe* (August 6, 1998), p. D1.

Holly, Noelle (July 25, 2007). Storytelling. In *Cancer Articles and Updates for Physicians*, nd.

HON Code of Conduct (HONcode) for medical and health web sites. *Health on the Net Foundation*. Retrieved on October 23, 2001, from www.hon.ch

Hood, Ann. *Comfort: A Journey Through Grief*. New York: W. W. Norton & Co., 2008.

Horne, Jo. *A caregiver's bill of rights*. Retrieved on May 3, 2002, from http://james.parkinsons.org.uk

Housden, Maria. *Hanna's Gift: Lessons from a Life Fully Lived*. New York: Bantam Books, 2002.

Houtzager, B. A., et al. Adjustment of siblings to childhood cancer: a literature review. *Supportive Care in Cancer*, vol. 7 (5) (August 11, 1999), pp. 302–320.

How you can help a family who has a child with cancer. The National Children's Cancer Society. Retrieved on August 4, 2001, from www.children-cancer.com

Hubert, Cynthia. A mother's journey. *Sacramento Bee*, 4 parts, July 9–12, 2006. Retrieved on July 13, 2006, from www.sacbee.com

Hudson, Melissa, et al. Health status of adult long-term survivors of childhood cancer: A report from the Childhood Cancer Survivor Study. JAMA the *Journal of the American Medical Association*, vol. 290 (12) (September 24, 2003), pp. 1583–1592.

Hughes, Deborah. Massage therapy as a supportive care intervention for children with cancer. *Oncology Nursing Forum*, vol. 35 (3) (May 2008), pp. 431–442.

Human, Katy. Deadly accuracy. *Cure*, vol. 6 (2) (Spring 2007), pp. 18–21.

Humor. Retrieved on November 5, 1999, from www.planetpsych.com

Hunt, Richard C. *Virology...oncogenic viruses*. Lecture retrieved on December 13, 2009, at http://pathmicro.med.sc.edu/lecture/retro.htm

I'm Still Me! Teens Coping with Cancer. Nashville, TN: American Cancer Society, Nashville/Davidson County Division, 1983.

Imai, A., et al. EST of the vagina in an infant: MRI evaluation. *Gynecology and Oncology*, vol. 48 (3) (March 1993), pp. 402–405.

Improvements needed for adolescents and young adults. *NCI National Cancer Bulletin*, vol. 5 (6) (March 8, 2008), p. 9.

Infante-Rivard, C., and Weichenthal, S. Pesticides and childhood cancer: an update of Zahm and Ward's 1998 review. *Journal of Toxicology and Environmental Health, B Critical Reviews*, vol. 10 (1–2) (January–March 2007), pp. 81–99.

Inhaled chemo for pediatric bone cancer (May 25, 2005). Retrieved on August 1, 2005, from www.mydna.com

Institute of Medicine. *When Children Die: Improving Palliative Care and End-of-Life Care for Children and Their Families*. Washington, DC: National Academy, 2002.

Issues for survivors of childhood cancer. *ASCO Online*. Retrieved on October 29, 2001, from www.asco.org

Jacobs, Sally. Survivor at a young age. *Boston Globe* (July 28, 1998), pp. C1.

Jacobsohn, D. S. Acute graft-versus-host disease in children. *Bone Marrow Transplantation*, vol. 41 (2008), pp. 215–221.

Janes-Hodder, Honna, & Nancy Keene. *Childhood Cancer: A Parents' Guide to Solid Tumor Cancers*. Sebastapol, CA: O'Reilly, 1998.

Jarvis, William T. How quackery harms cancer patients. Retrieved on July 16, 2001, from www.quackwatch.com

Jasper, Margaret C. *Healthcare and Your Rights Under the Law*. Dobbs Ferry, NY: Oceana Publications, 2002.

Jérémie, R., et al. Childhood hematopoietic malignancies and parental use of tobacco and alcohol. *Cancer Causes and Control*, posted at www.springerlink.com, 7/11/2008

Jerome, Marty. Beware of unhealthy sites. *Boston Globe* (March 19, 2000), p. C9.

Ji, B T., et al. Paternal cigarette smoking and the risk of childhood cancer among offspring of nonsmoking mothers. *Journal of the National Cancer Institute*, vol. 89 (3) (February 5, 1997), pp. 238–244.

Johnson, Christopher M. *Your Critically Ill Child: Life and Death Choices Parents Must Face*. Far Hills, NJ: New Horizon Press, 2007.

Jordan, Jerie. Erma Bombeck: touting the triumphs. *Childhood Cancer Today* (American Cancer Society), August 1989, pp. 5–6.

Joslin, Mary. *The Goodbye Boat*. Grand Rapids, MI: Eerdman's Books for Young Readers, 1998.

Kadohata, Cynthia. *Kira-Kira*. New York: Atheneum Books for Young Readers, 2004.

Kaplan, Karen. Stem cell treatment used for diabetes. *Boston Globe* (April 11, 2007), p. A5.

Katz, E. R., et al. School and social reintegration of children with cancer. *Journal of Psychosocial Oncology*, vol. 6 (3–4) (1988), pp. 123–140.

Kaushel, Rainu, et al. Medication errors and adverse drug events in pediatric inpatients. *JAMA the Journal of the American Medical Association*, vol. 285 (April 25, 2001), pp. 2114–2120.

Keane, Maureen, and Danielle Chace. *What to Eat If You Have Cancer: A Guide to Adding Nutritional Therapy to Your Treatment Plan.* Chicago, IL: Contemporary Books, 1996.

Keating, Armand, MD. (February 21, 2008). Stem cell transplantation: current trends and future directions. Telephone Education Program from the Leukemia and Lymphoma Society.

Keating, Dan. The doctor is in on the computer, but beware of biased information. *Philadelphia Inquirer* (October 2, 1997), p. F3.

Keene, Nancy, and Kevin Oeffinger. Bone health after childhood cancer. *Candlelighters National Journal*, Spring 2002, pp. 3.

Keene, Nancy. *Chemo, Craziness & Comfort, My Book About Childhood Cancer.* Bethesda, MD: Candlelighters Childhood Cancer Foundation, 2002.

Keene, Nancy, and Kevin Oeffinger. Comprehensive follow-up programs: a necessity not a luxury. *Candlelighters National Journal*, Fall 2002, pp. 3.

Keene, Nancy, and Kevin Oeffinger. Cognitive late effects to the brain [parts I and II]. *Candlelighters Childhood Cancer Foundation Newsletter*, Summer and Fall 2001.

Keene, Nancy, ed. *Educating the Child with Cancer: A Guide for Parents and Teachers*, Bethesda, MD: Candlelighters Childhood Cancer Foundation, 2003.

Keene, Nancy, and Kevin Oeffinger. Late effects of treatment to the teeth. *Candlelighters National Journal*, Spring 2003, pp. 3.

Keene, Nancy. Making hospital stays easier for children. *The Exceptional Parent*, vol. 29 (10) (October 1999), pp. 81.

Keene, Nancy. *Working with Your Doctor: Getting the Healthcare You Deserve.* Sebastapol, CA: O'Reilly, 1998.

Keene, Nancy, and Rachel Prentice. *Your Child in the Hospital, A practical guide for parents.* Sebastopol, CA: O'Reilly & Associates, 2d ed., 1999.

Keim, Rachel, and Ginny Smith. *What to Eat Now: The Cancer Lifeline Cookbook.* Seattle, WA: Sasquatch Books, 1996.

Kelly, Kara. Complementary and alternative medicines for use in supportive care in pediatric cancer. *Supportive Care in Cancer*, vol. 15 (4) (April 2007), pp. 457–460.

Kelly, Pat. *Cancer Self-Help Groups: A Guide.* Buffalo, NY: Firefly Books, 2000.

Kenney, Lisa B, MD. Increased incidence of cancer in infants in the U.S.: 1980–1990. *Cancer*, vol. 279 (21) (June 3, 1998), p. 1678F.

Keough, Althea. Temperature takers. *Baby Talk*, vol. 68 (7) (September 1, 2003), p. 74.

Kidney cancer: renal cell carcinoma. *Urology Notes.* Retrieved on May 29, 2002, from www.urologyinstitute.com

KidsAid, a safe place for kids to grieve. Retrieved on December 9, 2009, from www.kidsaid.org

Kingman, Sharon. Thyroid cancer rises after Chernobyl. *British Medical Journal*, vol. 305 (6854) (September 12, 1992), pp. 601.

Klein, Nancy C. *Healing Images for Children: Activity Book.* Watertown, WI: Inner Coaching, 2001.

Klein, Nancy. *Healing Images for Children: Teaching Relaxation and Guided Imagery to Children Facing Cancer and Other Serious Illnesses.* Watertown, WI: Inner Coaching, 2001.

Klein, Nancy. *Healing Images for Children: Relax and Imagine, Music and Relaxation to Promote Healing [CD].* Watertown, WI: Inner Coaching, 2001.

Kleinerman, R. A. Risk of new cancers after radiotherapy in long-term survivors of retinoblastoma: an extended follow-up. *Journal of Clinical Oncology*, vol. 23 (10) (April 1, 2005), pp. 2272–2279.

Klett, Amy. *The Amazing Hannah: Look at Everything I Can Do!* Bethesda, MD: Candlelighters Childhood Cancer Foundation, 2002.

Knox, Richard. Drugs offer new hope for cancer patients. *Boston Globe*, September 9, 1988, p. 7.

Kodish, Eric. Improving informed consent in childhood cancer trials. *Candlelighters National Journal*, Fall 2003, pp. 10.

Kohorn, E. I. EST of the infant vagina. *Gynecological Oncology*, vol. 20 (2) (February 1985), pp. 196–203.

Koifman, S., et al. High birth weight is associated with increased risk of infant leukemia. *British Journal of Cancer*, vol. 98 (3) (February 12, 2008), pp. 664–667.

Komp, Diane M. *A Child Shall Lead Them: Lessons in Hope from Children with Cancer*. San Francisco: Zondervan Publishing House, 1998.

Komp, Diane M. *Hope Springs from Mended Places*. San Francisco: Zondervan/ Harper SF, 1994.

Kony, Sabine J., et al. Radiation and genetic factors in the risk of second malignant neoplasms after a first cancer in childhood. *Lancet*, vol. 350 (9071) (July 12, 1997), pp. 91.

Koocher, Gerald P., and John J. O'Malley. *The Damocles Syndrome*. New York: McGraw-Hill, 1981.

Kornmehl, Carol L. *The Best News About Radiation Therapy: How to Cope and Survive*. Howell, NJ: Academic Radiation Oncology Press, 2003.

Kovacs, Diane. Information evaluation criteria and practical application of information evaluation criteria to internet information. in *Building Electronic Library Collections*. New York: Neal Schuman, 2000, pp. 16–27.

Kowalczyk, Liz. The birth of a tumor. Health Science section, *Boston Globe* (December 4, 2006), pp. C1.

Krisher, Trudy. *Kathy's Hats: A Story of Hope*. Dayton, OH: Marianist Press, 1990.

Kunze, Ursula, et al. Childhood cancer mortality in Austria. *European Journal of Epidemiology*, vol. 13 (1) (February 1, 1997), pp. 41–44.

Lacayo, Richard. And a little child shall lead them. *People Weekly*, October 24, 1991, pp. 64–65.

Lamb, Linda. An Interview with Author-Advocate Nancy Keene. *Patient-Centered Guides*. Retrieved on November 29, 2003, from www.patientcenters.com

Landers, Susan J. Complicated history: What happens when cancer survivors grow up? *AMedNews*. Retrieved on July 31, 2003, from www.ama-assn.org

Landier, Wendy, and Smita Bhatia. Cancer survivorship: a pediatric perspective. *The Oncologist*, vol. 13, (11) (November 2008), pp. 1181–1192.

Landier, Wendy. Keeping your single kidney healthy. *CureSearch Health Link*, 2008. Retrieved on November 30, 2009, from www.childrensoncologygroupp.org

LaTour, Kathy. Creating community online. *Cure*, vol. 4 (4) (Winter 2005), pp. 68.

Learning and Living with Cancer: Advocating for your child's educational needs. New York: Leukemia & Lymphoma Society, 2005.

Lee, S. H. Tandem high-dose chemotherapy and autologous stem cell rescue in children with bilateral advanced retinoblastoma. *Bone Marrow Transplantation*, vol. 42 (6) (September 2008), pp. 385–391.

Less-intense chemo effective in children with intermediate-risk neuroblastoma. American Society of Clinical Oncology annual meeting, Chicago, June 4, 2007. Retrieved on June 27, 2007, from www.cancer.gov

'Less is more' in new studies of germ cell cancer cures. *Childhood Cancerline*, vol. 8 (1) (July 2002), p. 3.

Lessons from antineoplaston [editorial]. *Lancet*, vol. 349 (9054) (March 15, 1997), p. 741.

Leukemia & the inheritance factor. St. Jude Children's Hospital, March 2005. Retrieved on April 21, 2005, from www.stjude.org

Liebermann, Laura Lee. Back to school. *The Main Vein (CCCF)*, Fall 1995, p. 4.

Linet, Martha S., et al. Cancer surveillance series: recent trends in childhood cancer incidence and mortality in the United States. *Journal of the National Cancer Institute*, vol. 91 (12) (June 16, 1999), pp. 1051–1058.

A Lion in the House: Community Engagement Campaign (2007). Independent Television Service. Retrieved March 29, 2007, from www.itvs.org/outreach

Liver tumors in children are rare, but not ignored by COG. *Friends of the Children's Oncology Group Newsletter*, November 2002.

Long-Term Follow-Up Program Resource Guide. CureSearch Children's Oncology Group. Retrieved from www.survivorshipguidelines.org, on February 26, 2009.

Lozowski-Sullivan, Sheryl. *Know Before You Go: The Childhood Cancer Journey.* Bethesda, MD: The Candlelighters Childhood Cancer Foundation, 1998.

Luhn, James. Mailing lists of interest. *The Main Vein (Candlelighters Network)*, (Summer-Fall 1997), p. 3.

The Lymphomas: Hodgkin Lymphoma and Non-Hodgkin Lymphomas. White Plains, NY: Leukemia & Lymphoma Society, 2006?

The Lymphomas: A Guide for Patients and Caregivers. White Plains, NY: Leukemia & Lymphoma Society, 2007.

Lynn, Allison. Buddy system. *People Weekly*, March 24, 1997, pp. 153–154.

Mack, J. W., et al. Understanding of prognosis among parents of children with cancer: parental optimism and the parent-physician interaction. *Journal of Clinical Oncology*, v. 25 (2007), pp. 1357–1362.

Magné, N., & C. Haie-Meder. Brachytherapy for genital-tract rhabdomyosarcoma in girls. *Lancet Oncology*, vol. 8 (8) (August 2007), pp. 725–729.

Major domains of complementary & alternative medicine. National Center for Complementary & Alternative Medicine. Retrieved on July 21, 2001, from http://nccam.nih.gov

Managing Your Child's Eating Problems During Cancer Treatment. U.S. Department of Health and Human Services, Public Health Service, National Institutes of Health, 1991.

Mangano, Joseph, et al. Elevated childhood cancer incidence proximate to U. S. nuclear power plants. *Archives of Environmental Health*, vol. 58 (2) (Feb. 2003) pp. 74.

Mantadakis, Elpisis, et al. A comprehensive review of acute promyelocytic leukemia in children. *Acta Haematologica*, vol. 119 (2) (2008), pp. 73–82.

Marcus, Erin. No evidence reactor leak caused cancer. *Washington Post*, September 1, 1990, p. A1.

Marcus, Mary Brophy. Kids who beat cancer may face later health challenges. *U.S. News & World Report*. Retrieved on August 4, 2001, from www.usnews.com

Masoorli, Sue. Tunneled catheters: their function and placement. *RN*, vol. 66 (12) (December 2003), p. 72.

Masucci, Maria G. Tumor viruses. in *McGraw-Hill Encyclopedia of Science and Technology*, 8th edition, 1997. Retrieved on March 16, 2001, from www. accessscience.com

Massachusetts Division, American Cancer Society. *Cancer Manual*, 9th edition, 1996. Framingham, MA: American Cancer Society, 1996.

Maule, M., et al. Risk of second malignant neoplasms after childhood leukemia and lymphoma: an international study. *Journal of the National Cancer Institute*, vol. 99 (10) (May 16, 2007), pp. 790–800.

Mauz-Korholz, Christine. Primary chemotherapy and conservative surgery for vaginal yolk-sac tumour. *Lancet*, vol. 355 (9204) (February 19, 2000), p. 625.

Maxwell, Bruce. *How to Find Health Information on the Internet*. Washington, DC: Congressional Quarterly, 1998.

Mayer, Nancy. Poison all around us: fouling our nests. *Oregonian*, May 14, 1995, pp. A1.

McClain, K. L., et al. Cancers in children with HIV infection. *Hematology and Oncology Clinics of North America*, vol. 10 (5) (1996), pp. 1189–1201.

McConnaughey, Janet. Approach in child cancers is questioned. *Boston Globe*, February 3, 2000, p. A4.

McDonald, Charles J., MD. Cancer trials debate [letter]. *U.S. News & World Report* (November 29, 1999), p. 6.

McElroy, Lisa Tucker. The right thermometer for your child. *Parenting*, vol. 19 (February 1, 2005), p. 42.

McGlynn, K. A., et al. Persistent organochlorine pesticides and risk of testicular germ cell tumors. *Journal of the National Cancer Institute*, vol. 100 (9) (May 7, 2008), pp. 663–671.

McGrath, Patrick J., et al. *Pain, Pain, Go Away: Helping Children with Pain*. Izaak Walton Killam Children's Hospital and Dalhousie University, Halifax, NS, Canada. Retrieved on August 4, 2001, from www.dal.ca

McGurk, Margaret A., ed. *The Lion in the House: Five Families, Six Years, True Stories from the War on Cancer*. Wilmington, OH: Orange Frazer Press, 2006.

McHenry, C. R., et al. Vaginal neoplasms in infancy: the combined role of chemo-therapy and conservative surgical resection. *Journal of Pediatric Surgery*, vol. 23 (9) (September 1988), pp. 842–845.

McKay, Judith, and Tamera Schacher. *The Chemotherapy Survival Guide*, 3rd ed. Oakland, CA: New Harbinger Publications, Inc., 2009.

McLean, Herbert E. A special camp for special kids. *American Forests*, vol. 96 (March-April 1990), pp. 28.

Mennes, M., et al. Attention and information processing in survivors of childhood acute lymphoblastic leukemia treated with chemotherapy only. *Pediatric Blood and Cancer*. Retrieved on October 18, 2004, from www3.interscience.wiley.com

Meltz, Barbara F. What about me? Managing emotion when a sibling feels left out. *Boston Globe*, November 26, 1998, pp. E1.

Meyer, Lacey, ed. Timeline: Milestones in cancer therapy. *Cure* (Special issue 2008), np.

Milch, Robert A., et al. *Palliative Pain and Symptom Management for Children and Adolescents*. Alexandria, VA: Children's Hospice International, 1985.

Minton, Lynn. Fresh voices: I want to be treated like a normal kid. *Parade Magazine*, January 9, 1994, p. 14.

Mishra, Raja. Children seen facing hospital drug errors. *Boston Globe* (April 25, 2001), p. A3.

Moldow, D. Gay, and Ida M. Martinson. *Home Care for Seriously Ill Children: A Manual for Parents*. Alexandria, VA: Children's Hospice International, 1991 [newer edition edited by Stacy Orloff and Susan M. Huff].

Morhmann, Margaret E. *Attending Children: A Doctor's Education*. Washington DC: Georgetown University Press, 2005.

Morris, H. H., et al. EST and embryonal carcinoma of the ovary in children. *Gynecological Oncology*, vol. 21 (1) (May 1985), pp. 7–17.

Morris, Jim. Small-time polluter, big-time problems. *U.S. News & World Report*, vol. 128 (8) (February 28, 2000), p. 57.

Morton, Carol Cruzan. Should you enroll in a clinical trial? New book offers guidance. *Boston Globe*, May 14, 2002, pp. C1.

Moulton, Gwen. NCI's childhood cancer monograph released on WEB. *Journal of the National Cancer Institute*, vol. 91 (15) (August 4, 1999), p. 1279.

Mulhern, Raymond, and Donna R. Copeland. Effect of cancer and cancer therapy on children's cognitive development. *Candlelighters Quarterly Newsletter*, vol. 22 (3) (Fall 1997), pp. 1.

Mulvihill, J. J., et al. Genetic disease in offspring of survivors of childhood and adolescent cancer. *American Journal of Human Genetics*, vol. 69 (4) (October 2001), p. 391.

Murray, Barbara. Doctor of last resort. *U.S. News & World Report*, vol. 122 (22) (June 9, 1997), p. 18.

Murray, Donald. *The Lively Shadow: Living with the Death of a Child*. New York: Ballantine Books, 2003.

Murray, Lisa. *Angels and Monsters: A Child's Eye View of Cancer*. Atlanta, GA: American Cancer Society, 2002.

Muse, Vance. Newman's own recipe for giving cheer to kids. *Life*, vol. 11 (September 1988), pp. 24.

Muth, Annemarie S., ed. *Death and Dying Sourcebook: Basic Consumer Health Information for the Layperson about End-of-Life Care and Related Ethical and Legal Issues*. Detroit, MI: Omnigraphics, 2000.

NCCF plays active advocacy role. *Childhood Cancerline*, vol. 3 (2) (1997?), p. 2.

NRPB [National Radiological Protection Board, UK] (study on parental preconception irradiation and subsequent cancer in the child). *Journal of Radiological Protection*, vol. 18 (1) (March 1, 1998), pp. 49–69.

Nagarajan, R., et al. Function and quality-of-life of survivors of pelvic and lower extremity osteosarcoma and Ewing's sarcoma. *British Journal of Cancer*, vol. 91 (2004), pp. 1858–1865.

Narod, S. A., et al. An estimate of the heritable fraction of childhood cancer. *British Journal of Cancer*, vol. 63 (6) (June 1991), pp. 993–999.

National Cancer Institute (August 3, 2004). Bone Marrow Transplantation and Peripheral Blood Stem Cell Transplantation: Questions and Answers. Retrieved June 21, 2007, from www.cancer.gov

National Cancer Institute. Cancer Facts: National Cancer Institute Research on Causes of Cancers in Children. Retrieved on March 30, 2001, from http://cis.nci.nih.gov

Nausea and Vomiting (PDQ©): Supportive Care—Patients. Cancer Net. Retrieved on November 20, 2009, from www.cancer.gov

Neergaard, Lauran. US cancer care uneven, policy panel concludes. *Boston Globe*, April 7, 1999, p. A5.

Neglia, J., et al. Second primary neoplasms (SPNs) of the central nervous system (CNS) in survivors of childhood cancer: a report from the Childhood Cancer Survivor Study (CCSS). ASCO Online. Retrieved on October 29, 2001, from www.asco.org

Neovastat information. Retrieved on October 29, 2009, from http://my.clevelandclinic.org/myeloma/education/neovastat.aspx

Ness, Kirsten, et al. Limitations on physical performance and daily activities among long-term survivors of childhood cancer. *Annals of Internal Medicine*, vol. 143 (9) (November 1, 2005), pp. 639–647.

Nessim-Keeney, Susan, and Judith Ellis. *Cancervive: The Challenge of Life after Cancer*. Boston, MA: Houghton-Mifflin Co., 1991.

Neudorf, S., et al. Autologous bone marrow transplantation for children with AML in first remission. *Bone Marrow Transplantation*, vol. 40 (4) (August 2007), pp. 313–318.

Neuroblastoma. Retrieved on August 4, 2001, from www.intelihealth.com

New Book: Educating a Child with Cancer: A guide for parents and teachers. *Candlelighters National Journal*, Fall 2003, p. 2.

Nkrumah, Gamal. Survival, and more. *Al-Ahram Weekly Online*, 521 (February 15–22, 2001). Retrieved on March 24, 2002, from www.ahram.org

Non-tunneled central lines. *CareNotes* [A Thomson Healthcare Company], December 2001, np.

Novakovic, B., et al. Experiences of cancer in children and adolescents. *Cancer Nursing*, vol. 19 (1) (1996), pp. 54–59.

Oeffinger, Kevin C., et al. Chronic health conditions in adult survivors of childhood cancer. *New England Journal of Medicine*, vol. 355 (15) (October 12, 2006), pp. 1572–1582.

Olness, Karen, MD and G. Gail Gardner, PhD. *Hypnosis and Hypnotherapy with Children*. New York: Gruen and Stratton, 2d edition, 1988 (newer edition not seen).

Olshan, A. F., et al. Neuroblastoma and parental occupation. *Cancer Causes and Control*, vol. 10 (6) (December 1999), pp. 539–549.

OncoLink Chemotherapy Drug Reference. University of Pennsylvania Cancer Center. Retrieved on July 21, 2001, from www.oncolink.org

OncoLink FAQ: Evaluating cancer web sites, an editorial by the OncoLink directors. University of Pennsylvania Cancer Center. Retrieved on July 21, 2001 from www.oncolink.net

O'Neill, Catherine. When a friend has cancer. *Washington Post*, July 20, 1993, pp. z18.

O'Neill, Catherine. When bad things happen to good kids. *Washington Post*, May 17, 1988, p. z26.

Oppenheim, Daniel, et al. Creative spirits. (Dissecting room). *Lancet*, vol. 30 (9329) (July 27, 2002), p. 345.

Oral Complications of Chemotherapy and Head/Neck Radiation PDQ. (nd). Cancer Net: A Service of the National Cancer Institute. Retrieved on July 21, 2001, from http://cancernet.nci.nih.gov

Osteen, Robert, et al. *Clinical Oncology*. Oxford: Blackwell 2001.

Osteosarcoma. Aetna InteliHealth. Retrieved on August 4, 2001, from www.intelihealth.com

Other resources. 411Cancer.com. Retrieved on August 16, 2001, from www. cancerconsultants.com

Oudot, C., et al. Prognostic factors for leukemic induction failure in children with acute lymphoblastic leukemia and outcome after salvage therapy: the FRALLE 93 study." *Journal of Clinical Oncology*, vol. 26 (9) (March 20, 2008), pp. 1496–1503.

Pacey, A. A. Fertility issues in survivors from adolescent cancers. *Cancer Treatment Reviews*, vol. 33 (2007), pp. 646–655.

Packer, Roger. New approaches for resistant brain tumors. *CCCF Newsletter* (Fall 2003), pp. 5–7. Available at www.candlelighters.org

Packer, Roger. Gene therapy for childhood brain tumors. Retrieved on December 13, 2009, from www.childhoodbraintumor.org

Pain Control: A Guide for People with Cancer and Their Families. National Institutes of Health, National Cancer Institute, 2000.

Parents' anxiety. Hershey Medical Center. Retrieved on August 4, 2001, from www.hmc.psu.edu

Parikh, Parag. OncoLink survivor story: Dear Normal People, An essay for adolescents with cancer. Retrieved on July 20, 1998, from http://oncolink.upenn.edu

Paternal smoking may increase childhood cancer risk. NIH News Release. National Institutes of Health, February 5, 1997.

A patient's guide to clinical trials. Pamphlet from *Cure*, nd.

Peckham, Virginia C. Cognitive late effects of treatment: Part I: Introduction to the research. *Candlelighters Childhood Cancer Foundation [Special Issue on Education]*, vol. 15 (4) (Fall 1991), pp. 1.

Pediatric Oncology Partnerships are models for success. *NCI Cancer Bulletin (Special Issue)*, vol. 5 (6) (March 18, 2008), pp. 1.

Pediatric Pain Sourcebook of Protocols, Policies, and Pamphlets. Retrieved on August 16, 2001, from http://painsourcebook.ca

Pediatrics experts study rise in U.S. childhood cancers. *Cancer Weekly Plus*, September 29, 1997. Retrieved on November 23, 2001, from http://library.bigchalk.com

Pelcovitz, D., et al. Posttraumatic stress disorder in mothers of pediatric cancer survivors. *Psychosomatics*, vol. 37 (2) (March 1996), pp. 116–126.

Perez-Saldivar, M. L., et al. Father's occupational exposure to carcinogenic agents and childhood acute leukemia. A new method to assess exposure. *BioMed Central Cancer*, vol. 8 (January 2008), pp. 7.

Peripherally inserted central catheters (PICCs). University of Michigan Section of Pediatric Surgery. Retrieved on April 15, 2004, from http://pediatric.um-surgery.org

Peripherally inserted central catheters and midline catheters. *CareNotes* [A Thomson Healthcare Company], December 2001, np.

Perry, J. D., and W. K. Flanagan. Pediatric psychology: applications to the schools [sic] needs of children with health disorders. *Techniques: A Journal for Remedial Education and Counseling*, vol. 2 (October 1986), pp. 333–340.

Pesmen, Curtis. Mistaken identity. *Cure*, vol. 5 (4) (Winter 2007), pp. 24–29.

Phillips, Ken, and Marie Phillips. A Grandma's and Grandpa's view of childhood cancer. *Candlelighters Childhood Cancer Foundation Quarterly Newsletter*, vol. 22 (1) (Spring 1997), pp. 1.

Picoult, Jodi. *My Sister's Keeper, a novel*. New York: Atria, 2004.

Plichart, M., et al. Parental smoking, maternal alcohol, coffee and tea consumption during pregnancy and childhood malignant central nervous system tumors. *European Journal of Cancer Prevention*, vol. 17 (4) (Aug. 2008) pp. 376–383.

Poetry relating to death. Retrieved on April 23, 2002, from www.photoaspects.com

Powered by Hope—Providence Cancer Center: building the new cancer center. Providence Health System. Retrieved on February 27, 2007, from www.providence.org

Prayer and Spirituality. Alternative and Complementary Therapies. American Cancer Society. Retrieved on February 4, 1999, from www.cancer.org

Primary cancerous bone tumors. *Merck Manual Home Edition*. Retrieved on November 30, 2001, from www.merckhomeedition.com

Prince vs. Massachusetts, 321, US 158 (1943).

Problems paying expenses. Hershey Medical Center. Retrieved on August 4, 2001, from www.hmc.psu.edu

Promoting independence. Hershey Medical Center. Retrieved on August 4, 2001, from www.hmc.psu.edu

Proton beam therapy: is it the future of radiation?" *Hematology/Oncology Today*, posted Dec. 10, 2008 at www.hemonctoday.com

Pryce, Deborah. *Cancer care for the future*. Testimony, House of Representatives Committee on Government Reform, Integrative Oncology, Cancer Care for the New Millennium. June 7, 2000.

Queasy-Pops Added to Website Store. *National Journal, Candlelighters Childhood Cancer Foundation*, (nd), p. 9.

Racadio, John M. Controlling radiation exposure during interventional procedures in childhood cancer patients. *Pediatric Radiology*, vol. 39 (Supp. 1) (February 2009), pp. 571–573.

Racial/Ethnic Patterns of Cancer in the United States 1988–1992. SEER Monograph, Barry A. Miller, editor-in-chief. Bethesda, MD: *The Cancer Control Program*, Division of Cancer Prevention and Control, National Cancer Institute, 1996.

Radiation Therapy and You: A Guide to Self-Help During Cancer Treatment. National Cancer Institute. Retrieved on May 16, 2002, from www.cancer.gov

Rafinski, Karen. Cancer and kids. *Miami Herald* (March 14, 1999), pp. 1L.

Raloff, Janet. Paternal smokers' cancer legacy. *Science News*, vol. 151 (9) (March 1, 1997), p. 135.

Recklitis, Christopher. Suicidal thoughts and attempts in adult survivors of childhood cancer. *Candlelighters Newsletter*, (Fall–Winter 2007). Retrieved on November 28, 2009, from www.candlelighters.org

Redd, W. H., et al. Behavioral intervention for cancer treatment side effects. *Journal of the National Cancer Institute*, vol. 93 (11) (June 1, 2001), pp. 810–823.

Relling, Mary. Genetics and anti-leukemia therapy: The TPMT story. *Candlelighters Childhood Cancer Foundation National Journal*, Fall 2003, pp. 3.

Renner, Gerald. Attitude all-important in surviving cancer, speaker says. *Hartford Courant* (April 22, 1995), p. F6.

Rescorla, F. J. Pediatric germ cell tumors. *Seminars in Surgical Oncology*, vol. 16 (2), pp. 144–158.

Resource directory (2005). Retrieved on April 13, 2005, from www.curesearch.org

Resource guide on children's environmental health. Retrieved on November 19, 2001, from www.cehn.org

Reulen, Raoul, et al. Pregnancy outcomes among adult survivors of childhood cancer in the British Childhood Cancer Survivor Study. *Cancer Epidemiology, Biomarkers and Prevention*, vol. 18 (8) (August 2009), pp. 2239–2247.

Rewards and challenges of cancer communication. *National Cancer Bulletin*, vol. 21 (28) (July 12, 2005), pp. 1.

Rhabdomyosarcoma. Aetna InteliHealth. Retrieved on August 4, 2001, from www.intelihealth.com

Richardson, Susan D., et al. Identification of drinking water contaminants in the course of a childhood cancer investigation in Toms River, New Jersey. *Journal of Exposure Analysis and Environmental Epidemiology*, vol. 9 (3) (June 1, 1999), pp. 200–216.

Robison, Leslie L. Second primary cancers after childhood cancer: low absolute risk, but prevention and monitoring are high priorities [Editorial]. *British Medical Journal*, vol. 312 (7035) (April 6, 1996), pp. 861.

Rodriguez, Rick. A 'raw and real' story of childhood cancer trauma. *Sacramento Bee*, July 8, 2006. Retrieved on July 13, 2006, from www.sacbee.com

Rogers, Ada. *Coping with Pain at Home: A Guide for Cancer Patients and Their Families*. Wilmington, DE: Du Pont Pharmaceuticals Biomedical Department, E.I. DuPont de Nemours & Co., Inc., 1986.

Ross, Irving B. Tax tips for parents of children with cancer. *Quarterly Newsletter of the Candlelighters Childhood Cancer Foundation*, vol. 23 (1) (Winter/Spring 1998), pp. 1.

Ross, Lone, et al. Psychiatric hospitalizations among survivors of cancer in childhood or adolescence. *New England Journal of Medicine*, vol. 349 (7) (August 14, 2003), pp. 650–657.

Rovner, Sandy. Discrimination on the job. *Washington Post*, December 3, 1991, pp. Z21.

Rudant, J., et al. Childhood hematopoietic malignancies and parental use of tobacco and alcohol: the ESCALE study (SFCE). *Cancer Causes and Control*, vol. 19 (10) (December 2008), pp. 1277–1290.

Rush, Morag, and Amanda Wetherall. Temperature measurement: practice guidelines. *Pediatric Nursing*, vol. 15 (9) (November 2003), pp. 25.

Sachdeva, Kush. Renal cell carcinoma. *Medicine: Instant Access to the Minds of Medicine*. Retrieved on May 29, 2002, from www.emedicine.com

Saltus, Richard. Cancer in the classroom. *Boston Globe Magazine*, October 31, 1999, p. 4.

Saltus, Richard. Key immune switch reported found. *Boston Globe*, November 5, 1993, p. 17.

Saltus, Richard. Tests show vaccine can shrink tumors. *Boston Globe*, February 29, 2000, pp. 1.

Sankila, R., et al. Risk of cancer among offspring of childhood cancer survivors. *New England Journal of Medicine*, vol. 338 (May 7, 1998), pp. 1339–1344.

Schmid, Randolph E. Little proof tying cancer to power lines, but study cites concern. *Boston Globe*, (June 16, 1999), p. A25.

School: Understanding the problem. *Hershey Home Medical Guide*. Retrieved on August 4, 2001, from www.hmc.psu.edu

School and the child with cancer. *Candlelighters Childhood Cancer Foundation [Special Issue]*, vol. 13 (3) (Summer 1989), pp. 1.

Schorr-Ribera, Hilda. Caring for siblings during diagnosis and treatment. *Candlelighters Childhood Cancer Foundation Quarterly Newsletter*, vol. 16 (2) (Summer 1992), pp. 1.

Scottish Intercollegiate Guidelines Network. Long-term follow-up of survivors of childhood cancer; Quick reference guide. *SIGN*, Edinburgh, January 2004.

Seam, P., et al. The role of FDG-PET scans in patients with lymphoma. *Blood*, vol. 110 (10) (November 15, 2007), pp. 3507–3516.

SEER Cancer Statistics Review 1973–1997, edited by Lynn A. Gloeckler Ries, et al. U.S. Department of Health and Human Services, Public Health Service, National Institutes of Health, National Cancer Institute, NIH 00-2789.

Shark cartilage. http://www.cancerhelpp.org.uk/about-cancer/treatment/complementary-alternative/therapies/shark-cartilage. Accessed October 29, 2009.

Shapiro, Margaret. Chernobyl's young victims pay toll. Thyroid, other cancers are Belarus' legacy of nuclear disaster. *Washington Post* (June 24, 1995), p. A1.

Shebib, S., et al. EST in infants and children: a clinical and pathology study: an 11-year review. *American Journal of Pediatric Hematology and Oncology*, vol. 11 (1) (Spring 1989), pp. 36–39,

Shenoy, S. *Late effects of therapy for cancer*. Retrieved on May 27, 2004, from www.webbugs.wustl.edu

Shih, C.-S., et al. High-dose chemotherapy with autologous stem cell rescue for children with recurrent malignant brain tumors. *Cancer*, vol. 112 (6) (2008), pp. 1345–1353.

Shimshock, Nikki. The new normal. *Dream* (Summer 2008). Retrieved on November 21, 2009 from www.childrenshospital.org

Shrout, Richard Neil. *Resource Directory for the Disabled*. New York: Facts on File, 1991.

Shurin, Susan. It's only a phase! Clinical trials Part II. *Candlelighters National Journal*, Spring 2003, pp. 6.

Sikorski, Robert, and Richard Peters. Oncology ASAP: Where to find reliable cancer information on the Internet. *Journal of the American Medical Association*, vol. 277 (18) (May 14, 1997), pp. 1431.

Sinopoli, Theresa, and Tara S. Manrique. Sperm banking issues for the testicular cancer patient. Oncology Nursing Service. Retrieved on November 18, 2001, from www.ons.org

Sloper, P. Needs and responses of parents following the diagnosis of childhood cancer. *Child: Care Health & Development*, vol. 22 (3) (May 1, 1996), pp. 187–202.

Smith, Malcolm, and Martha L. Hare. An overview of progress in childhood cancer survival. *Journal of Pediatric Oncology Nursing*, vol. 21 (3) (May–June 2004), pp. 160–164.

Sorahan, Tom. Smoking men may raise risk to offspring. *Washington Post* (November 19, 1997), p. A7.

Sovinz, Petra, et al. Tunneled femoral central venous catheters in children with cancer. *Pediatrics*, vol. 107 (6) (June 2001), p. 1417.

Speak Up: Help Prevent Errors in Your Care. A Joint Commission on Accreditation of Healthcare Organizations Publication, distributed by St. Elizabeth's Health Care at Brighton Marine, nd.

Specialove for Children with Cancer Information Links. Retrieved on April 19, 2007, from www.speciallove.org

Spence, A. M., et al. The role of PET in the management of brain tumors. *Applied Radiology Online*, vol. 36 (6) (June 2007). Retrieved on June 27, 2007, from www.appliedradiology.com

Spotlight on conformal radiation. (2005). St. Jude Children's Research Hospital. Retrieved on April 21, 2005 from www.stjude.org. [Reprint from Promise magazine, Winter 2005.]

Spunt, S., et al. Pediatric nonrhabdomyosarcoma soft tissue sarcomas. *The Oncologist*, vol. 13 (6) (June 2008), pp. 668–678.

Standish, Mary. From a working mom. *Candlelighters Childhood Cancer Foundation Quarterly Newsletter*, vol. 14 (1) (Winter-Spring 1990), p. 5.

Starer, Daniel. *Who to Call: The Parent's Source Book*. New York: W. Morrow, 1992.

Steen, Grant, and Joseph Mirro, eds. *Childhood Cancer: A Handbook from St. Jude Children's Research Hospital*. Cambridge, MA: Perseus Books, 2000.

Stem Cell Transplant Coloring Book. New York: Leukemia and Lymphoma Society, 2005?

Steiner, M., et al. Trends in infant leukaemia in West Germany in relation to in utero exposure due to the Chernobyl accident. *Radiation and Environmental Biophysics*, vol. 37 (2) (July 30, 1998), pp. 87–93.

Stem cell transplantation treatment by disease type (2007). Cancer Treatment Centers of America. Retrieved May 1, 2007 from www.cancercenter.com

Stereotactic radiosurgery. American Brain Tumor Association, 2007. Retrieved on November 12, 2009, from www.abta.org

Stevenson, Robert G. Chemotherapy: Its impact in the classroom. *Loss, Grief & Care*, vol. 1 (3–4) (June 1987), pp. 111–116.

Still going strong: After 18 years, Katie and her doctor are still a team. Beyond the Cure/Dana-Farber Cancer Institute, 2001.

Stiller, Charles. *Childhood Cancer in Britain: Incidence, Survival and Mortality*. New York: Oxford University Press, 2007.

Stolberg, Sheryl Gay. Childhood cancer patients find survival has price. *New York Times*, January 3, 1999, pp. 1.

Storb, Rainer F, MD (June 21, 2007). *New Perspectives on Stem Cell Transplantation*. Telephone Education Program from the Leukemia and Lymphoma Society.

Strutin, Michele. Family: going to the hospitable. *In Health*, November–December 1990, pp. 36–37.

Study seen to bolster drug's benefit in skin, kidney cancers. *Boston Globe*, March 23, 1994, p. 54.

Subclavian venous infusion catheter with implantable target. *Clinical Reference Systems Annual*, 2001, p. 1869.

Sugar, Jan. SuperSibs aims to help families. *Bone Marrow and Transplant Newsletter*, vol. 14 (March 2003), p. 3.

Sugarman, Barry, and Lainie Sugarman. Selecting your doctor or hospital: Procedures to follow and questions to ask. The Cure Our Children Foundation. Retrieved on July 21, 2001, from www.cureourchildren.org

Sugarman, Barry, and Lainie Sugarman. Treatments for nausea and vomiting for cancer patients—drugs, devices, dietary supplements, and herbs. The Cure Our Children Foundation. Retrieved on January 27, 2005, from www.cureourchildren.org

Suicidal behavior is risk for teenagers with cancer. *The Brown University Child and Adolescent Behavior Letter*, vol. 11 (6) (June 1995), pp. 5.

Summary of medical literature [Complementary or alternative medicine]. *Columbia Information*. Retrieved on June 11, 2001 from http://carolann.hs.columbia.edu

Suplee, Curt. No greater cancer risk found in children living near power lines; federal study tries to shed light on high-voltage debate. *Washington Post* (July 3, 1997), p. A3.

Support groups available for families of children with cancer. *Candlelighters Childhood Cancer Foundation* press release, Bethesda, MD, June 12, 1997.

Support in the fight against child cancer. *Middle East Health Magazine*. Retrieved on March 24, 2002, from www.middleeasthealthmag.com

Supporting children and families through grief. Fernside, An Affiliate of Cincinnati, Inc. Retrieved on December 9, 2009, from www.fernside.org

Surveillance Epidemiology and End Results [SEER], 2009, National Cancer Institute (cancer statistics). http://seer.cancer.gov/statistics. Retrieved on November 12, 2009

Surviving childhood cancer. Long-term follow-up study. University of Minnesota Cancer Center. Retrieved on August 1, 2003, from www.cancer.umn.edu

Survivors—follow-up clinics. Pediatric Oncology Resource Center. Retrieved on May 17, 2002, from www.acor.org

Survivor's Guide to a Bone Marrow Transplant. Southfield, MI: National BMT Link. Retrieved from www.nbmtlink.org on November 12, 2009.

Susan Butcher Family Center Program description. *Providence Health System*. Retrieved on February 17, 2007, from www.providence.org

Taking Time: Support for People with Cancer and the People Who Care About Them. National Institutes of Health, National Cancer Institute, 1999.

Talbott, E. O., et al. Mortality among the residents of the Three Mile Island accident area: 1979–1992. *Environmental Health Perspectives* vol. 108 (6) (June 2000), pp. 545–552.

Talking With Your Child About Cancer. U.S. Department of Health and Human Services, Public Health Service, National Institutes of Health, 1990. Also retrieved on July 20, 1998, from http://cancernet.nci.nih.gov

Talvensaari, Kimmo, and Mikael Knip. Childhood cancer and later development of the metabolic syndrome. *Annals of Medicine*, vol. 29 (5) (October 1, 1997), pp. 353–355.

Tangley, Laura. A winning verdict for power lines. *U.S. News & World Report*, vol. 123 (2) (July 14, 1997), p. 30.

Tarbell, Nancy, et al. Cancers in children. In *American Cancer Society Massachusetts Division Cancer Manual*, 9th edition, 1996, pp. 567–577.

Taubes, Gary. Fields of fear. *Atlantic Monthly*, vol. 274 (November 1994), pp. 94.

Teenagers with cancer do not always get the best care. *National Childhood Cancer Foundation Childhood Cancerline*, vol. 5 (2) (nd), pp. 1.

Templeton, Sara-Kate. Doctors freeze eggs of girls, 5. *Sunday Times (London)* July 1, 2007. Accessed at www.timesonline.co.uk, July 25, 2008.

Texas Children's Cancer Center. *Cancer Pain Management in Children* (1999). Retrieved from www.childcancerpain.org, November 12, 2009.

This Battle Which I Must Fight: Cancer in Canada's Children and Teenagers. Ottawa, ON: Minister of Supply and Services Canada, 1996.

Thomas, Jay. How do you treat constipation caused by pain-relieving opioid use? *Cure*, vol. 5 (2) (Summer 2006), p. 19.

Thornton, A. J., and P. N. Lee. Parental smoking and risk of childhood cancer: a review of the evidence. *Indoor and Built Environment*, vol. 7 (2) (January 1, 1998), pp. 65–86.

Treatment aftershocks: survivors guided through territory of long-term and late effects. *Cure*, vol. 5 (special issue 2006), pp. 58–61.

Treatment of pediatric melanoma. St. Jude Children's Research Hospital. Retrieved on August 13, 2001, from www.stjude.org

Trillin, Alice. *Dear Bruno*. New York: New Press, 1996.

Tuladhar, R., et al. Sacrococcygeal teratoma in the perinatal period. *Postgraduate Medical Journal*, vol. 76 (902) (December 2000), pp. 754–759.

Tuma, Rabiya. Future risk for survivors. *Cure*, vol. 5 (2) (Summer 2006), pp. 60–64.

Tumors of the liver. Chapter 29, p. 957, in *Pediatric Oncology*, 5th ed., edited by Philip Pizzo and David Poplack. Philadelphia: Lippincott Williams & Wilkins, 2006.

Tunneled central lines child [sic]. *CareNotes* [A Thomson Healthcare Company], December 2001, np.

Turner, Barbara. *A Little Bit of Rob*. Morton Grove, IL: A. Whitman, 1996.

Understanding Clinical Trials for Blood Cancers. White Plains, NY: Leukemia & Lymphoma Society, 2006?

Understanding Drug Therapy and Managing Side Effects. White Plains, NY: Leukemia & Lymphoma Society, 2007.

University of Utah Health Sciences Center Chemotherapy Overview. Retrieved on January 20, 2005, from www.uuhsc.utah.edu

Varley, Susan. *Badger's Parting Gifts* New York: Lothrop, Lee and Shepard Books, 1984.

Video games seen to relax patients. *Boston Globe*, December 10, 2004, np.

Vitamin E. *Facts About Dietary Supplements*. Clinical Nutrition Service, Warren Grant Magnuson Clinical Center, Office of Dietary Supplements, National Institutes of Health. March 2001.

Wallace, Karin. Keep the light. *Candlelighters Childhood Cancer Foundation Quarterly Newsletter*, vol. 21 (1) (Spring 1996), p. 8.

Wallace, W. H. B. and D. M. Green, eds. *Late Effects of Childhood Cancer*. London: Arnold, 2004.

Wanebo, Harold J., et al. Preoperative regional therapy for extremity sarcoma: a tricenter update. *Cancer*, vol. 75 (9) (May 1, 1995), pp. 2299.

Wang, S-M., and Zeen N. Kain. P6 acupoint injections are as effective as droperidol in controlling early postoperative nausea and vomiting in children. *Anesthesiology* vol. 97 (2) (Aug. 2002), pp. 359–366.

Ward, Jennifer Dawn. Pediatric cancer survivors: assessment of late effects. *Nurse Practitioner*, vol. 25 (12) (December 2000), pp. 18.

Weber, Melissa. Medical marijuana use in oncology. *Cure*, vol. 4 (3) (Fall 2005), p. 33.

Weiner, Susan Lipschitz, and Joseph V. Simone, eds. *Childhood Cancer Survivorship*. Washington, DC: National Academies Press, 2003.

Wiens, B. A., and B. O. Gilbert. A reexamination of a childhood cancer stereotype. *Journal of Pediatric Psychology*, vol. 25 (3) (April 1, 2000), pp. 151–159.

Welcome Message (October 18, 2004). Pediatric Oncology Resource Center. Retrieved October 18, 2004 from www.acor.org

What is a 'clinical trial'? From lab to bedside. Retrieved on May 14, 2002, from www.nccf.org

What is the Partnership for Prescription Assistance? Retrieved on April 16, 2005, from www.pparx.org

When Someone in Your Family Has Cancer. U.S. Department of Health and Human Services, Public Health Service, National Institutes of Health, Office of Cancer Communications, National Cancer Institute, 1985.

Where to begin. Looking for reliable medical information?" *AARP* (March/April 2007), p. 42.

White-Konig, Mélanie. Compliance to treatment of adolescents with cancer. *Bulletin du Cancer*, vol. 94 (4) (April 2007), pp. 349–356.

Whitaker, Julian. This family is fighting for their son's life. *Dr. Julian Whitaker's Health & Healing, Special Supplement*, February 2000.

Whittington, Elizabeth. Tips for preventing infection. *Cure*, vol. 5 (2) (Summer 2006), p. 57.

Whittington, Elizabeth. Keeping hydrated during therapy is essential for cancer patients. *Cure*, vol. 5 (2) (Summer 2006), p. 47.

Whittington, Elizabeth. Quick relief for breakthrough pain. *Cure*, vol. 5 (1) (Spring 2006), p. 55.

Whittington, Elizabeth. Blood counts may predict survival. *Cure*, vol. 5 (4) (Winter 2007). Retrieved November 12, 2009, from www.curetoday.com

Whittington, Elizabeth. The choice to work [with sidebars]. *Cure*, vol. 5 (Fall 2006), pp. 56.

Williamson, David. Study suggests Three Mile Island radiation may have injured people living near reactor. Carolina News Services. Retrieved on March 27, 2009, from www.unc.edu/news

Windebank, Kevin P., and John J. Spinetta. Do as I say or die: Compliance in adolescents with cancer. *Pediatric Blood & Cancer*, vol. 50 (S5) (May 2008), pp. 1099–1100.

Wing S., et al. A reevaluation of cancer incidence near the Three Mile Island nuclear plant: the collision of evidence and assumptions. *Environmental Health Perspectives*, vol. 105 (1997), pp. 52–57.

Wish with Wings, Inc. Advice to educators: the best teachers (a parent's view)...the worst teachers (a parent's view). *Candlelighters Childhood Cancer Foundation Quarterly Newsletter*, vol. 16, (1) (Spring 1992), p. 5.

Wogrin, Carol. *Matters of Life and Death: Finding the Words to Say Goodbye*. New York: Broadway Books, 2001.

Wolf, Buck. Living life in a cancer cluster. ABC News. Retrieved on February 4, 1999, from http://abcnews.go.com

Wolf, Buck. Putting the 'Civil' into *Civil Action*. ABC News. Retrieved on February 4, 1999, from http://abcnews.go.com

Wolfe, J., et al. Symptoms and suffering at the end of life in children with cancer. *New England Journal of Medicine*, vol. 342 (5) (February 3, 2000), pp. 326–333.

Wood, Debra. Into the brain: unlocking new brain cancer treatments. *Cure*, Spring 2004, pp. 23.

Woodgate, R. L. Life is never the same: childhood cancer narratives. *European Journal of Cancer Care*, vol. 15 (1) (March 2006), pp. 8–18.

Woolhandler, Steffie, et al. Costs of health care administration in the United States and Canada. *New England Journal of Medicine*, vol. 349 (8) (August 21, 2003), pp. 768–775.

Wooten, Patty. *Compassionate Laughter: Jest for Your Health*. Salt Lake City, UT: Commune-A-Key Publishing, 1996.

World of Understanding (2000). CancerSource Kids. Retrieved July 21, 2001 from www.cancersourcekids.com

World without cancer. www.vitaminb17.net, accessed July 1, 2008

Woznick, Leigh H., and Carol D. Goodheart. *Living with Childhood Cancer: A Practical Guide for Helping Families Cope*. Washington DC: American Psychological Association, 2002.

Yasko, Alan W. Limb-salvage strategies to optimize quality of life: The M. D. Anderson Center Experience. *CA*, vol. 47 (4) (July–August 1997), pp. 226.

Young People with Cancer: A Handbook for Parents. U.S. Department of Health and Human Services, National Institutes of Health, National Cancer Institute, 2001.

Zeltzer, Lonnie & Linda Zame. The problem of pain in childhood cancer survivors. *Candlelighters Childhood Cancer Foundation National Journal* (Fall 2005), pp. 2–4.

Zwartjes, G. M., et al. Students with cancer. *Today's Education*, vol. 70 (4) (November–December 1981), pp. 20–25.

Glossary

Terms and Common Abbreviations

For additional terms, see the excellent Dictionary of Cancer Terms at the US National Cancer Institute Web site: www.cancer.gov.

ABMT: Autologous bone marrow transplant

ACTH: Adrenocorticotropic hormone

Acute: Appearing suddenly, having a rapid and severe course

Adrenal glands: Two glands in the upper rear portion of the abdomen atop the kidneys; they secrete hormones, including adrenaline and cortisone

Alopecia: Hair loss, baldness

Alpha-fetoprotein (AFP): An antigen identified in some types of cancer as a "tumor marker." AFP is normal in fetuses. AFP is found in the blood of patients with some ovarian, testicular, and pineal gland tumors.

Analgesic: Drug that relieves pain. Aspirin is one.

Anemia: Reduction in the number of red blood cells. Symptoms are weakness and fatigue.

Antibody: An important part of the immune system. Produced by blood cells, it is an individualized weapon against specific germs or viruses. The antibody molecule reacts only to the antigen that produced it or a very similar one. Immunizations like polio vaccine stimulate the body to produce antibodies, which will attack polio virus if there is subsequent exposure.

Antiemetic: A medicine to prevent or stop vomiting

Antigen: A substance important to the body's immunity. Capable of triggering the body's immune response, causing antibodies to be produced to fight invading infection or disease. Antigens are injected for active immunization against diseases like polio.

Apoptosis: Cell suicide, the body's normal method of getting rid of abnormal or no-longer-needed cells. May not work properly in cancer cells.

Aspiration: Removal of sample cells and fluid by needle. Also refers to food particles or fluid accidently sucked into the lungs.

BCG: Bacillus Calmette-Guérin, a strain of tuberculosis bacteria used in Europe as an anti-TB vaccine. Has been under investigation as an immunotherapy agent.

BID: *bis in die,* twice a day

B lymphocyte: A white blood cell that makes antibodies and is an important part of the immune system. B lymphocytes come from bone marrow. Also known as a *B cell.*

BM: Bowel movement

BMR: Basal metabolic rate

BP: Blood pressure

BPM: Beats per minute

BUN: Blood urea nitrogen; the part of a blood test that assesses kidney function

Beckwith-Wiedemann syndrome: A rare genetic disorder characterized by overgrowth of certain body parts like the tongue. Can be a risk factor for Wilms tumor.

Benign: Not malignant; with generally favorable chances for recovery, although there are some exceptions

Beta hCG: Human chorionic gonadotropin, a hormone produced in pregnancy. Measurement of hCG is used for early pregnancy testing. Also a tumor marker for some cancers, such as germ cell tumors.

Bilateral: On both sides. Tumors in both kidneys, eyes, etc., are called bilateral.

Biopsy: Removal of sample cells, whether tissue or fluid, for microscopic study to identify any disease present

Bladder: An organ like a sac that stores liquid. The word is usually used to refer to the urinary bladder.

"Blast": Short for *lymphoblast, myeloblast, erythroblast,* etc. An immature white blood cell (WBC). The bone marrow normally has less than 5% blasts, but in leukemia they accumulate in a high percentage until they crowd out other cells. Blasts do not perform the work of mature WBCs and look abnormal under a microscope.

Blood: Liquid that circulates throughout the body carrying nutrients and oxygen to the cells. Contains red and white blood cells and platelets suspended in a pale yellow liquid called plasma. *Peripheral blood* is the blood in circulation in arteries and veins throughout the body outside of the organs and tissues.

Blood–brain barrier: A natural barrier that prevents foreign substances from reaching and possibly damaging the brain. The layer of tissue lining the blood vessels of the brain is less permeable than the tissue lining other blood vessels, which stops some substances from passing through into the brain. This mechanism prevents many chemotherapy drugs from being effective on brain tumors.

Bone marrow: Spongy material in the hollows of some bones where the body makes blood cells. Because these cells are fast-growing, they are especially sensitive to chemotherapy drugs. In healthy adults only a few bones contain red marrow for manufacturing blood cells, whereas in infants most bones contain blood-cell-producing marrow.

Brain stem: The lower part of the brain lying between the brain proper and the spinal cord

C&S: Culture and sensitivity

CBC: Complete blood count. Blood tests to diagnose illness and to follow the course of treatments. See *blood count* in Appendix D for more discussion.

Cancer: One of a class of diseases characterized by abnormal tissue growth in the body. This growth invades surrounding organs and spreads elsewhere in the body via the blood or lymph system to form new colonies or tumors.

Carcinogen: A substance that either causes or advances the development of cancer (adjective: carcinogenic)

Carcinoma: Malignant growth that arises from tissues lining the body—skin and tissue lining hollow organs of the urinary, digestive, and respiratory systems. Carcinomas are the major types of cancers that strike adults but they are rare in children.

Cartilage: Tough elastic tissues at the ends of bones

Catheter: A tube inserted into the body to put in or remove fluids. May be flexible or rigid. The most familiar type of catheter is used to drain the urinary bladder.

cc: Cubic centimeter

CCU: Critical care unit (may be used instead of ICU)

Central nervous system (CNS): The brain and spinal cord

Cerebrospinal fluid (CSF): The fluid in the cavities of the brain and between the layers of tissue covering it and surrounding the spinal column

Cerebrum: The main part of the brain, composed of right and left hemispheres. Controls voluntary processes of the body.

Chemotherapy: A broad term that means treatment by drugs of any kind, even aspirin and vitamins. In the context of cancer, "chemo" means powerful medications used to fight malignancies.

Chromosome: Material found in the nucleus of each cell, containing the DNA or genetic information

Chronic: Long-term, perhaps with no cure on the horizon. A chronic illness may become acute as it progresses.

Cirrhosis: A chronic liver disease (not necessarily related to alcoholism)

CNS: Central nervous system

Colony-stimulating factor: A substance that stimulates the production of specific blood cells, whether as a prelude to a peripheral blood stem cell transplant or to counteract the side effects of some chemotherapy drugs

Colostomy: Surgery to bring the large intestine to the abdomen and create an opening there for it to empty. This is done when there is a bowel obstruction; in some cases it is only a temporary measure, and normal function is restored through later surgery.

Connective tissue: Body structures that connect, support, or surround other tissues and organs. Includes mucus, bone, and cartilage.

Conscious sedation: A type of anesthesia using drugs in which patients are sedated but not unconscious, are pain-free and able to respond to some verbal directions. Used when the patient must be able to respond to the surgical team or when full anesthesia is not required for a procedure. Carries less risk than full anesthesia.

Contrast medium: A radiopaque substance used to help distinguish various body tissues on x-rays

Creatinine: Results from the normal breakdown of certain muscle substances; measured in the blood and urine, an indication of kidney function

"Crit": Hematocrit, the volume percentage of red blood cells in whole blood. An indication of the presence or absence of anemia.

CSF: Cerebrospinal fluid

CV: Cardiovascular

CVU: Clean voided urine

Cystitis: Inflammation of the urinary bladder.

Cytomegalovirus (CMV): A serious infection common after transfusions of large volumes of blood. It can be detected in body fluids like blood, urine, and tears, and a large proportion of the population apparently carries the virus without symptoms, as antibodies detectable on cell surfaces but not within the cells themselves. CMV may become active if the patient's immune system is impaired, for instance by chemotherapy or the preparation for a bone marrow transplant. The test for the virus is performed after transplants to watch for a change in the CMV antibody level over the course of time. If it becomes active, it can cause a devastating illness.

DC or D/C: Discontinue

DNA: Deoxyribonucleic acid, a substance found in the nucleus of a cell in a twisted ladder shape, which contains hereditary information. Has a role in the manufacture of protein and transfer of genetic traits from mother to daughter cells during reproduction.

"Diff": Differential white count. Shows the proportion of different kinds of white blood cells (WBCs) in blood count.

Distal: Away from the point of origin. In limbs or bones, the end away from the trunk. Opposite of proximal.

Drsng, drsg: Dressing

Dx: Diagnosis

Dysembryoma: A teratoma

Dyspnea: Pain when breathing or shortness of breath. Can be a drug side effect or caused by a tumor or metastasis.

ECG, EKG: Electrocardiogram

EEG: Electroencephalogram

Encapsulated: Enclosed within a capsule or membrane covering. An encapsulated tumor is still completely contained in the primary, original sac.

Endocrine system: Pituitary, thyroid, ovaries, and other ductless glands that secrete their hormones directly into the bloodstream to control body functions like sweating, digestive juice production, and milk production for breastfeeding

Endothelium: A layer of cells that lines the cavities of the heart, blood, and lymph vessels as well as other body cavities

Enzyme: A protein made in a living cell and capable of stimulating certain chemical activity within the body, without itself being changed or destroyed

Epstein-Barr virus (EBV): A common virus that causes infectious mononucleosis; also associated with some cancers like Burkitt lymphoma

Erythrocyte: Red blood cell. Carries oxygen to the body tissues.

ESR: Erythrocyte sedimentation rate (sed rate), a laboratory finding

ET: Endotracheal

Femur: Thigh bone, extending from the pelvis to the knee. The longest, strongest, and largest bone in the human body.

Fever: A temperature more than 2 degrees Fahrenheit above normal. 98.6 degrees Fahrenheit (37 degrees centigrade) usually is normal, but that can vary for different people. Fever usually indicates an infection and is a natural defense, since many organisms that cause disease are killed by higher temperatures. The degree of fever doesn't necessarily indicate the seriousness of the illness.

Fibula: The outer and thinner of the two lower leg bones, extending from the knee to the ankle

Fluoroscope: Piece of equipment used to examine the body by radiation with an image projected on a fluorescent screen. See *fluoroscopy* in Appendix D.

F/U: Follow-up

FUO: Fever of unknown origin

Gamma globulin: A natural body substance containing antibodies to fight disease. It can be removed from one person's blood and given to someone who has no natural immunity and needs temporary protection against chickenpox or certain other diseases. Each disease requires a specific gamma globulin.

Gene: Carriers of the hereditary message contained in chromosomes, passed from parent to offspring through genes in sperm and egg cells (adjective: genetic)

Genitourinary: Body parts that play a role in reproduction, urine production for waste removal, or both

Genome: The complete genetic makeup of an organism

GI: Gastrointestinal

Graft-versus-host-disease (GvHD): A potentially lethal problem that may follow transplants. The transplanted organ or material recognizes its new home as foreign and goes on the attack.

G-tube: Gastrostomy tube

H/a: Headache

Hematocrit (Hct): See *crit*.

Hematology: The study of the blood and blood-forming organs. Doctors who specialize in this field are called hematologists.

Hemihypertrophy: A condition where one side of the body is larger than the other. Children with this problem are at greater risk for Wilms tumor and liver cancer.

Hemisphere: One half of the brain, the right or the left side

Hemoglobin (Hgb): The red substance in the red blood cells that carries oxygen to all the tissues of the body.

H&H: Hemoglobin and hematocrit

Histiocyte: Cell important to the immune system. Most often histiocytes are fixed in a single place, perhaps in the wall of a blood vessel, but when stimulated by an inflammation they wander through the body gobbling up foreign particles like bacteria.

Histology: The structure of tissue as seen under a microscope; also called *microscopical anatomy*

H/O: History of

Hormone: A chemical substance produced by an organ that regulates the activity of specific organs. Insulin is one example.

Hs: *hora somni,* hour of sleep or at bedtime

Hx: History

Humerus: The long bone of the upper arm, extending from the shoulder to the elbow

Hydrocephalus: Accumulation of abnormal amounts of fluid in the brain

Hypothalamus: A part of the brain that regulates body temperature, sleep, food intake, and development of some sex characteristics, among other functions

I & O: Fluid intake and output

ICU: Intensive care unit. Also called *CCU.*

Ig (Immunoglobulin): Proteins made by B cells and plasma cells that act as antibodies

Ilium: The upper part of the pelvis bone

IM: Intramuscular injection

Immune: Not susceptible to disease, having immunity

Immunophenotyping: A process used to identify cells, based on the type of antigens or markers on the surface of the cell. This process is used to diagnose specific types of leukemia and lymphoma by comparing the cancer cells to normal cells of the immune system. Think of antigens as baseball players are identified by their uniforms, showing which team they're on!

Immunosuppression: The lack of natural immunity, possibly as a result of drugs. May be deliberately caused, as after a transplant, or a side effect, as from some chemotherapy.

Inc: Incontinent

Infection: Invasion of the body by disease germs, whether bacteria, viruses, or parasites

Intrathecal: Injection of a substance into the spinal fluid. This is a route for introducing methotrexate, for example, into the central nervous system to prevent leukemic spread.

Intravenous (IV): The giving of nutrients or medication directly into a vein. In common usage, the term also refers to the needle, tubing, and other equipment required for the procedure.

Ionizing radiation: X-rays and gamma rays beamed at a tumor to destroy the cells

Isotopes: Slightly different forms of a single element like iodine. Radioactive isotopes break up spontaneously, giving off energy that can be tracked with special equipment.

IVP: Intravenous pyelogram

Kidneys: A pair of bean-shaped organs at the rear of the abdomen that filter the blood to remove waste products and water, which are excreted as urine

KUB: X-ray of the kidneys, ureter, and bladder

Laparotomy ("lap"): An operation involving an abdominal incision. A *staging* laparotomy is a surgical procedure in which the doctors look into the abdomen to determine if or how far the disease has spread (its stage).

Li-Fraumeni: A syndrome susceptible to cancer with a genetic p53 mutation

LOC: Level (or loss of) consciousness

Lumbar puncture: Spinal tap. See *lumbar puncture* in Appendix D.

Lymph: A clear yellowish liquid containing cells, fat, and protein derived from body fluids. Lymph is returned to the bloodstream by the lymphatic system (channels and nodes or glands).

Lymphocyte: A type of white blood cell

Malaise: Vague feeling of not being well

Malignancy: Cancerous tumor

Malignant: Cancerous. Dangerous to life. Having the capacity to worsen and result in death. Capable of metastasizing.

Mediastinum: The space between the lungs, containing the heart and its major blood vessels, the esophagus, the thymus, and other lymph nodes

Metastases: Tumors that grow when cancer cells leave the primary tumor and migrate elsewhere in the body by the blood or lymph system. *Metastases* is the plural form of *metastasis*. The adjective is metastatic. *Metastasis* is also the term for the spread of cancer from the original or primary site.

Microliter: A thousandth of a milliliter or one millionth of a liter, used to measure platelets as part of a CBC

MRI: Magnetic resonance imaging

Mucus: A slippery fluid made by the linings of body parts like the mouth and vagina

Mucositis: Inflammation of the soft tissue of the mouth and other linings in the digestive system. Also called *stomatitis*. A side effect of some chemotherapy drugs and radiation.

N&V: Nausea and vomiting

Neuropathy: A painful nerve problem, often starting in the hands and feet with tingling, swelling, or muscle weakness. Can be caused by cancer, diabetes, and chemotherapy drugs.

NG (nasogastric) tube: A tube slid into the nose and down into the stomach to drain its contents or to feed the patient. Often used after abdominal surgery to allow the digestive system to recuperate.

Noc: At night (nocturnal)

NPO: *nil per os*, nothing by mouth. A child who is NPO isn't allowed any food or drink at all, usually in preparation for tests or anesthesia.

Oncogenes: Genes important to daily growth and division of cells. When activated by environmental agents, chemicals, or chromosome damage, cells become malignant, grow out of control, and become cancer. Oncogenes may stimulate growth of other cells as well.

Oncology: The field of medicine concerned with tumors; a doctor with this specialty is an oncologist.

Palliative: Giving relief of some or all symptoms but not a cure. Noun: palliation.

Pc: *Post cibos*, after meals

Palpable: Capable of being felt or touched

Papilledema: Swelling of the optic nerve

P/E: Physical examination

Philadelphia chromosome: A detectable genetic abnormality in which specific chromosomes switch locations. Bone marrow cells with the Philadelphia chromosome are found in some malignancies like chronic myelogenous leukemia.

PICU: Pediatric intensive care unit

Plasma: The liquid portion of the blood. What's left after the red and white blood cells and platelets are filtered out.

Platelets: Thrombocytes, or small colorless discs in the circulating blood that, like sticky corks, aid in clotting

Polyp: An abnormal mucous membrane growth in the nose, etc.

Pons: A section of the brain stem, the lowest part of the brain that connects to the spinal cord

Primary tumor: The original tumor, the site where the cancer began before it spread (metastasized)

PRN: *pro re nata,* as needed

Prognosis: A forecast of the outcome of an illness, an assessment of the patient's chances for recovery

Protocol: A detailed and precise formal treatment plan

Proximal: Toward or nearer the beginning or point of origin, as the end of the femur closer to the hip joint. Opposite of distal.

Px: Physical examination or past history

Q2h: *quaque seconda hora,* every 2 hours

QAM: *quaque* (every) morning

QD: quaque die, every day

QID: *quarter in die,* four times a day

QOD: *quoque alternis die,* every other day

Radioresistant: Not especially susceptible to radiation

Red blood cell: Erythrocyte. Carries oxygen to the body tissues.

Remission: Not having any detectable remaining disease

R/o: Rule out

Sarcoma: A type of malignant tumor arising from connective tissue like bone and muscle. More likely than carcinoma to strike children.

SGOT: serum glutamic-oxalocetic transaminase (a blood value determined in the laboratory)

Shunt: Bypass. A tube surgically implanted to drain fluid from the brain, for example, is called a shunt. Surgeons also create shunts, like detours, to bypass blood clots.

SICU: Surgical intensive care unit

Side effect: An effect that a drug or other therapy has in addition to the intended effect. Most but not all side effects are harmful or unpleasant.

Sign: An objective indication of a disease or injury, one that the doctor can detect. Fever is a sign, for example, of some infections. See also *symptom*.

Spleen: An abdominal lymph organ that manufactures and replaces blood cells

Sq or sub-q: Subcutaneous, beneath the skin

S/S: Signs and symptoms

Staging: Determining the extent (or spread, if it has grown beyond an original site) of the cancer in the body; allows the physician to select the most effective treatment

Stem cell: A cell from which other types of cells can develop

Stomatitis: See *mucositis*

Sublingual (SL): Route of drug administration beneath the tongue

Supp: Suppository

Sx: Symptoms

Symptom: A subjective sensation that the patient feels due to a disease or injury. Pain, for example, is a *symptom* of a broken bone, as opposed to swelling, which may be a *sign* of the broken bone. A child's headache is a *symptom* of illness, while swollen lymph nodes are a *sign* that the doctor can use to find the cause of the headache. See *sign*.

T: Temperature

T cell: One type of white blood cell that attacks virus-infected cells, foreign cells, and cancer cells. T cells also produce a number of substances that regulate the immune response.

T-cell receptor (TCR): Molecule on the surface of T cells that recognizes antigens

Teratoma: Tumors formed of misplaced embryonic tissue. For example, an ovarian teratoma may include stomach tissue. Most often ovarian or testicular.

Thymus: Lymph organ located under the breastbone in the midchest between the lungs. The two lobes taper upward toward the lungs. Plays an important role in the development of the immune system. Most important in prenatal life, it reaches maximum size around puberty, then shrinks in adulthood and is replaced by fat.

Tibia: Shin bone. The larger and inner of the two lower leg bones.

TID: *ter in die,* three times a day

Trisomy: A genetic abnormality in which there are three chromosomes where there normally would be only two. Down syndrome is caused by an extra chromosome number 21.

Tumor: A swelling or growth. May be benign (noncancerous) or malignant (cancerous).

Tumor marker: Substances secreted by certain tumors, measurable by blood tests. The presence or absence of these markers indicates whether the tumor has reactivated after therapy. Alpha-fetoprotein is a tumor marker.

Tumor suppressor genes: Normal genes that regulate a cell's division rate and that can repair DNA errors, blocking the development of cancer or tumors. These may lead to new forms of therapy.

Tx: Therapy or treatment

U/A: Urinalysis

Unilateral: On one side only. A unilateral Wilms tumor affects only one kidney, for example.

Venipuncture: Blood draw. See *venipuncture* in Appendix D.

Vital signs (VS): Pulse rate, breathing, and temperature, which nurses monitor as general indicators of the patient's condition

VSS: Vital signs stable

Von Recklinghausen's disease: Neurofibromatosis, or "elephant man's disease." A hereditary disorder marked by developmental difficulties in the nervous system, muscles, skin, and bones. The patient has many (perhaps thousands) of benign tumors in nerves under the skin.

WBC: White blood cell

White cells: White blood cells, leukocytes, or WBCs. Used to be called corpuscles. Several types of cells (lymphocytes, granulocytes, neutrophils, monocytes, eosinophils, basophils) important to the body's immune system. Made in the bone marrow.

Wt: Weight

x: Times

Xeroderma pigmentosum: A rare hereditary disease in which the skin and eyes are extremely sensitive to light. It can lead to carcinoma and melanoma. Complete protection from the sun is required to help prevent tumor growth.

X-rays: Roentgen rays. Short light rays passed through a glass vacuum tube by an electric generator. These rays are capable of penetrating the body's tissues. The term also refers to a radiograph made with the rays.

Index

A few words of explanation are in order regarding the preparation of this index. Since the material in the appendices is easily accessible, it has not been included in this index, nor are subtopics (chemotherapy, surgery) in specific disease situations. Among the chapter end citations, only the book authors have been indexed.